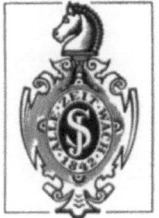

S. S. Hayreh

Anterior Ischemic Optic Neuropathy

With 139 Figures and
16 Stereoscopic Illustrations

Springer-Verlag Berlin Heidelberg GmbH 1975

SOHAN SINGH HAYREH, Professor of Ophthalmology, University of Iowa, Iowa City, IA 52242/USA

A stereopticon viewer for the stereo pair figures 14d, 15a and f, 16a, f and j, 17h, 21a, 22a and d, 23b, 25a, 26a and b, 27i and m is attached inside the back cover

ISBN 978-3-642-65959-1   ISBN 978-3-642-65957-7 (eBook)
DOI 10.1007/978-3-642-65957-7

© Springer-Verlag Berlin Heidelberg 1975
Originally published by Springer-Verlag Berlin Heidelberg New York in 1975
Softcover reprint of the hardcover 1st edition 1975

Library of Congress Cataloging in Publication Data. Hayreh, Sohan Singh, 1928-   . Anterior ischemic optic neuropathy. Bibliography: p.   . Includes index. 1. Optic nerve—Diseases. 2. Eye—Blood-vessels—Diseases. 3. Ocular manifestations of general diseases. I. Title. [DNLM: 1. Cardiovascular diseases—Complications. 2. Eye diseases. 3. Eye manifestations. 4. Ischemia. 5. Optic nerve—Blood supply. WW 280 H424a] RE 701.H 39. 617.7'1. 74-23702.

*Dedicated to my parents
as a small token
of my gratitude to them*

Preface

Vascular disorders of the optic disc and nerve are important not only to the ophthalmologist but also to the neurologist and the internist. To the first specialty group they represent one cause of blindness or severe visual impairment; to the second group the optic disc edema and optic atrophy seen in these disorders can pose serious problems of diagnosis, or give indications of the involvement of the cerebral circulation; while to the last group they are frequently indicative of systemic disease, particularly of the cardiovascular system. Recent advances in our knowledge of the blood supply of the optic nerve head have shed a significant new light on the subject. With the recent advent of fluorescein fundus angiography, an extra dimension has been added to the study of the ocular and optic disc circulations, and we have entered into a new era in the understanding of ocular vascular disorders *"in vivo"*. In the pre-angiography era, postmortem injection studies, although very valuable, did not completely reveal the vascular pattern of the optic disc in the living, in health, and disease. The ophthalmoscope, without doubt, has been valuable in assessing optic disc lesions, but could not give us information on the circulation of the eye and optic disc *"in vivo"*. This lack of information on the ocular and optic nerve head circulations has in the past resulted in confusion, ignorance, and misconceptions about the ischemic disorders of the optic nerve head, as is evident from the numerous names used to describe anterior ischemic optic neuropathy and the controversy about its pathogenesis.

One common and dangerous misconception is that anterior ischemic optic neuropathy is a rare condition. This lack of awareness has resulted from insufficient information on the subject, and unfortunately, leads to many patients with anterior ischemic optic neuropathy being misdiagnosed, particularly when they present for the first time with optic atrophy. Even when these patients are correctly diagnosed during early stages of the disease, the condition is almost always considered to be untreatable, and the patients are sent away with the advice that they should accept the visual loss as a natural calamity or "act of God". Recent studies, however, have indicated that a significant number of patients can be helped to regain fairly useful visual function, provided they are diagnosed early enough and adequate therapy instituted immediately. Recent studies have also suggested that anterior ischemic optic neuropathy, glaucoma, and low-tension glaucoma represent ischemic disorders of the anterior part of the optic nerve—the ischemia being of an acute and sudden onset in anterior ischemic optic neuropathy and of a chronic nature in the other two.

In this book, I have not only tried to describe fully the clinical picture, diagnosis, and management of anterior ischemic optic neuropathy, but also have laid out in some detail, the basic background information which has led us to a better understanding of this by no means uncommon disorder. The subjects discussed include the vascular pattern and histology of the optic nerve head in health and ischemia, and the pathogenesis of anterior ischemic optic neuropathy—information which has shed a significant light on the pathogenesis of a variety of visual field defects and of the optic disc cupping seen not only in anterior ischemic optic neuropathy but also in glaucoma and low-tension glaucoma. As anterior ischemic optic neuropathy, like optic disc edema, is not a disease in itself but a manifestation of a large number of systemic cardiovascular diseases and some ocular disorder (a fact not generally appreciated up to now), a brief account of these disorders has been considered desirable for a better understanding of their association with anterior ischemic optic neuropathy. Even though it is impossible to cover the entire literature, an attempt has also been made to review relevant literature on the various topics discussed in this book, to provide historic background information, and to place the present studies in their true perspective. I hope that the information provided in this book may help clinical ophthalmologists, neurologists, and internists to become more aware of anterior ischemic optic neuropathy and to assist them not only in its early diagnosis and better management, but also the other vascular disorders of the optic nerve head. I also hope that it will be of assistance to all those interested in the study of vascular disorders of the optic disc and nerve from a purely scientific viewpoint.

University of Iowa Hospitals and Clinics,   SOHAN SINGH HAYREH
Iowa City, Iowa

Acknowledgements

It is a pleasure to acknowledge my indebtedness to many ophthalmologists for referring patients to me and to a host of colleagues for their invaluable help in this study—it would be invidious to make special mention of any one of them. I also wish to thank my wife, SHELAGH, for her help in the preparation of this manuscript, to Mrs. MARIA WARBASSE and Miss ELIZABETH CONKLIN for their secretarial help, to the British Journal of Ophthalmology, the American Academy of Ophthalmology and Otolaryngology, and to Butterworths and Company Publishers Ltd., for permission to reproduce illustrations from my various publications and to the American Journal of Ophthalmology for Figure 13c. I am grateful to the Medical Research Council of Great Britain and the National Institutes of Health of the United States (Program Project Grant No. NS-03354) for their research grants under which this study was carried out.

Contents

Introduction

In anterior ischemic optic neuropathy there is a comparatively sudden loss of vision in the entire eye or in one sector of the field of vision, initially associated with edema of the optic disc, which resolves to optic atrophy within a month or two, leaving a permanent visual defect. A large number of such cases have been reported in the literature, but, although this clinical entity is well-known under different names, its pathogenesis and management have, until recently, been ill-understood. An attempt is made to give a comprehensive clinical description of the condition, its management, and its pathogenesis, based on my own as well as on studies previously reported in the literature.

Terminology

This condition has been given different eponyms by various authors because its pathogenesis is controversial:

1. Optic neuritis [81, 454],
2. Acute optic neuritis of hypertension or arteriosclerosis [58, 59, 124, 125],
3. Arteriosclerotic papillitis [124, 125, 329, 339, 342, 473],
4. Papillary apoplexy [458],
5. Senile papillitis or senile papillopathy [35],
6. Pseudo-papillitis [342],
7. Vascular pseudo-papillitis [173, 182, 183, 185, 186, 201, 398],
8. Optico-malacia [325],
9. Infarction of the optic nerve [151],
10. Ischemic retrobulbar neuritis [70, 71],
11. Ischemic neuritis of Papilla [548],
12. Ischemic papillopathy [471],
13. Acute ischemia of the disc [498],
14. Ischemic edema of the disc [40, 309],
15. Ischemic optic neuritis [44, 285],
16. Ischemic optic neuropathy [88, 388].

The most popular term in the European literature has been "Vascular pseudo-papillitis". As will be evident from the pathogenesis of this condition, perhaps the most suitable term is "Anterior Ischemic Optic Neuropathy" because the condition is ischemic, involves both the optic nerve head and retrolaminar optic nerve (hence terms defining it as a disease only of the optic disc are not correct), is noninflammatory (therefore all terms with the suffix -itis are incorrect), and there is nothing "pseudo-" about it.

Part I Pathogenesis

A proper understanding of the pathogenesis of anterior ischemic optic neuropathy would make its clinical pattern and management easier to follow. A brief account of the anatomy and blood supply of the anterior part of the optic nerve, which consists of the optic nerve head and retrolaminar optic nerve, is an essential prerequisite. As far as the arterial blood supply of the optic nerve is concerned, the optic nerve head and retrolaminar region form a single unit. Hence, it is appropriate to study their structure and blood supply together.

A. Structure of the Anterior Part of the Optic Nerve

This has been discussed in detail elsewhere [254, 265]. Most authors divide the optic nerve head into the retinal, choroidal, and scleral parts, from the front backwards. For descriptive purposes, I have divided the optic nerve head into the following three parts (Figs. 1, 34) [250].

a) Surface Nerve Fiber Layer

This is the most superficial layer, containing the compact optic nerve fibers as they converge here from all parts of the retina and bend backward. The surface nerve fiber layer is covered by the inner limiting membrane of Elschnig, which is composed of astrocytes and which separates the nerve fiber layer from the vitreous [7, 465].

b) Prelaminar Region

This region has been called glial, choroidal, or, more commonly, the anterior part of the lamina

cribrosa [6, 61, 144, 265, 354, 573, 575], resulting in a certain amount of confusion. Sometimes even the very existence of this glial region, as a distinct entity, has been ignored [575].

The prelaminar region consists of nerve fibers arranged in bundles surrounded by tube-like glial channels, formed by specialized astrocytes ("spider cells" [6, 575]). The loose glial tissue between the nerve fiber bundles forms trabeculae. Capillaries are located within the glial septa. A narrow, perivascular, connective tissue space accompanies most of the capillaries [6]. The capillaries are surrounded by a glial limiting membrane, built up from the foot-plates of the glial cells [265].

WOLTER [575] described the presence of a shallow, cap-like "wicker basket" (composed of the "spider cells" lying in this part of the optic nerve head) which is closely connected to the lamina cribrosa at its base, with its rounded convexity towards the vitreal surface of the optic nerve head. According to WOLTER, the basket acts as an important supporting, protective, and nutritive organ to the nerve fibers. In our studies we did not observe an anterior limit of this basket [265]. The only connective tissue seen in this part is that accompanying the capillaries [6, 265]. WOLTER [575] described glial fibers surrounding both the nerve fiber bundles and the individual nerve fibers in the bundle; ANDERSON [6], in studies with an electron-microscope, found that while the bundles are surrounded by glial cells, only an occasional astrocyte crosses through the bundle at right angles to the nerve fibers.

At its edge the prelaminar region is separated by a layer of glial tissue from the adjacent deeper layer of the retina ("Intermediary tissue of Kuhnt" [326]) and from the adjacent choroid ("Border tissue of Jacoby" [303]).

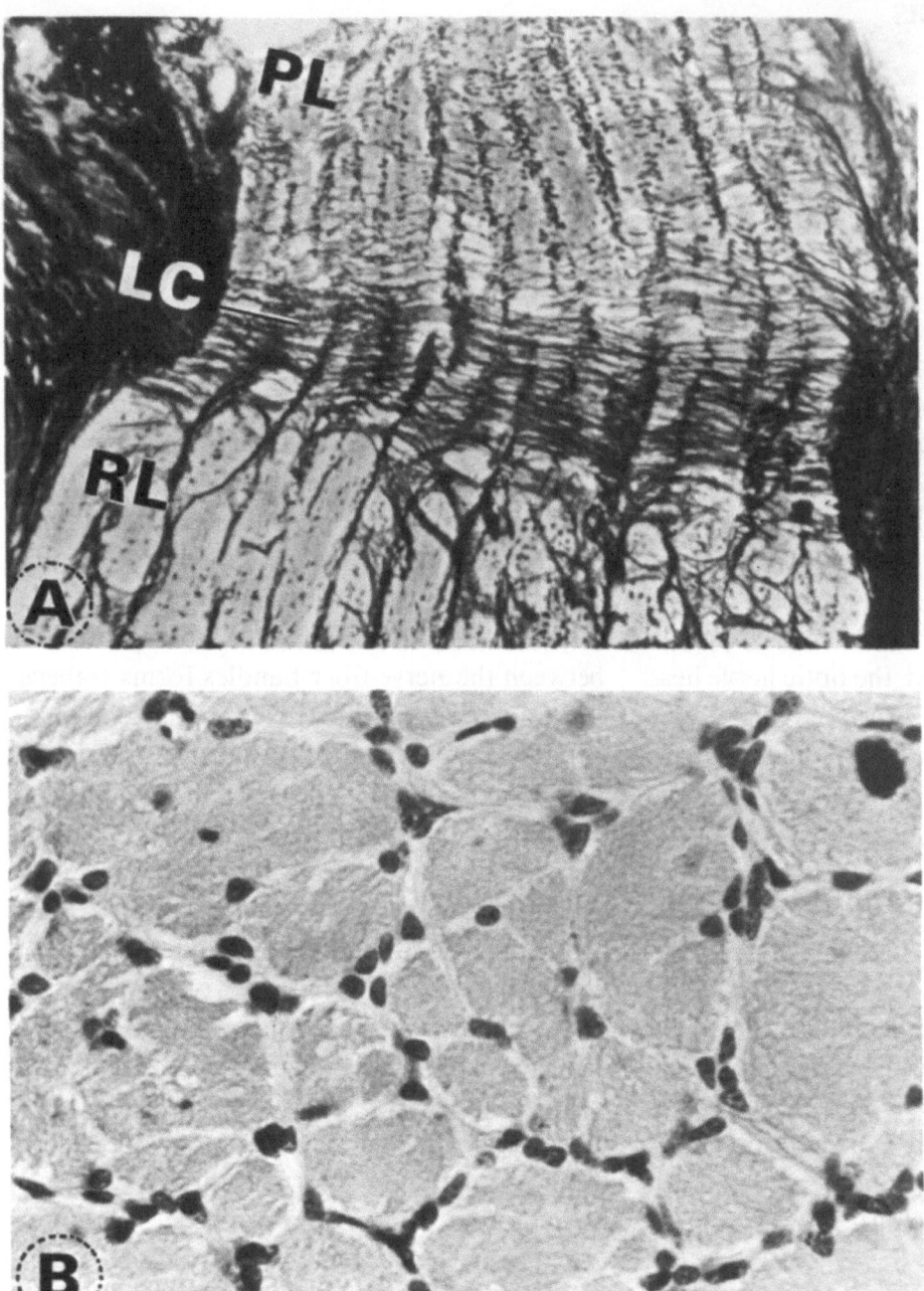

Fig. 1A–D. Histological section of the optic nerve head and adjacent retrolaminar optic nerve in rhesus monkeys.
A) Longitudinal section (*LC* Lamina cribrosa, *PL* Prelaminar region, *RL* Retrolaminar region).
B, C, D) Transverse sections in (B) prelaminar, (C) lamina cribrosa, and (D) retrolaminar regions

The optic nerve fibers make a 90° bend and their main support is the glial tissue of the prelaminar region.

c) Lamina Cribrosa Region

This region has been described as the scleral or posterior part of the lamina cribrosa, which, as mentioned previously, is confusing terminology. I have restricted the term *lamina cribrosa* to only this part of the optic nerve head.

The lamina cribrosa region forms a band of dense, compact connective tissue that bridges across the scleral canal. In addition to an opening in the center for the central retinal vessels, this band contains many oval or rounded open-

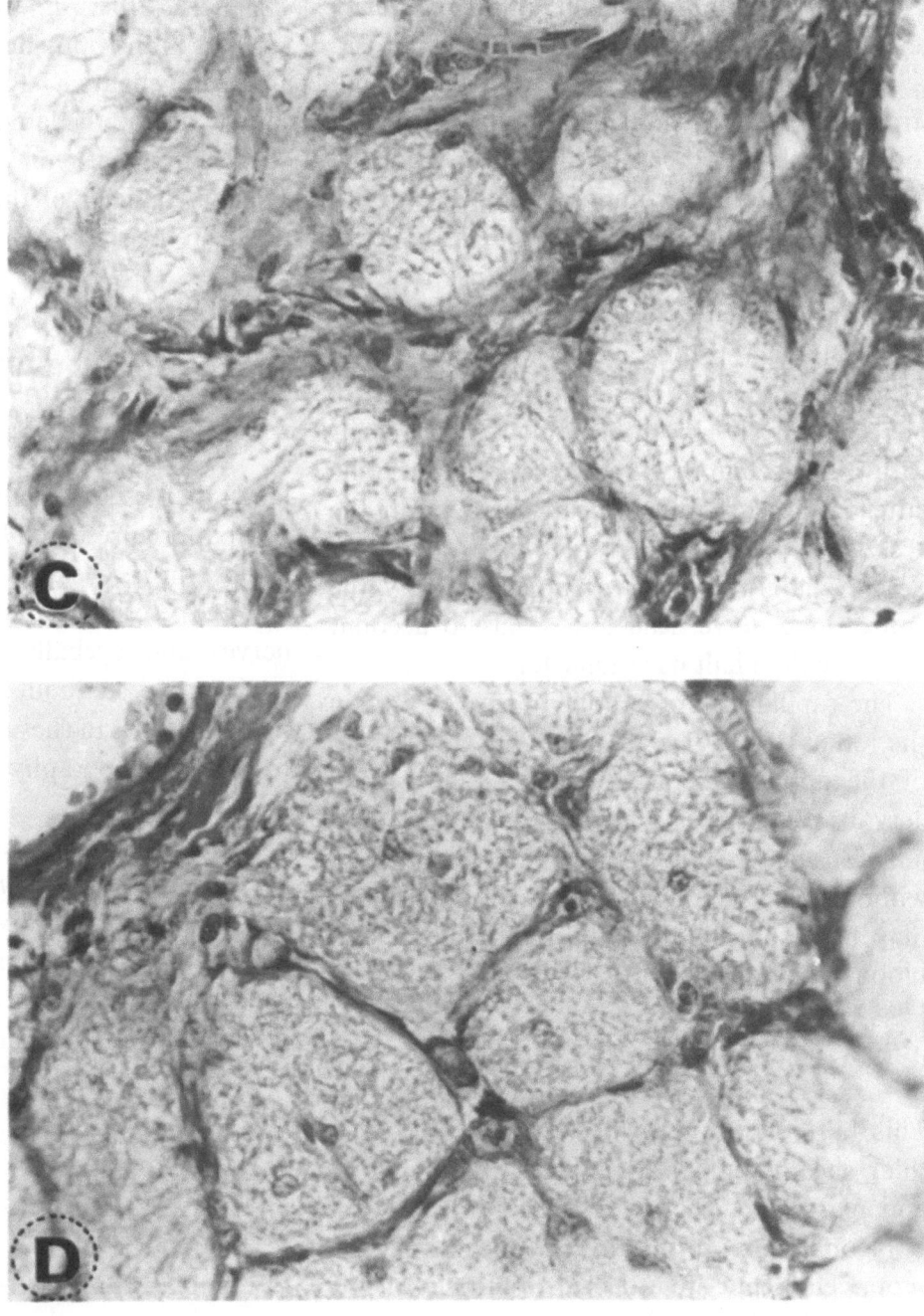

Fig. 1 (continued)

ings for the transmission of nerve fiber bundles. The lamina cribrosa shows a lamellar nature, with connective tissue alternating with glial sheets [6, 573]. Posteriorly the connective tissue sheets become more and more prominent. Connective tissue septa of the retrolaminar part of the optic nerve are attached to the posterior surface of the lamina cribrosa. WOLFF [573] and

HOGAN *et al.* [282] found a large amount of elastic tissue in the lamina cribrosa, but ANDERSON [6] found it varied greatly from one eye to another. The openings in the lamina cribrosa are lined by astrocytes, which form a continuous glial membrane that surrounds each nerve fiber bundle, as in the prelaminar region. Thus nerve fiber bundles are separated from adjacent connective tissue. Each trabecula has a capillary in its center. Most authors include the prelaminar region in their description of the lamina cribrosa.

The border tissue of Elschnig, which is more strongly developed on the temporal as compared to the nasal side, separates the sclera from the nerve fibers and is composed of dense collagenous tissue, with many glial and elastic fibers and some pigment [470]. It continues forward to separate the choroid from nervous tissue.

The lamina cribrosa and the prelaminar regions, throughout their entire thickness, are pierced centrally by the central retinal vessels with their accompanying connective tissue. The latter forms a cylindrical sheath surrounding the vessels.

The glial framework occupies virtually the entire optic nerve head and seems to account for more than half its volume [6].

The capillaries in the optic nerve head, as in the retina [110, 301, 340, 341, 493], other parts of the optic nerve [5, 10], and in the central nervous system [21, 401, 456, 514, 574] have tight junctions between the adjacent endothelial cells, without fenestration [6]. These tight junctions may be responsible for the retinal-blood and blood-brain [456] barrier.

d) Retrolaminar Part of the Optic Nerve

This part of the optic nerve is enclosed in a thick sheath composed of the dura, arachnoid, and pia mater. The nerve fiber bundles lie in polygonal spaces formed by the connective tissue septa. The septa are attached to the pia on the surface, to the envelope around the central retinal vessels centrally, and to the lamina cribrosa in front. They contain blood vessels. As in the rest of the central nervous system, at the neuroectodermal-mesodermal junction the nerve fibers are always separated from collagenous tissue and blood vessels by an astroglial layer throughout the course of the optic nerve. Within the nerve fiber bundles lie astrocytes (which form the supporting glial framework), rows of oligodendroglia (responsible for the formation of myelin sheaths), and scattered microglial cells (reticuloendothelial cells); the latter

are also seen in other parts of the optic nerve. The nerve fibers in this part are myelinated, whereas in the optic nerve head and retina, they are unmyelinated. The myelin sheaths stop shortly behind the lamina cribrosa. The absence of myelin sheath may be responsible for the smaller diameter of the optic nerve head compared to the retrolaminar optic nerve.

B. The Blood Supply of the Anterior Part of the Optic Nerve

I have discussed this subject fully elsewhere [245]. The pattern presented here is based on my studies in human eyes (neoprene latex injection in 100 eyes, serial histologic sections of 10 optic nerves and eyeballs, and fluorescein fundus angiography in about 500 eyes), and my experimental studies in rhesus monkey eyes (fluorescein fundus angiography and latex injection studies in over 200 eyes).

I would like to stress that *the pattern of blood supply varies greatly between individuals*. The following pattern usually is seen in most individuals. The blood supply in different parts of the optic nerve head is discussed using the divisions described for structure.

1. Arterial Supply

a) Lamina Cribrosa Region

Centripetal branches from the short posterior ciliary arteries and, in a few cases, by the so-called circle of Zinn and Haller supply this region in its entirety. I want to emphasize that a typical circle of Zinn-Haller is an uncommon finding and, when present, is quite often an incomplete circle; this finding also has been confirmed by others [354]. ANDERSON [8] never found this circle. It is unfortunate that the circle of Zinn and Haller is usually the only structure mentioned when the blood supply of the optic nerve head is discussed, attaching tremendous significance

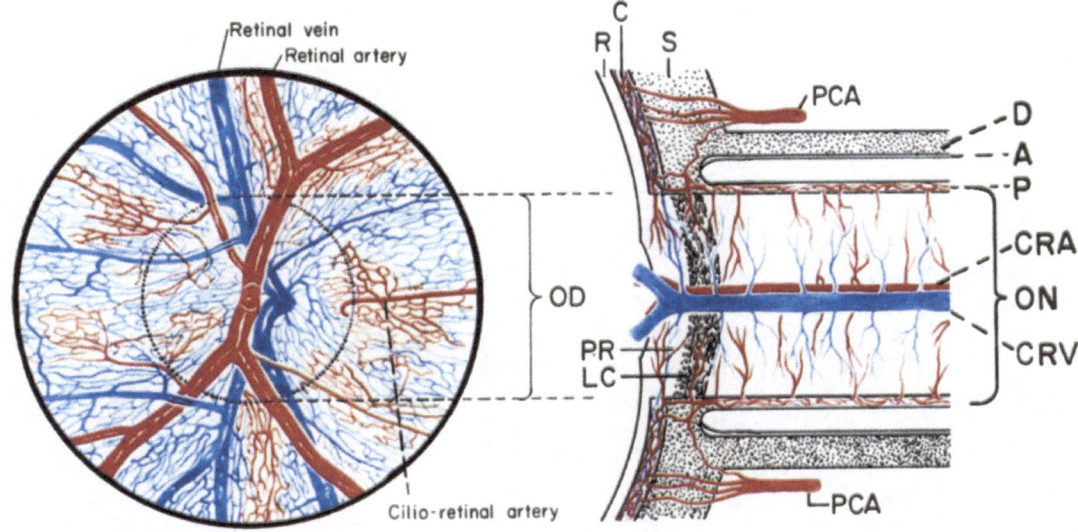

Fig. 2. Diagrammatic representation of blood supply of the optic nerve head:

A	Arachnoid	*D*	Dura	*P*	Pia
C	Choroid	*LC*	Lamina cribrosa	*PCA*	Posterior ciliary artery
CRA	Central retinal artery	*OD*	Optic disc	*PR*	Prelaminar region
CRV	Central retinal vein	*ON*	Optic nerve	*R*	Retina
				S	Sclera

to this uncommon structure. This reflects the widely-prevailing ignorance about the vasculature of this part of the optic nerve.

The blood vessels lie in the fibrous septa and form a dense capillary plexus. The central retinal artery gives no branch in this region.

b) Prelaminar Region

This region is supplied mainly by centripetal branches from the peripapillary pre-choriocapillaris choroidal vessels with no communication between the capillaries in the optic nerve head and peripapillary choriocapillaris. This choroidal supply to this region has been further confirmed by other workes [8, 273, 354, 532]. The distribution of these vessels, as revealed by fluorescein angiography, is sectoral (Fig. 3). Vessels in the region of the lamina cribrosa may also contribute to the blood supply in this region. Angiographic studies strongly suggest that the temporal part of this region is the most vascular and receives maximum contribution from the adjacent peripapillary choroid (Figs. 4–6). ERNEST and ARCHER [158], based on fluorescein angiography in one patient with a subtotal loss

of peripapillary choroid and on a few questionable experiments on monkey eyes, concluded that the peripapillary choroid does not significantly contribute to the vasculature of the optic nerve head in man. My results, based on studies of many hundreds of eyes, completely refute their conclusions. Their finding represents one of the rare variations seen in the pattern of the blood supply of this region; however, a rare occurrence does not constitute a classic pattern. I have observed more than one similar instance in my studies. The central retinal artery does not contribute branches to this region.

c) Surface Nerve Fiber Layer

Blood to this area is supplied mainly by branches of the retinal arterioles. These branches commonly arise from the main retinal arterioles in the circumpapillary region and less often on the disc. Capillaries on the surface of the disc are continuous with capillaries of the peripapillary retina and with the long radial peripapillary capillary network described by MICHAELSON and CAMPBELL [387], TOUSSAINT *et al.* [539] and HENKIND [271]. On the disc the capillaries usually

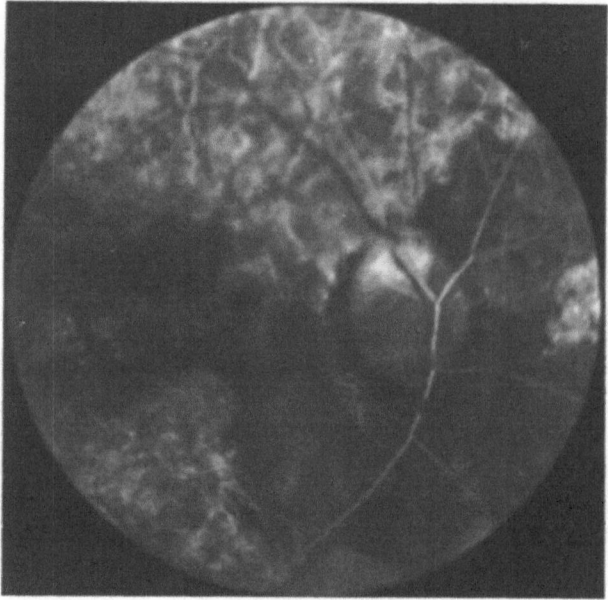

Fig. 3. Fluorescein fundus angiogram of a normal human right eye, showing sectoral filling of the choroid and the adjacent prelaminar region of the optic nerve head

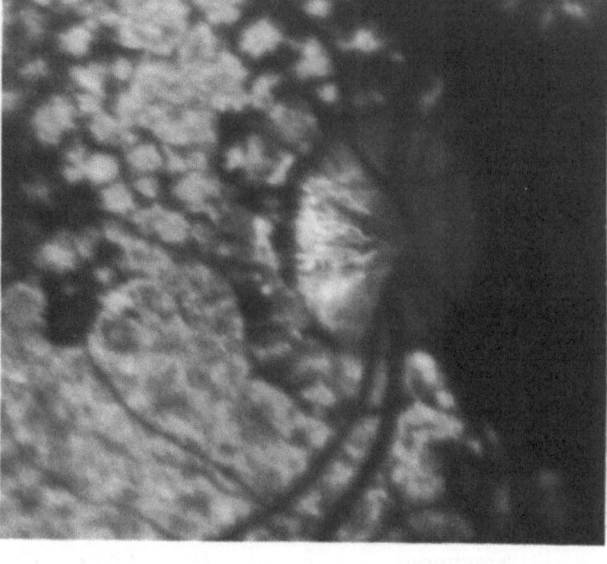

Fig. 4. Fluorescein fundus angiogram of right eye of a monkey during the preretinal-arterial phase, showing filling of temporal half of the choroid and prelaminar vessels in temporal part of the optic disc

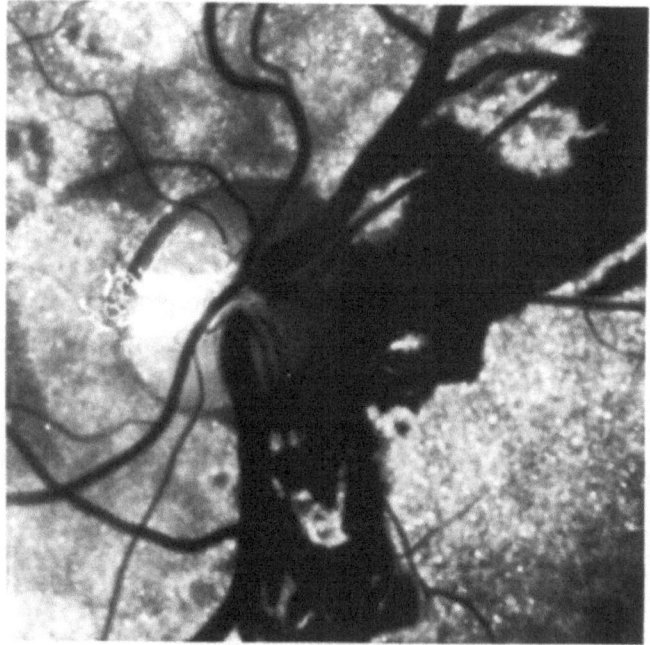

Fig. 5. Fluorescein fundus angiogram of right eye of a monkey after experimental occlusion of the central retinal artery in the orbit. The lateral posterior ciliary artery supplies the temporal half and the superior nasal part of the choroid. Filling of the medial posterior ciliary artery is seen in the inferior nasal sector of the choroid. The border zone between the two and the nasal peripapillary region is still not filled. Part of the optic disc supplied by the lateral posterior ciliary artery is filled

are venous in nature and drain into the central retinal vein or its tributaries. The capillaries in this region are continuous with those in the prelaminar region.

It is not uncommon to find vessels of choroidal origin, derived from the adjacent prelaminar part of the disc, in the surface nerve fiber layer. These vessels are seen most often in the temporal sector of the disc, and one may enlarge to form the cilioretinal artery.

d) Retrolaminar Region of the Optic Nerve

On the basis of blood supply, this region forms an integral part of the optic nerve head. It is

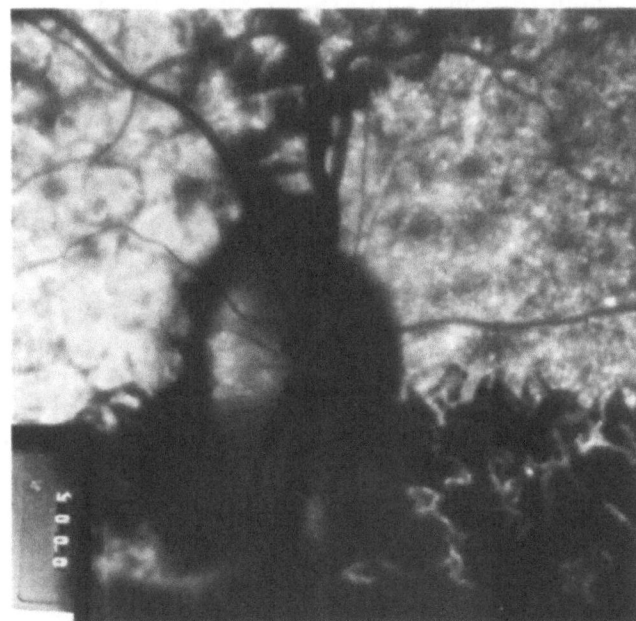

Fig. 6. Fluorescein fundus angiogram of right eye of a monkey after experimental occlusion of the central retinal artery in the orbit, showing filling of the upper half of the choroid and optic disc, with a well demarcated horizontal border

supplied mainly by centripetal branches from the pial vessels, which most often are recurrent pial branches from the peripapillary choroid, although some are from the circle of Zinn (or usually its substitute, i.e., direct branches from the short posterior ciliary arteries [241]). Although in 75 percent of optic nerves the central retinal artery gives out centrifugal branches during its intraneural course in the optic nerve [240–244, 503], in many instances there may be no branch from the artery in the region immediately behind the lamina cribrosa. In such cases the pial supply from the posterior ciliary arteries may be the only or the major source of blood to the retrolaminar region.

From this description of the blood supply of the optic nerve head and retrolaminar region, it is evident that the *posterior ciliary arteries are the only source to 'a' and 'b' and the main (if not the only) source of 'd', and they may supply the temporal part of 'c'*. Other workers also have described the choroid and posterior ciliary arteries as the major source of blood to the optic nerve head [34, 159, 273, 354]. The posterior ciliary arteries have a segmental distribution, the main artery supplying the nasal or temporal half or the superior or inferior half of the choroid and optic nerve head [247, 249, 259]. The short

posterior ciliary arteries may supply smaller sectors. All capillaries in the optic nerve head are interconnected, being continuous posteriorly with those of the retrolaminar region and anteriorly with the adjoining retina but no connection is seen with the choriocapillaris.

I have never seen the so-called "central artery of the optic nerve" [174–177, 180, 571] in any of my specimens [238, 239, 503]. This experience has been confirmed by others [26, 513].

Usually there are two to three posterior ciliary arteries, arising from the ophthalmic artery [239], that supply the choroid and optic nerve head (Fig. 7). These are designated medial and lateral posterior ciliary arteries, depending on their relationship to the optic nerve near their site of entry into the sclera. The main lateral or medial posterior ciliary artery usually supplies half of the choroid and optic nerve head, the distribution being either vertical (Figs. 4, 5, 24n, 27b) or horizontal (Fig. 6) [247]. If there are three posterior ciliary arteries, a smaller sector may be supplied by each artery (Fig. 3). Smaller divisions of the main posterior ciliary arteries would supply smaller sectors.

Venous Drainage. The optic nerve head and retrolaminar region are drained by the central retinal vein. The prelaminar region also drains into the choroidal veins and, via these channels, the central retinal vein communicates with the choroidal veins.

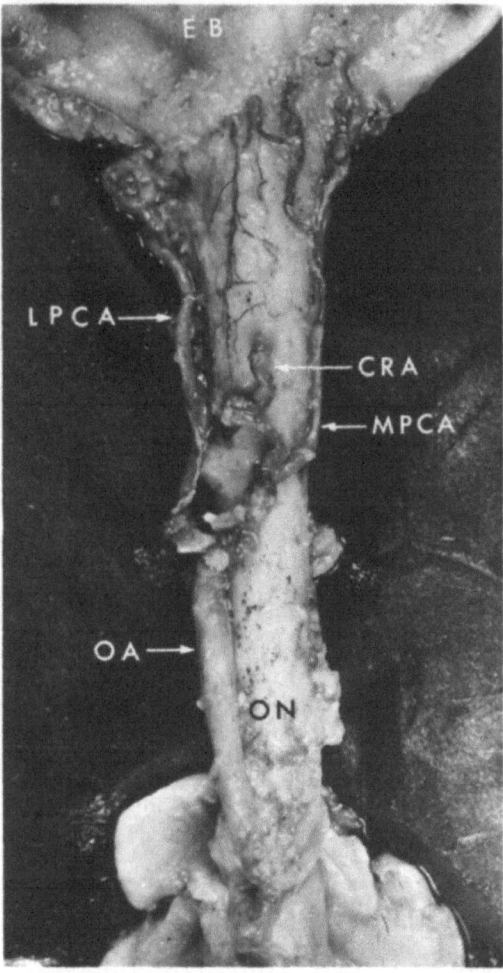

Fig. 7. Photograph of inferior surface of human right eyeball (*EB*) and optic nerve (*ON*), showing ophthalmic (*OA*), central retinal (*CRA*), lateral posterior ciliary (*LPCA*) and medial posterior ciliary (*MPCA*) arteries

C. Fluorescein Angiography Pattern of Normal Optic Disc

Fluorescein angiography plays an important role in studies of the blood supply of the optic nerve head in health and disease. It is therefore essential to know the normal pattern of fluorescence

of the optic disc. The subject has been discussed fully elsewhere [245, 251, 262].

Usually, the optic disc starts to show fluorescence before the retinal arteries show any filling, because the posterior ciliary artery (and choroidal) circulation is slightly faster than the retinal arterial circulation (Figs. 3, 4). However, the reverse is also common. Frequently, a large number of vessels in the prelaminar region fill from the adjacent choroid. In the disc this initial filling usually is prominent in the temporal sector.

Preretinal-arterial or initial filling of the optic disc represents the posterior ciliary artery's contribution to the optic nerve head; it is due most often to prelaminar filling, but also is frequently due to the filling of vessels in the lamina cribrosa, which is a very vascular structure. ERNEST and ARCHER [158] attributed preretinal-arterial fluorescence of the optic disc to fluorescein in the retrobulbar vessels and theorized that "the greater the atrophy (of the optic disc) the more the fluorescence will be transmitted. This is because the decrease in the plexus of small vessels—and thus the amount of blood in the optic nerve—may offer less impediment to the light from the extraocular vasculature which does contain fluorescein." The interpretation and assumption of ERNEST and ARCHER seem to be wrong, because a) the connective tissue of the lamina cribrosa is opaque like sclera, and one does not expect to see immediate and significant fluorescence from retrobulbar tissue; b) fluorescence of the optic disc always is reduced in optic atrophy and frequently is nonexistent [61, 245, 262, 263, 412].

Fluorescence of the optic disc peaks at the early retinal arteriovenous phase. The peak is due in part to the contribution by the posterior ciliary artery to the optic disc, but is due most often to filling of the dense capillary plexus in the surface nerve fiber layer, which represents a retinal arterial contribution (Fig. 8) [251].

Fluorescence of the disc then fades rapidly, but a certain amount of well-defined staining of the optic disc is seen in the late phases (10–15 minutes after the dye is injected), usually more marked near the margin of the disc, and prob-

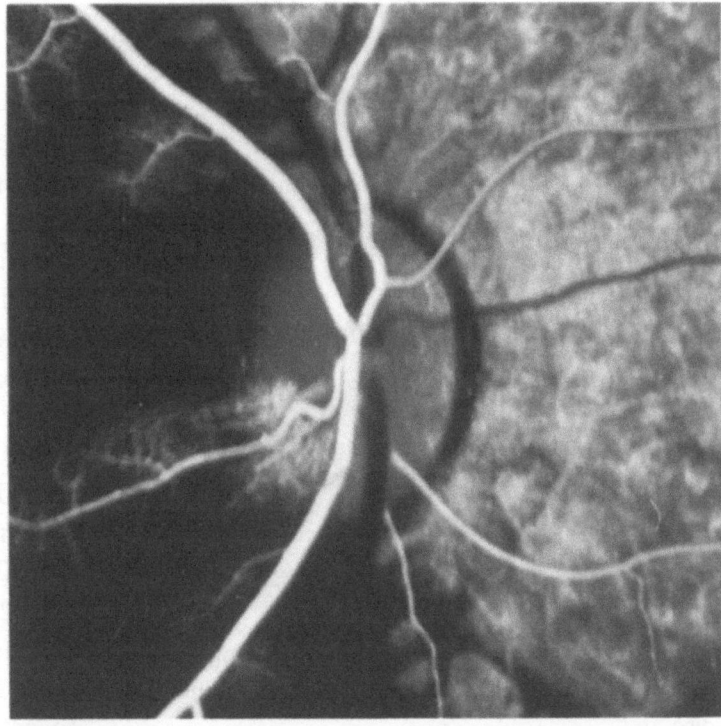

a

b

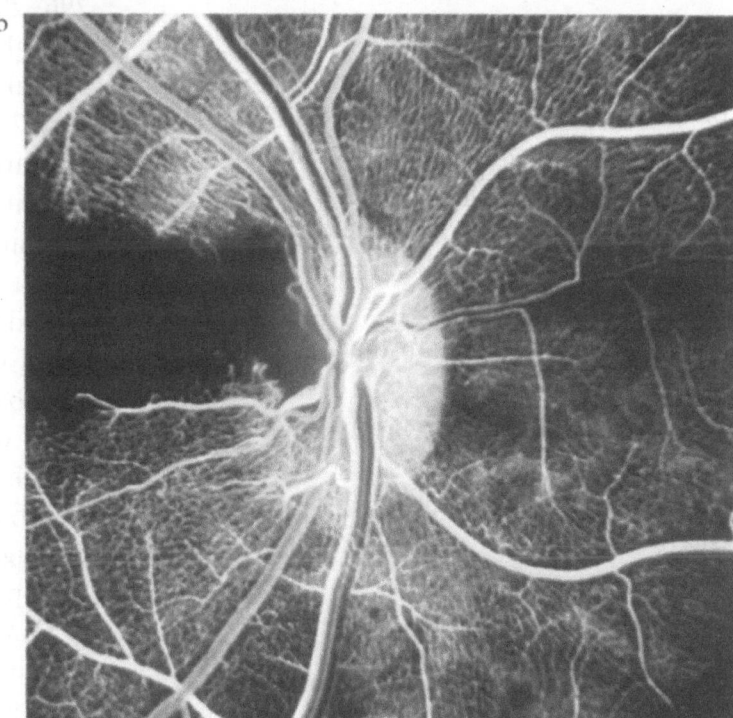

Fig. 8a and b. Fluorescein fundus angiograms of a rhesus monkey after experimental occlusion of the lateral posterior ciliary artery: Note the complete absence of filling of the temporal part of choroid and optic disc (a) as well as of the retinal vasculature in a sector of the retinal capillary bed supplied by a cilioretinal artery on the temporal side (b)

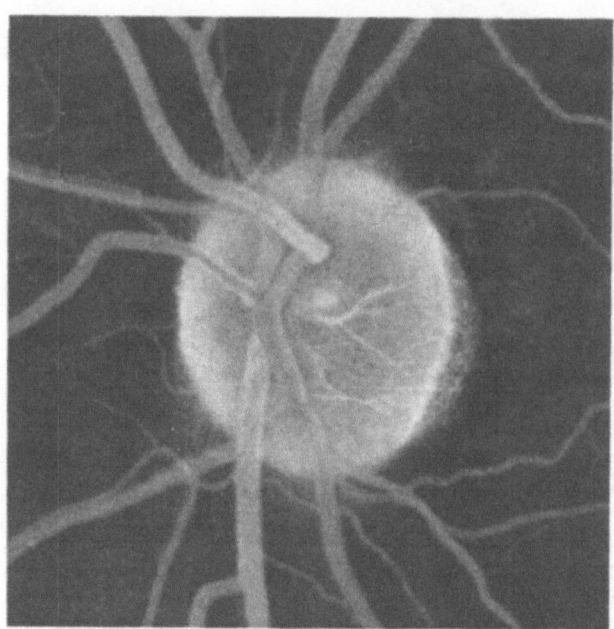

Fig. 9. Fluorescein fundus angiogram of a human eye showing normal late fluorescence pattern of the optic disc

ably because of a diffusion from the choroid of the dye which stains the connective tissue of the lamina cribrosa in a manner similar to that seen in the sclera (Fig. 9).

Fluorescein angiographic studies of the optic disc have shown that the temporal part of the optic disc, in spite of its paler appearance, usually is more vascular than the nasal part. This indicates that redness is not a true index of the vascularity of the normal disc [245, 251, 262]. Possible explanations for this phenomenon are discussed elsewhere [245, 251].

D. Pathogenesis of Anterior Ischemic Optic Neuropathy

Many theories have been proposed to explain the pathogenesis of anterior ischemic optic neuropathy.

Review of the Literature

The site of the lesion in anterior ischemic optic neuropathy is thought to lie in the optic nerve,

although some authors considered it to be due to involvement of the retina. It is almost universally agreed that it is due to interference with the circulation of either of these structures. SKILLERN and LOCKHART [505], however, thought that anterior ischemic optic neuropathy in diabetes is due to the toxic effect of prolonged hyperglycemia and failure of glucose utilization, and did not consider arterial circulatory disorders a significant factor.

Most authors, while describing a circulatory lesion in the optic nerve, have made nonspecific, vague statements as to the exact lesion. It was considered to be a circulatory disturbance in the optic nerve [309, 433] due to pathologic changes [193, 296, 297, 457, 515] or occlusive disease [40, 81, 329, 473] of the small vessels of the nerve. Occlusion of the small nutrient vessels of the optic nerve was generally considered to be due to arteriosclerosis [39, 76, 119, 183, 193, 274, 296, 297, 352, 359, 433, 457, 515, 543]; others thought the change mainly affected the central retinal artery [1, 43, 227, 466] although IGERSHEIMER [297] and RINTELEN [457] were of the opinion that arteriosclerosis of the central retinal artery has little effect on the optic nerve. The possibility that arteritis of vessels of the optic nerve and retina is responsible for this has also been mentioned [506]. Some authors have stated that these small vessel changes are located in the anterior retrobulbar part of the optic nerve [39, 68, 300, 462]; while according to others these are in the vessels of the optic disc [103, 170, 382, 471]. MEADOWS [384] mentioned that there is ischemic damage to the papilla and anterior portion of the optic nerve.

FRANÇOIS and co-workers [173, 180, 183, 185, 186] and others [441, 442, 473] postulated that anterior ischemic optic neuropathy was due to occlusion of a "central artery of the optic nerve", an artery whose existence they assumed. According to them, this artery arises directly from the ophthalmic artery, proximal to the origin of the central retinal artery [174], enters the optic nerve behind the central retinal artery, and divides into anterior and posterior branches on reaching the center of the optic nerve; the anterior and posterior branches run to the lamina cribrosa and optic foramen respectively in the center of the optic nerve. The anterior branch anastomoses with the circle of Zinn and Haller. They state that it is "impossible to explain the symptoms without the presence of an individualized axial arterial system in the optic nerve" and concluded that "a central optic nerve vascular system always exists" [180]. My anatomic studies on the blood supply of the optic nerve and branches of the ophthalmic artery in about 100 human specimens [238, 239, 241, 243, 502, 503] and those of BEAUVIEUX and RISTITCH [26] and STEELE and BLUNT [408] failed to reveal a "central artery of the optic nerve" corresponding to the description mentioned by FRANÇOIS et al. [174, 175, 176, 177, 180]. Hence, occlusion of the "central artery of the optic nerve" cannot be significant in the etiology of anterior ischemic optic neuropathy.

Interference with the blood supply to the retina as the cause of anterior ischemic optic neuropathy has been considered by some workers [44, 416, 506] because central retinal artery pressure fell, as judged by ophthalmodynamometry. UHTHOFF [543] and SMITH and GREEN [506] thought it was due to the involvement of vessels in both the optic nerve and retina.

There are many histopathologic studies on patients with anterior ischemic optic neuropathy [79, 88, 94, 103, 105, 221, 272, 275, 322, 325, 363, 364, 369, 382, 462, 490, 511, 576]. The area of greatest involvement in the optic nerve is at the retrolaminar and optic nerve head (mentioned as lamina cribrosa in reports pertinent to the lamina cribrosa and prelaminar regions) [88, 103, 272, 322, 325, 363, 364, 462, 511]. The lesion begins with infarction and evolves through liquefaction necrosis (in four weeks, Fig. 13a) [364], a reactive increase in astrocytes and lymphocytes in eight weeks [103], and finally to retrolaminar fibrosis in four months (Fig. 13c) [272]. The involved part of the optic nerve usually is well-defined and circumscribed. All but two of these reports are of patients with temporal arteritis; the remaining two are of anterior ischemic optic neuropathy due to arteriosclerosis [88, 322]. In 16 reports of temporal arteritis [79, 94, 103, 105, 221, 272, 275, 325, 363,

364, 369, 382, 462, 490, 511, 576], the central retinal artery was involved in 11 [88, 94, 103, 105, 221, 325, 363, 369, 462, 511, 576], the posterior ciliary artery in 10 [88, 103, 105, 221, 325, 363, 364, 462, 511, 576], and the ophthalmic artery in 7 [88, 103, 105, 275, 325, 363, 511]. There is only one case in which none of these arteries was involved [272], and this finding was explained as due either to the long-term use of corticosteroids before the patient died, or to the self-limiting nature of the disease. RODENHAUSER [462] is the only investigator to report arteritis in the choroidal arteries and retinal arterioles. KNOX and DUKE [322] reported focal necrosis of the temporal half of the optic nerve head and retrolaminar optic nerve, with some distension of the lamina cribrosa in that region, in a patient with occlusion of the left common carotid artery and generalized arteriosclerosis, two weeks after the onset of visual disturbance. COGAN [88] also reported a case of anterior ischemic optic neuropathy with well-defined infarction of the retrolaminar optic nerve in the entire temporal half (Fig. 13b).

It is interesting to note that ELLENBERGER et al. [151] examined 40 optic nerves of people older than 45 years for atherosclerosis and arteriosclerosis and found that changes in the optic nerve vessels were similar to those seen elsewhere in the body, suggesting that the optic nerve vessels were constantly involved in systemic atherosclerosis and arteriosclerosis. In anterior ischemic optic neuropathy, vascular changes in the optic nerve correlated slightly or not at all with those in the retina [296, 433]. WOLTER et al. [576] and MACFAUL [363] reported that temporal arteritis involves only the extraocular parts of the short posterior ciliary arteries and not the choroid, which is contrary to the opinion expressed by RODENHAUSER [462].

Various mechanisms for the production of ischemic necrosis in the anterior part of the optic nerve have been postulated. KREIBIG [325] considered it to be due to combined involvement of the axial and peripheral (from short posterior ciliary arteries) vascular system due to occlusion of the ophthalmic artery and short posterior ciliary arteries. SPENCER et al. [511] agreed with

KREIBIG's hypothesis [325]. MEADOWS [382], WAGNER *et al.* [552], and MACFAUL [363] thought that ischemic necrosis is due to involvement of the short posterior ciliary arteries as they form the circle of Zinn and Haller. According to BIRKHEAD *et al.* [44], anoxic damage of the optic nerve is probably due to extreme narrowing of the lumen of the ophthalmic artery or central retinal artery.

Recent Studies

The concept of pathogenesis of anterior ischemic optic neuropathy, which is presented below, is based on:

a) Pattern of Arterial Supply of the Anterior Part of the Optic Nerve

This was studied in man and experimentally in rhesus monkeys and is summarized on p. 6.

b) Clinical Studies

These consisted of ophthalmoscopic and fluorescein fundus angiographic studies on more than 75 patients with anterior ischemic optic neuropathy of different etiologies (mainly due to arteriosclerosis and temporal arteritis [256], p. 31, 71).

c) Experimental Studies

Anterior ischemic optic neuropathy was produced in rhesus monkeys and its evolution studied by ophthalmoscopy, fluorescein fundus angiography, and histopathology [261].

d) Histopathologic Studies on Eyes with Anterior Ischemic Optic Neuropathy

These were obtained from cases reported in the literature and are summarized on p. 13.

From my studies of the blood supply of the optic nerve head, I [245, 246] pointed out that the basic lesion in anterior ischemic optic neuro-

pathy is the occlusion of the posterior ciliary arteries, which produces infarction not only of the optic nerve head but also of the retrolaminar part of the optic nerve, by virtue of their distribution to the prelaminar, lamina cribrosa, and retrolaminar regions. In patients with cilioretinal arteries, the retinal area supplied by these vessels is also infarcted (Figs. 10, 17). FOULDS [171] also attributed anterior ischemic optic neuropathy to interference with posterior ciliary artery circulation.

Fluorescein angiographic studies in patients with anterior ischemic optic neuropathy confirmed the presence of occlusive disorder of the posterior ciliary arteries [256] (p. 71). These eyes showed very slow and poor filling of the choroid, or on occasion, complete absence of filling and also nonfilling of the optic disc.

Experimental studies were conducted in rhesus monkeys to investigate the pathogenesis of anterior ischemic optic neuropathy, in which the various posterior ciliary arteries were occluded [261]. These eyes developed anterior ischemic optic neuropathy that ophthalmoscopically showed swelling of the optic disc soon after occlusion of the posterior ciliary arteries (Fig. 11) and within 5–6 weeks, optic atrophy. Histologic examination of these eyes showed that the optic nerve head and retrolaminar region were involved (Fig. 12). LESSELL [352a] in a recent review of our experimental anterior ischemic optic neuropathy paper [261] pointed out that, according to him, there are obvious differences between the clinical picture of anterior ischemic optic neuropathy in humans and the lesions produced by us by occlusion of the posterior ciliary arteries in monkeys [261]. I fail to understand the basis for his erroneous impression. Recently, ANDERSON and DAVIS [9a], from experimental occlusion of the posterior ciliary arteries in eleven squirrel monkeys, concluded that anterior ischemic optic neuropathy must represent disease of more than just the posterior ciliary arteries, because in their study they found only minute areas of atrophy in the optic nerve head. The fallacy of such a statement can be readily perceived if one considers the following factors:

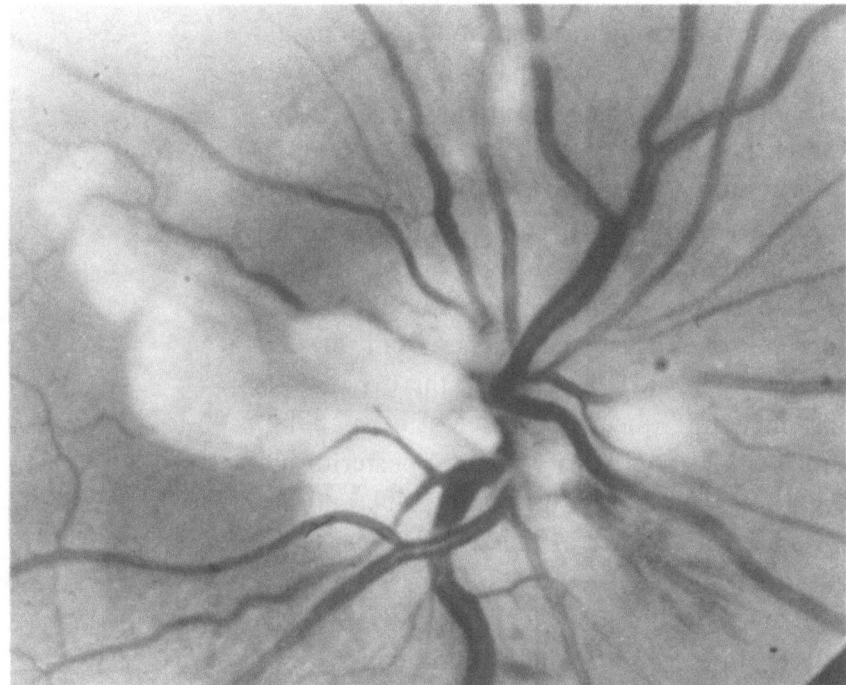

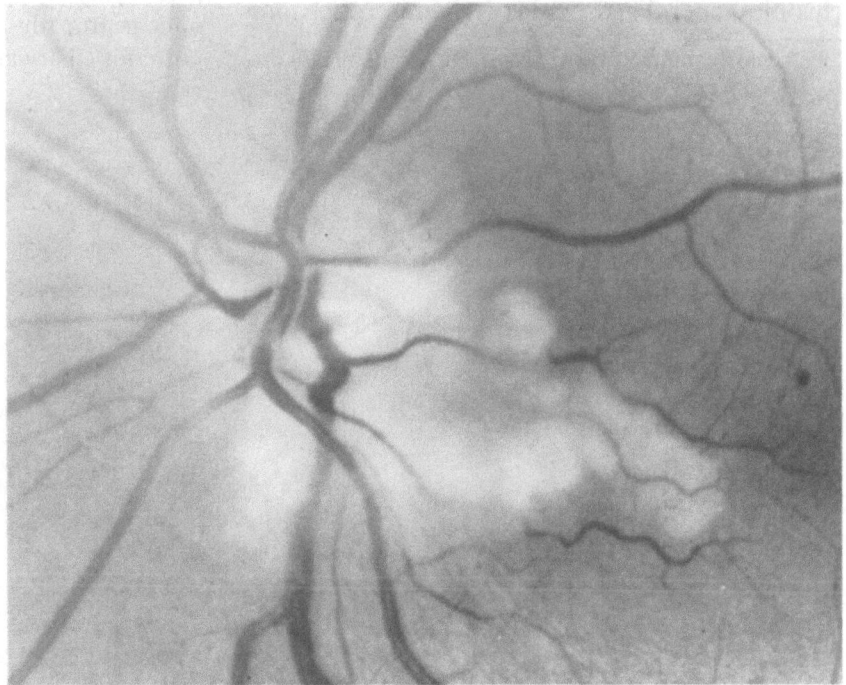

Fig. 10a and b. Right (a) and left (b) fundi of a 68-year-old woman with temporal arteritis. Sudden loss of vision occurred in both eyes at an interval of 4 days. Note the pale edema of the disc and the retinal infarct on the temporal side of the optic disc in both eyes. The area of the retinal infarct is that supplied by the cilioretinal artery in each eye.

1. The age of the monkeys used in experimental posterior ciliary artery occlusion by us [261] and by ANDERSON *et al.* [9a] is comparable to an age of 10–15 years at the maximum in humans. Anterior ischemic optic neuropathy, however, is predominantly a disease of persons past middle age. It is well-established that in young healthy persons of 10-15 years age all the possible anastomotic channels are available and good potentials exist for the quick establish-

ment of such anastomotic channels; thus an arterial occlusion would produce much less damage in them than in a man past middle age with extremely poor potentials for anastomoses. This applies particularly to persons with arteriosclerosis and other vascular diseases. Posterior ciliary artery occlusion in young animals immediately opens up the anastomoses between the peripapillary choroid and the pial plexus on the optic nerve via the recurrent branches from the peripapillary choroid (Fig. 2) [259]; this explains the extremely infrequent occurence of peripapillary choroidal lesions in experimental posterior ciliary artery occlusion in primates [260], and also the frequent absence of massive damage to the anterior optic nerve. A similar or even much less severe occlusion of the posterior ciliary arteries in elderly persons would produce massive infarction. In an experiment* to produce chronic generalized ocular ischemia, one com-

* Personal communication from Dr. PAUL HENKIND.

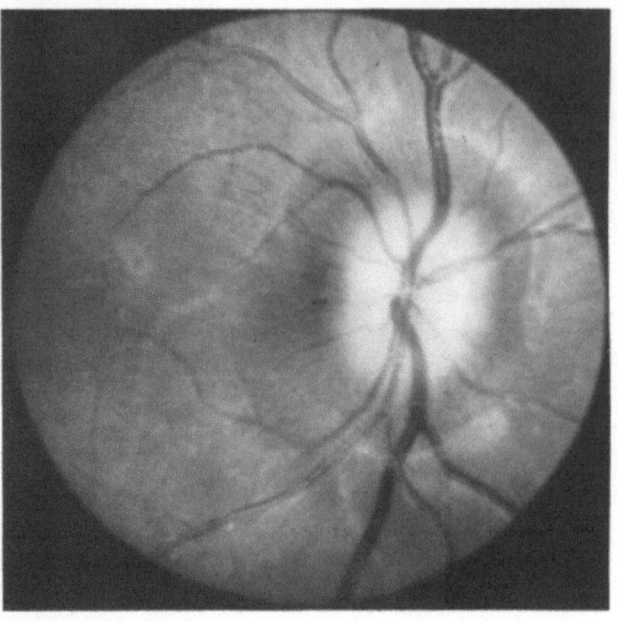

Fig. 11. Fundus picture of a rhesus monkey, showing pale edema of the optic disc (due to anterior ischemic optic neuropathy) 2 days after occlusion of the lateral posterior ciliary artery

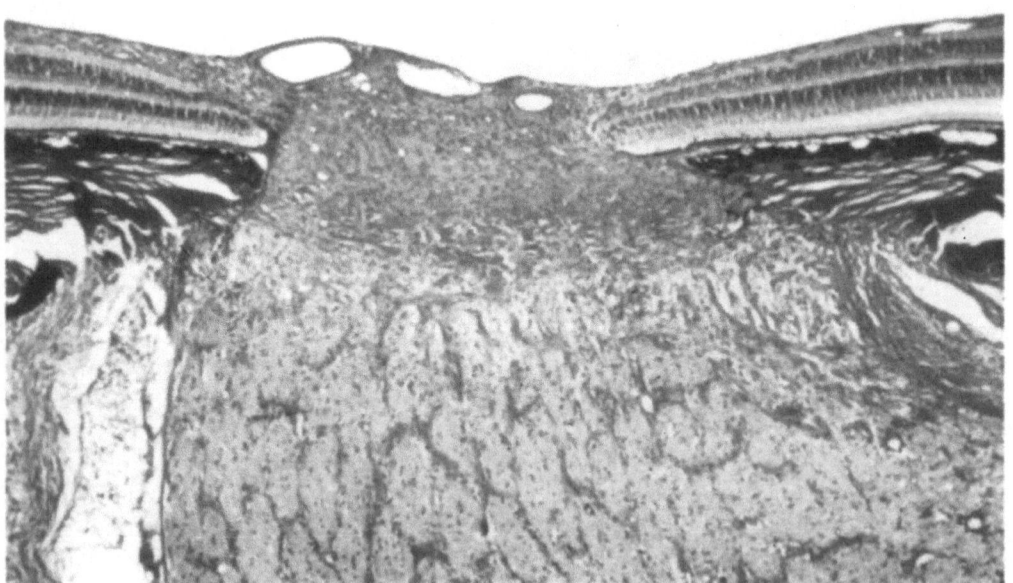

Fig. 12a–c. Photomicrographs of the optic nerve head and retrolaminar optic nerve in rhesus monkeys.
a) 36 days after occlusion of all the posterior ciliary arteries (Masson's Trichrome stain) showing atrophy and degenerative changes in retrolaminar region.
b) Higher magnification of a part of (a) showing marked degeneration of neural tissue in retrolaminar region, producing an appearance resembling cavernous degeneration.
c) 42 days after occlusion of the lateral posterior ciliary artery (Masson's Trichrome stain) showing degenerative changes involving the temporal half of the optic nerve, with nasal half normal

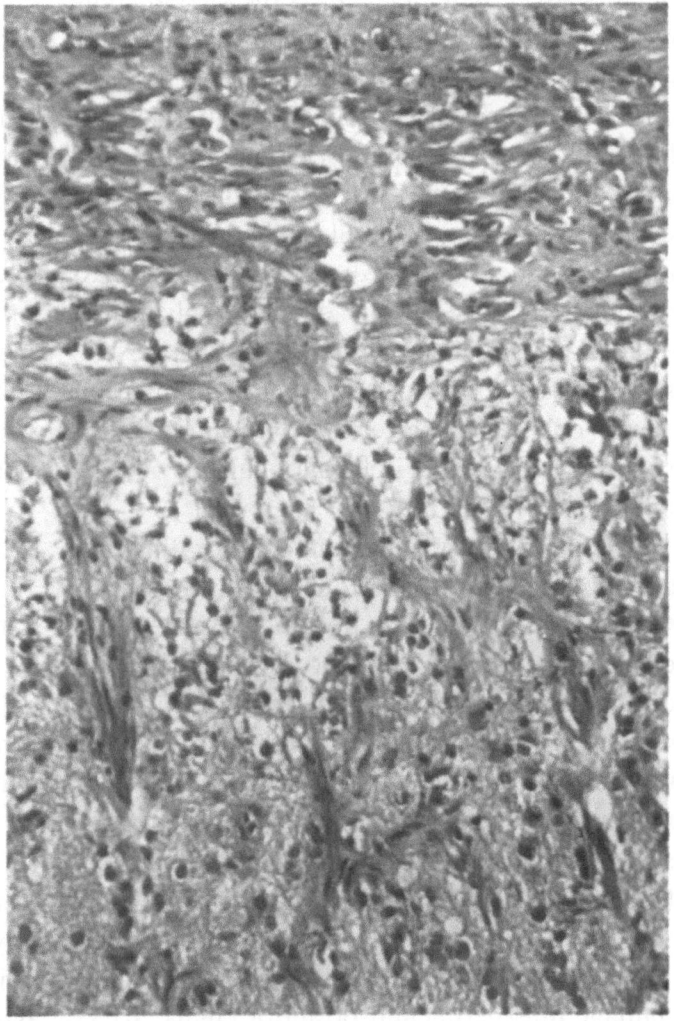

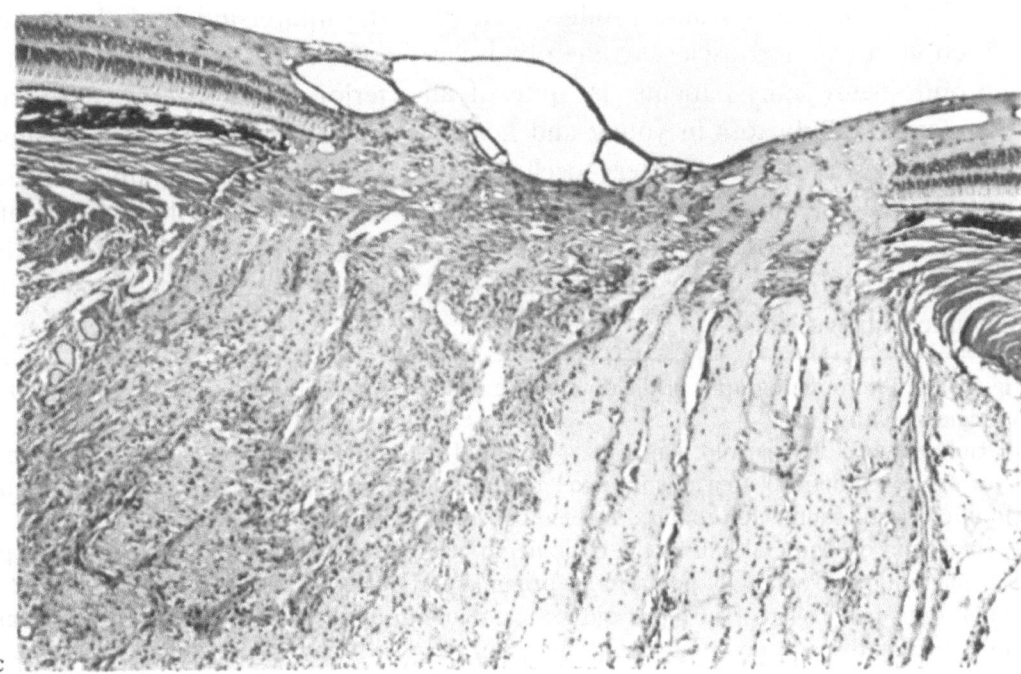

Fig. 12 (continued)

mon carotid artery was ligated in an animal without any effect. After a few days the second common carotid artery was ligated and still no ocular ischemia was produced. Then after some time one vertebral artery was ligated, but this also failed to produce ocular ischemia. Finally the second vertebral artery was also ligated. The animal showed no sign of ocular or brain ischemia in spite of ligation of all the four arteries to the head, because of the quick establishment of good collateral circulation. In an arteriosclerotic elderly human, on the other hand, ligation of any one of these arteries would immediately produce significant ischemic damage in the majority.

2. The other very important complicating factor in experimental posterior ciliary artery occlusion as compared to the posterior ciliary artery occlusion occuring in patients is the marked fall of intra-ocular pressure after lateral orbitotomy in the former [258a, 260]. In the patients the intraocular pressure is usually normal. This marked fall of intraocular pressure in animals significantly improves the perfusion of vessels of the optic nerve head and peripapillary choroid, and reduces the degree of ischemia still further.

Thus the development of minor ischemic damage in experimental posterior ciliary artery occlusion in young healthy animals indicates that similar occlusion would produce massive infarction in old arteriosclerotic anterior ischemic optic neuropathy patients. In spite of all these favourable factors in young and healthy monkeys posterior ciliary artery occlusion in some animals of our series did cause anterior ischemic optic neuropathy identical to that in man, while in others there were less marked ischemic changes.

3. Complete filling of the main choroidal vascular bed (supplied by the posterior ciliary arteries) on fluorescein fundus angiography is no guide to the circulation in the anterior optic nerve (which is also mainly supplied by the posterior ciliary arteries, mainly via the peripapillary choroid. p. 7) as is clearly shown in Fig. 16d; unfortunately far too much stress has been laid on the choroidal filling as an index of circulation in the anterior part of the optic nerve, because both happen to be derived from the posterior ciliary arteries. The vessels in the prelaminar region of the optic nerve head and peripapillary choroid are much more susceptible to obliteration on a fall of perfusion pressure than the main choroid, in spite of all these structures being supplied by the posterior ciliary arteries (p. 21).

Thus, evidently ANDERSON et al. [9a] have not taken these additional factors into consideration when making the allegation that anterior ischemic optic neuropathy must represent a disease of more than just the posterior ciliary arteries.

The fluorescein angiographic studies in patients and experimental studies in rhesus monkeys, established the role of occluded posterior ciliary arteries in anterior ischemic optic neuropathy. Histopathologic studies, mentioned above (p. 13), further confirmed this, because the infarct involved the optic nerve head and retrobulbar region (Fig. 13) in all eyes. The posterior ciliary arteries were frequently involved in these eyes (10 of 16 case reports mention posterior ciliary artery involvement, while five make no mention of the absence of posterior ciliary artery involvement; presumably changes in the posterior ciliary arteries were not recorded. Only one case showed no changes in the posterior

Fig. 13a–f. Photomicrographs of the optic nerve head and retrolaminar optic nerve in man in anterior ischemic ▷ optic neuropathy.

a) Right eye of a 74-year-old man with 4-week-old anterior ischemic optic neuropathy and temporal arteritis, showing a well-defined area of infarction of the optic nerve head and retrolaminar optic nerve (Verhoeff's modified elastic stain). (Reproduced by kind courtesy of Dr. I.M. MacMichael).

b) Infarction of temporal half of the optic nerve head and retrolaminar optic nerve in a patient with anterior ischemic optic neuropathy of non-arteritis origin (Reproduced by kind courtesy of Dr. D.G. Cogan).

c) Left optic nerve head of a 67-year-old woman 4 months after onset of temporal arteritis and anterior ischemic optic neuropathy and no perception of light. It shows atrophy of prelaminar tissue and fibrosis and gliosis of lamina cribrosa and retrolaminar tissue (Verhoeff elastic stain) (Reproduced by kind courtesy of Dr. Paul Henkind)

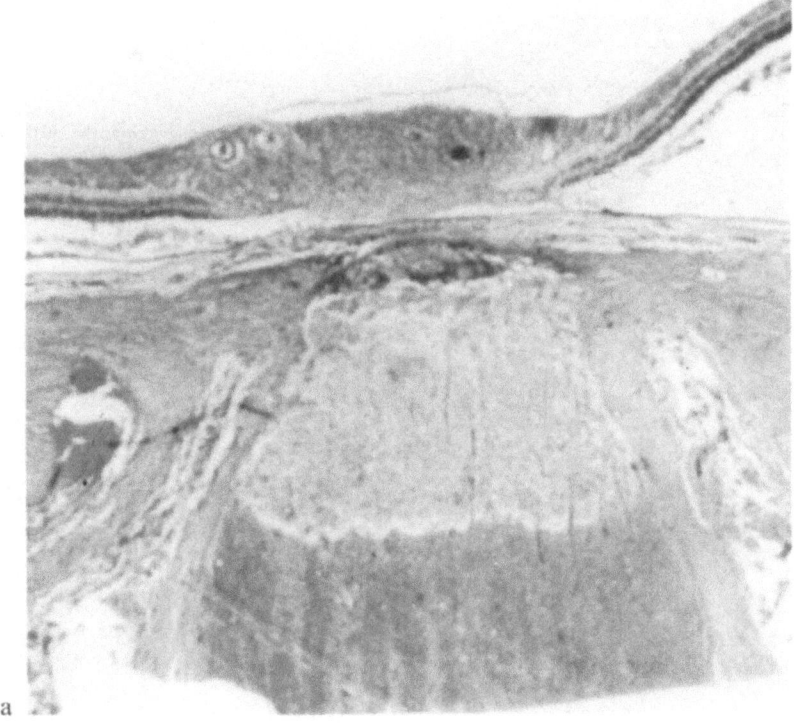

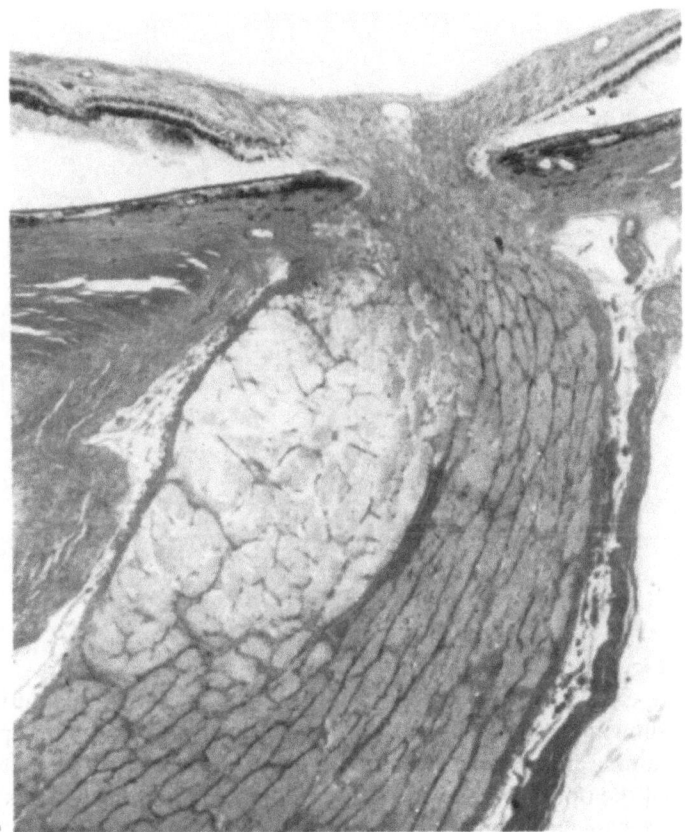

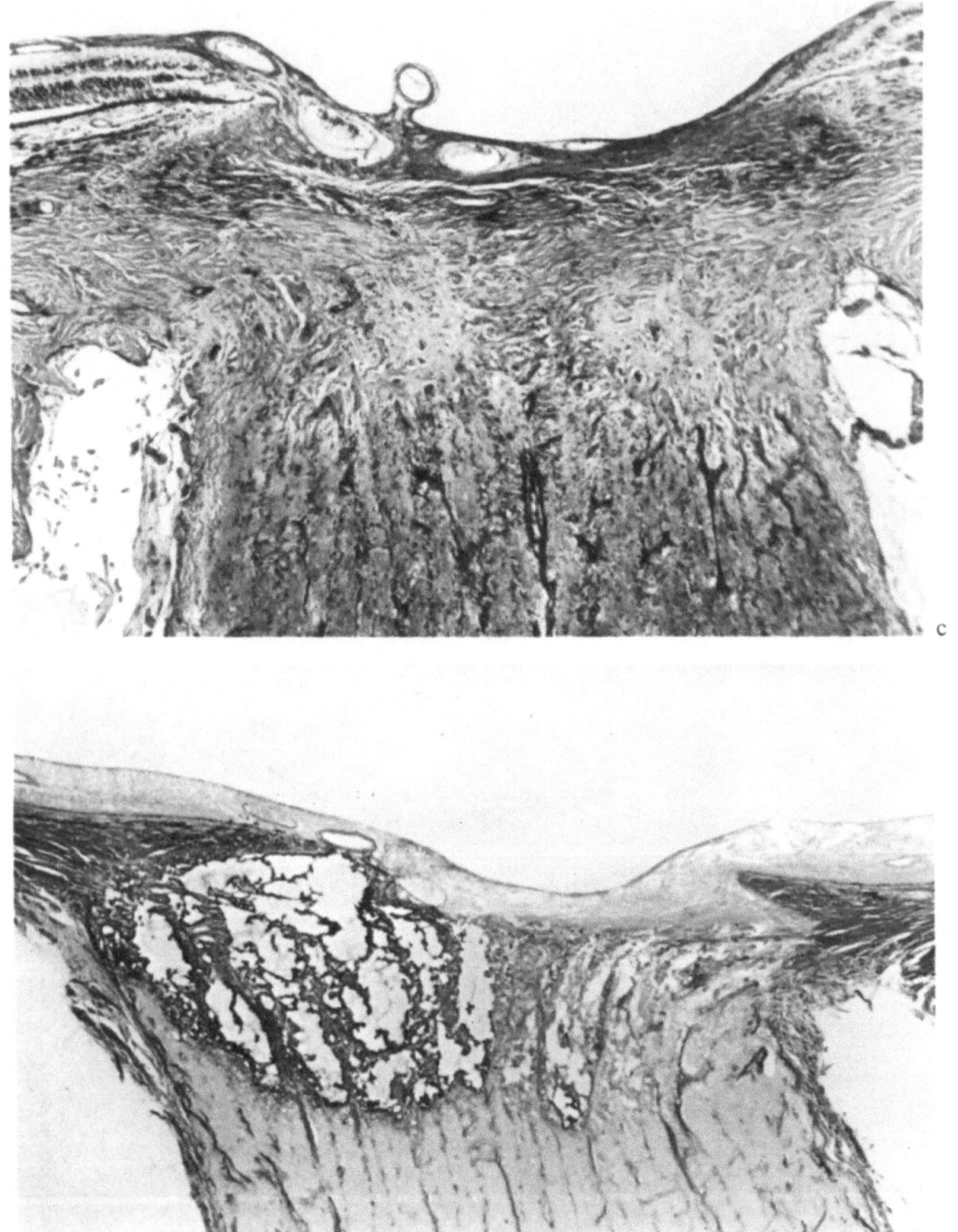

Fig. 13 (continued)

d, e, f) Left eye of a 68-year-old man, with 18-day-old anterior ischemic optic neuropathy and temporal arteritis, showing a sharply defined area of necrosis in the anterior part of the optic nerve and a partially disintegrated lamina cribrosa. The presence of hyaluronidase-sensitive material, similar to that found in cavernous degeneration of the optic nerve (as demonstrated by colloidal iron stains), was demonstrated within the area of retrolaminar ischemic necrosis.

d) stained with Alcian blue for acid mucopolysaccharides.

e and f) stained with hematoxylin-eosin. Fig. f is a magnified view of the area marked in Fig. e. (Reproduced by kind courtesy of Dr. E.N. HINZPETER)

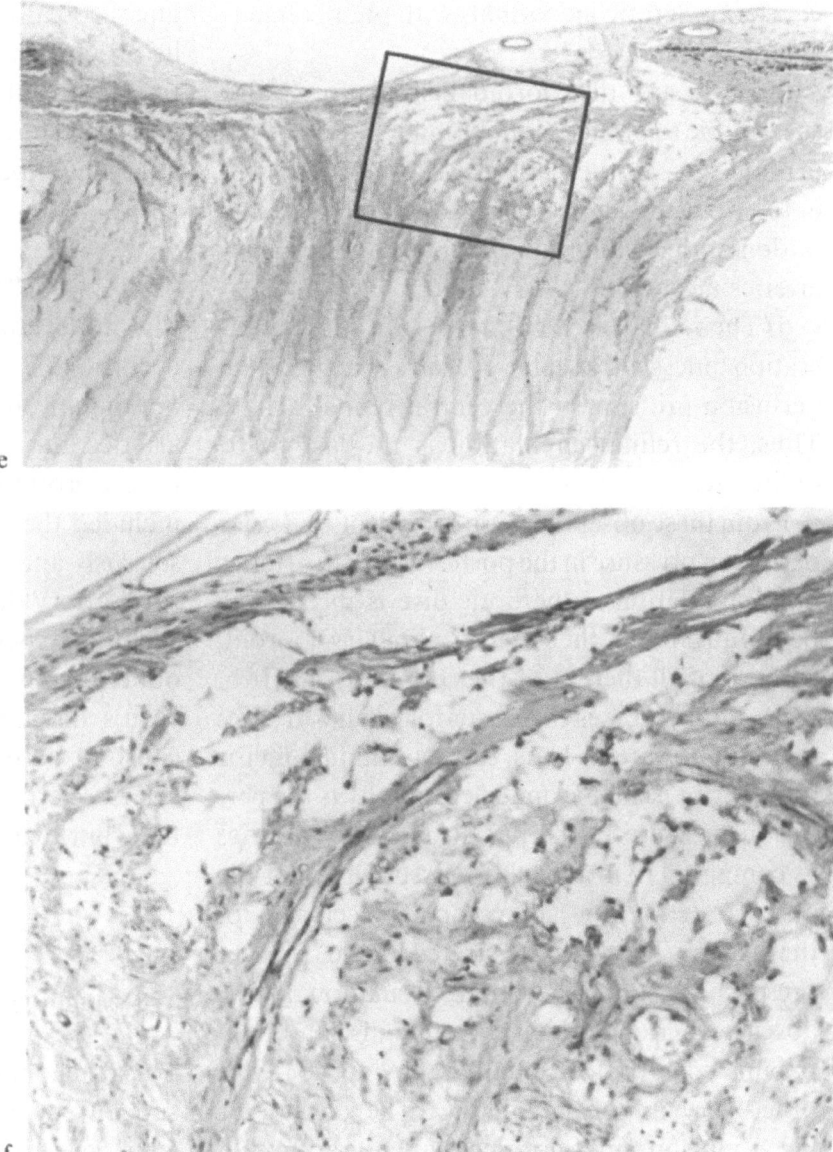

Fig. 13 (continued)

ciliary arteries and the explanation for the absence of these changes is given on p. 13. The possible role of posterior ciliary artery occlusion in the etiology of anterior ischemic optic neuropathy was also speculated by some workers who found these obstructed histopathologically [325, 363, 382, 552].

One point to be stressed is that the posterior ciliary arteries need not be occluded completely to produce anterior ischemic optic neuropathy. In fact, I feel that the posterior ciliary arteries are never occluded completely in most eyes. We [264] demonstrated that circulation in the optic disc, peripapillary choroid, and choroid depends upon the difference between intraocular and perfusion pressures in the posterior ciliary arteries. When imbalance is produced between perfusion and intraocular pressure, either by lowering perfusion pressure or raising intraocular pressure, the susceptibility of intraocular blood vessels to obliteration varies considerably:

a) Vessels in the prelaminar part of the optic disc are most susceptible to obliteration and are usually the first to be obliterated.

b) The peripapillary choroid is either equally or slightly less susceptible to obliteration. Obliteration of the peripapillary choroid itself would, in turn, involve the blood supply to the prelaminar region of the disc and retrolaminar optic nerve as well (Figs. 2, 16d, 32, 33), particularly in arteriosclerotic individuals with poor collateral circulation.

c) The rest of the choroidal circulation is also susceptible to obliteration, but much less so than (a) and (b). In the choroid it is most marked in the watershed areas where territories of distribution of the medial and lateral posterior ciliary arteries meet (Figs. 17, 27, 33).

d) The retinal circulation does not show obliteration unless intraocular pressure is higher than perfusion pressure in the central retinal artery. Thus, the retinal circulation is the last to be obliterated.

From these observations it is evident that once perfusion pressure in the posterior ciliary arteries falls, circulation in the optic disc is the first to be compromised, then the peripapillary choroid, and last of all the rest of the choroid (Figs. 16b, c, d). In these cases the posterior ciliary arteries may still be patent. Thus, the determining factor for anterior ischemic optic neuropathy is the perfusion pressure in the posterior ciliary arteries as compared to intraocular pressure and not the absence or presence of complete occlusion of the arteries. This is demonstrated by the frequent presence of some choroidal circulation in the absence of circulation in the optic disc and peripapillary choroid on angiography (p. 73). The other very important factor to be considered when interpreting fluorescein angiographic filling of the posterior ciliary artery circulation is the time-lapse between the onset of anterior ischemic optic neuropathy and fluorescein angiographic examination. Even in eyes in which the posterior ciliary artery is not filled at the onset of the disease, circulation is restored fairly soon so that a significant filling defect is not seen within a few days or weeks (p. 73). Thus, the absence of a filling defect in posterior ciliary artery circulation on intravenous fluorescein angiography is not a true guide to an earlier occurrence of a filling defect. I have demonstrated this also in retinal vascular occlusions [248].

Imbalance between perfusion pressure in the posterior ciliary artery circulation and intraocular pressure also has been pointed out by FOULDS [170, 171]. If the imbalance is chronic, it produces so-called *low-tension glaucoma,* but when its onset is sudden, anterior ischemic optic neuropathy results. The fall in perfusion pressure in the posterior ciliary arteries may be due to a large number of causes.

1. Local Vascular Causes

The important factors in this category include occlusion or stenosis of posterior ciliary arteries, ophthalmic, internal carotid, or common carotid arteries due to any cause, particularly in an arteriosclerotic individual. In this group may be included the temporal arteritis, marked atherosclerosis and arteriosclerosis, hypertension, carotid artery disease, diabetes, collagen diseases, syphilis, hypercholesterolemia, thromboangiitis obliterans, Raynaud's disease, migraine, Takayasu's disease, etc. By far the most common cause of anterior ischemic optic neuropathy is arteriosclerosis. Temporal arteritis is an important, but by no means common, cause.

2. Systemic Causes

a) Systemic Arterial Hypotension

This category includes any disease that produces sudden and marked systemic arterial hypotension, e.g., shock of any etiology, surgical hypotension, heart failure, myocardial infarction, ischemic heart disease, severe hemorrhages, recurrent hemorrhages, etc. In a patient with poor perfusion pressure in the posterior ciliary arteries due to local vascular factors, even a slight drop in systemic blood pressure may be enough to produce anterior ischemic optic neuropathy. It is common to find that anterior ischemic optic neuropathy is noticed by a patient as he wakens in the morning because systemic hypotension during sleep can be enough to produce the imbalance between perfusion and intraocular pressure in already diseased and narrowed posterior ciliary arteries. Thus systemic arterial hypotension is an important precipitating factor.

b) Embolic Phenomenon

An embolus originating anywhere in the cardiovascular system may get lodged in the posterior ciliary arteries.

c) Hematologic Disorders

These may produce vascular occlusion, e.g., in polycythemia, sickle cell disease, thrombocytopenic purpura, leukemia, and, possibly, the contraceptive pill. In this category severe anemias can also be included, because oxygenation of the optic nerve head depends not only upon the amount of blood flow but also upon the oxygen-carrying capacity of the blood [171]. Low-grade optic disc edema and fall of central vision in severe anemias and chlorosis, resembling anterior ischemic optic neuropathy, was described nearly a century ago by GOWERS [212]. Unrecognized visual disturbances in severe anemia may be due to some degree of anterior ischemic optic neuropathy [171]. In chronic bronchitis with polycythemia, poor oxygenation of the blood and slow circulation because of increased viscosity may produce anterior ischemic optic neuropathy [171].

3. Ocular Causes

To produce anterior ischemic optic neuropathy the most important factor in the eye itself is elevated intraocular pressure, compromising circulation in the optic disc. Thus, a patient with chronic simple glaucoma has a higher chance of developing anterior ischemic optic neuropathy than does a person with a low intraocular pressure. This has been reported by FOULDS [170, 171], BEGG et al. [31, 32], DRANCE and BEGG [132], and SANDERS [471]. Drusen in the optic nerve head could produce anterior ischemic optic neuropathy by direct pressure on vessels.

While discussing the blood supply of the optic nerve head, it was pointed out that usually two to three posterior ciliary arteries arise from the ophthalmic artery and each posterior ciliary artery then subdivides into multiple short ones. The occlusive disorder may involve only one posterior ciliary artery or a short one, thus producing only a sectoral and not a generalized anterior ischemic optic neuropathy. The anterior ischemic optic neuropathy may start as a sectoral change but soon progresses to complete anterior ischemic optic neuropathy because edema in one part of the optic nerve may, by raising the pressure in tissue, slowly compromise small blood vessels in parts adjoining the edematous one. Thus the edema may gradually creep to involve other parts. Similarly, FOULDS [171] postulated that optic disc edema may occur before symptoms appear because anoxic damage might be severe enough to cause capillary dilatation and increased permeability without interrupting the function of optic nerve fibers: increased permeability → a rise of local tissue pressure → either damage of the optic nerve fibers directly or further impairing of the circulation in the optic nerve head → anterior ischemic optic neuropathy.

Thus, anterior ischemic optic neuropathy, glaucoma, and low-tension glaucoma are manifestations of ischemia of the optic nerve head and retrolaminar optic nerve due to interference with posterior ciliary artery circulation as a result of an imbalance between perfusion pressure in the posterior ciliary arteries and intraocular pressure. If the process is sudden, it produces anterior ischemic optic neuropathy with infarction of the optic nerve head and retrolaminar region. If it is chronic (as in glaucoma and low-tension glaucoma), it produces slow degeneration of neural tissue in the optic nerve head and retrobulbar region, resulting in cupping of the optic disc and cavernous degeneration of the retrolaminar optic nerve.

Part II   The Clinical Picture of Anterior Ischemic Optic Neuropathy

A clinical description of anterior ischemic optic neuropathy, based on my own studies and what is revealed by a review of the literature on the subject, is presented and discussed in this section.

Material and Methods of Present Study

Category I. Twenty-five patients with complete or partial anterior ischemic optic neuropathy were studied. All had a detailed initial ophthalmic examination. Erythrocyte sedimentation rate (ESR) was estimated by the Westergren method as an emergency. If the ESR was higher than 20 mm in the first hour, a temporal artery biopsy was performed to look for the evidence of temporal arteritis (giant cell arteritis). A routine hematologic and systemic examination was performed. A stereoscopic fundus color photograph was taken and intravenous fluorescein angiography of the fundus was performed at the first examination, or at the earliest possible time, in all eyes.

Systemic prednisolone, 40 to 80 mg daily, frequently with an initial dose of 40 units of adrenocorticotropic hormone (ACTH) intramuscularly, was given to 19 patients, and none to six patients. In six patients with progressive deterioration of visual acuity or fields at a later date, long-acting acetazolamide (Diamox) (500 mg twice daily) was given.

All patients were reviewed, for the first few days as in-patients, and thereafter as outpatients, at various intervals. Review studies included: recording of visual acuities, visual fields (when possible), ophthalmoscopic examination, ESR in patients with temporal arteritis, and

regulation of the patient's therapy. At different intervals, in ten eyes with anterior ischemic optic neuropathy, angiography was repeated to assess ocular circulation. Periodic stereoscopic color photographs of the fundus were taken in all eyes. In eyes with recordable visual fields, these were recorded on a Bjerrum screen or on a Goldmann perimeter.

Electro-oculograms and electroretinograms were recorded in 16 patients of this series. Table 11 summarizes the frequency of and the interval of time between such recordings and the onset of anterior ischemic optic neuropathy in various patients; the last or the only recording in all except one (Case 5) was taken at the end of the follow-up period. The electro-oculogram was recorded in the standard manner, described by ARDEN et al. [16], during 12 minutes of dark adaptation, followed by 12 minutes of light adaptation (luminance = 1,700 milli-lamberts). The scotopic electroretinogram, after 15 minutes of dark adaptation, was recorded by contact lens electrodes [148] in response to a brief flash stimulus from a Flash Tac Stroboscope (Electronic Applications Commercial Ltd.). The recording system incorporated a computer of average transients. The electroretinograms were measured in millimicrons, the maximum *b-wave* being measured from the trough of the *a-wave* to the peak of the *b-wave*. Flicker Fusion Frequency of the electroretinogram was recorded to determine whether the response was scotopic (20 Hertz or less), photopic (60 Hertz) or mixed (40 Hertz).

The follow-up period in these patients varied from three months to three years, most being between 1 and $2^{1}/_{2}$ years (mean 15 ± 9 months).

Category II. In addition to these 25 cases, I have seen more than 50 patients with anterior ischemic optic neuropathy over the years. These were not investigated as systematically and thoroughly as the ones mentioned above, although fluorescein angiographic studies were performed in all. Some data from these additional cases are cited in the text to further substantiate observations without giving statistical data.

Since the evaluation of the 25 cases in Category I above, I have started to treat all of my patients with non arteritis type of ischemic optic neuropathy with an initial dose of 60 to 80 mg of prednisolone daily and very gradually tapering off. The systemic corticosteroid is given so long as edema of the optic disc is present. There were 22 patients in Category II, all of whom underwent the above-mentioned investigations and follow-up studies.

The Clinical Picture of Anterior Ischemic Optic Neuropathy

Age

Anterior ischemic optic neuropathy generally affects persons in later life, although some patients, with anterior ischemic optic neuropathy caused by other than temporal arteritis, may be young. In my series, although the overall age varied between 59 and 88 (mean 72 ± 8) years, patients with temporal arteritis tended to be older than those with no temporal arteritis, i.e., 75 ± 9 years and 69 ± 8 years respectively. In the literature, although the age incidence for anterior ischemic optic neuropathy due to temporal arteritis is somewhat similar to that for my series (54 to 84 years [500], 55 to 80 years [94], 60 to 83 years [552], 61 to 86 years [50, 51], 67 to 85 years [486], 69 to 81 years [106], 80 percent 70 years or more [384], 78 to 81 years [185]) for cases with no temporal arteritis, much younger patients have been reported to suffer from anterior ischemic optic neuropathy (29 to 52 years [151], 34 years and over [170], maximum incidence in fifth and sixth decades [73], 44 to

61 years [471], 45 to 52 years [339], 46 to 65 years [388], 50 to 75 years [60, 536], 50 to 78 years [185], 54 to 69 years [81], 55 years [322], 64 to 81 years [486]). These findings establish that anterior ischemic optic neuropathy due to temporal arteritis occurs in a comparatively older age group than anterior ischemic optic neuropathy due to other causes.

Sex

In the present series there were 10 men and 15 women with anterior ischemic optic neuropathy, but further analysis revealed that anterior ischemic optic neuropathy due to temporal arteritis affected eight females and three males of this group; the group with no temporal arteritis comprised seven males and seven females. In the literature, the incidence of females was high (13 females and 4 males [107]) in the group with anterior ischemic optic neuropathy due to temporal arteritis, as compared to an inconsistent pattern seen in the group with no temporal arteritis (5 females and 15 males [185], 13 females and 6 males [486]). These findings suggest that anterior ischemic optic neuropathy due to temporal arteritis occurs much more commonly in females (in about 75 percent) than in males, but no such preponderance of any one sex is seen in the group with no temporal arteritis. (This could be explained simply by the larger number of females in the 70 + age group in the general population.)

Laterality

Bilateral anterior ischemic optic neuropathy is frequently reported in both with and without temporal arteritis. In the former category, the reported incidence varies between 22 percent and 40 percent (22 percent [44], 33 percent [50, 51, 108], 36 percent [107, 486], 40 percent [400]) although it may be as low as only 12 percent [552]. In the category without arteritis the reported incidence of the bilateral disease varies widely from 18 percent to 73 percent (18 percent [50, 51], 20 percent [185], 30 percent [170], 57 percent [505], 73 percent [388]). However the incidence is mentioned as being usually [81] or as a rule unilateral [474]. In my series, it was bilateral in 27 percent of cases with temporal arteritic anterior ischemic optic neuropathy, and bilateral in 14 percent of non-arteritic anterior ischemic optic neuropathy.

The reported time interval between the involvement of the two eyes varies widely. In the group with temporal arteritis it can occur almost simultaneously [108, 384] or after a period of 1 to 21 days [552], 3 days to 2 weeks [107], up to 12 days and, occasionally, several weeks [384], up to 3 to 4 weeks [108], or a few days or weeks [466]. It is reported that if the second eye in temporal arteritis is not involved within 6 weeks [384] to 2 months [552], the prognosis is good for that eye. In the group with non-arteritic anterior ischemic optic neuropathy, this time interval has been reported as weeks or months [505], a few months [399], one year [35], several weeks to one year [61], 2 weeks to 17 years [388], one month to 7 years [73], and 15 years [201]. In my series, in the group with temporal arteritis involvement of the two eyes was simultaneous in one patient; after an interval of two days and several days in three patients; more-or-less simultaneous in one patient with arteriosclerotic anterior ischemic optic neuropathy, and after one day in one patient. An important factor to bear in mind is that it is not always possible to get exact information regarding this time gap because some patients may not be aware that vision in one eye is either partially or completely absent until the second eye is involved. Such patients may report that visual loss in both eyes occurred simultaneously.

These findings suggest that bilateral anterior ischemic optic neuropathy can occur in about one-quarter to one-third of those cases due to temporal arteritis; no definite incidence can be given for non-arteritic category as that reported varies from 14 percent to 73 percent. The time interval in which anterior ischemic optic neuropathy involved both eyes also varied in the two groups. In the group with temporal arteritis it was most often 3 to 4 weeks, with a slight chance after two months. In non-arteritic category however, this time interval may vary from almost nil to 17 years [388]. This is quite understandable because temporal arteritis is an active disease with a self-limiting course; the causative vascular disease in non-arteritic category is unequal in the two eyes, progressive, and constantly present, with no acute self-limiting course, although some of the precipitating factors of the original disease process may be transitory and recurring.

When anterior ischemic optic neuropathy was unilateral, it involved the right eye in 13 and the left eye in seven of the present series.

Symptoms

These are always ocular and sometimes may be associated with systemic symptoms.

a) Prodromal Ocular Symptoms

In my series prodromal symptoms were present in about half of the patients. They were far more common in the temporal arteritis cases (in about three-quarters of the patients) than in the group without arteritis (in about one-quarter of the patients). In the former group, it was mainly transient blurring (varying from gray to blurred vision) or loss of vision, involving the entire vision in the eye or an altitudinal hemianopic defect (frequently in the inferior field only); this preceded permanent loss by an interval ranging from a few hours to several days. Transiently obscured vision preceding complete loss is frequently described in anterior ischemic optic neuropathy, particularly when the neuropathy is due to temporal arteritis [44, 106, 107, 384]. In addition, other visual symptoms, e.g., difficulty with focusing, flickers and flashes of light, photophobia, distorted or color-tinted vision also were seen. Patients with no temporal arteritis complained of flashing and flickering light more often than did those with temporal arteritis, and vice versa with photophobia. Persistent loss of vision may occur suddenly or gradually and spread like a curtain or progress concentrically from the periphery. One patient with temporal arteritis complained of intermittent pain around the eye for a day. This symptom was also mentioned by FRANÇOIS et al. [185].

b) Systemic Symptoms

Headache. In my series about one-half of the patients with temporal arteritis complained of headache and/or tenderness of the temporomandibular joint and pain on chewing. One patient who developed anterior ischemic optic neuropathy in the right eye and transient blurring of vision in the left complained of pain on the left side. The headache was more often in the fronto-temporal than in the occipital region. The side of headache, etc., did not seem to be related to the side of ocular involvement. These symptoms usually started about two weeks before the onset of anterior ischemic optic neuropathy. Although absent in the "occult" variety and in anterior ischemic optic neuropathy originating from no temporal arteritis, headache is a well-documented phenomenon in temporal arteritis. Headaches are common in the general population and must not be confused with the headaches of temporal arteritis.

General. In this series some patients with temporal arteritis complained of being generally unwell and lost weight. One patient had fainting attacks. Some of these patients experienced euphoria, showing little concern about their loss of vision; in such cases it was common to find that even with no perception of light in an eye, patients insisted that they could see "not too badly". This may completely mislead a person not aware of it. General systemic symptoms of temporal arteritis are mentioned on p.114.

In the group with no temporal arteritis there was a high incidence of cardiovascular symptoms, e.g., hypertension, heart failure, paroxysmal tachycardia, collapse and, in one case, intermittent claudication.

c) Presenting Ocular Symptoms

In my series the presenting ocular symptoms were:

Bilateral. Two of the five patients in this group complained of sudden and complete loss of vision in both eyes, more or less simultaneously (Patients 1 and 4 in Table 1). In the remaining three patients visual disturbance in one eye preceded symptoms in the other (Patients 2, 3 and 5 in Table 1).

Table 1. Initial visual acuity in bilateral anterior ischemic optic neuropathy

Patient number	Age (years)	Visual acuity		Temporal arteritis	Time interval between onset of visual disorder and consulting ophthalmologist	
		Right eye	Left eye		Right eye	Left eye
1	88	NPL	NPL	+	1 day	1 day
2	71	NPL	HM	+	Several days	5 days
3	65	NPL	6/18 [a]	+	2 days	few hours
4	60	NPL	NPL	−	2 days	2 days
5	78	6/12	6/18	−	18 days	19 days

[a] NPL next morning while in the hospital.

Abbreviations used in all tables: AION Anterior ischemic optic neuropathy, *art.* artery, *CRAO* Central retinal artery occlusion, *CF* Counts fingers, *C/D* Cup/disc, *EOG* Electro-oculogram, *ERG* Electroretinogram, *FFF* Flicker fusion frequency, *HM* Hand motion, *HZ* Hertz, *Lt.* Left, *NPL* No perception of light, *No.* Number, *Occ.* Occlusion, *OD* Optic disc, *Pt(s)* Patient(s), *PL* Perception of light, *ret.* retinal, *Rt.* right, *T.A.* Temporal arteritis, *VA* Visual acuity

Unilateral. Table 2 summarizes the presenting ocular symptoms in these cases.

The time interval between the onset of visual disturbance and the first consultation with an ophthalmologist was considered in the present study. Findings for bilateral anterior ischemic optic neuropathy (in five patients) are summarized in Table 1. In 20 cases of unilateral anterior ischemic optic neuropathy, two patients reported for consultation within 24 hours (with no perception of light in one and perception of light in the second); about a quarter reported to the hospital within a week, about a third within 2 to 3 weeks, and the remainder took up to three months, except one who was seen after $1^1/_2$ years (with central scotoma and nasal hemianopia).

These findings show that the presenting symptom was almost invariably the sudden onset of a significant degree of visual disturbance, sometimes amounting to complete blindness.

Most of the patients with bilateral anterior ischemic optic neuropathy reported for an ophthalmic opinion significantly earlier than did those with unilateral anterior ischemic optic neuropathy, because in the latter group the visual disturbance was not as severe. In uniocular anterior ischemic optic neuropathy patients, there was no significant association between the degree of visual loss and the time lapse between the onset of visual disturbance and the first consultation with an ophthalmologist.

Visual Acuity

In my series visual acuity at the time of first ophthalmic consultation was as follows:

a) Table 1 summarizes the visual acuity of patients with bilateral anterior ischemic optic neuropathy.

b) Visual acuity of patients with uniocular anterior ischemic optic neuropathy is summarized in Table 3.

These findings suggest that:

1. In anterior ischemic optic neuropathy due to temporal arteritis, visual loss is much more marked than in non-arteritic category. CULLEN [108] and BLODI [50, 51] also showed marked loss of vision due to temporal arteritis, it being better than counting fingers (CF) in about 20 percent of the eyes; in my series it was in 7 percent. In anterior ischemic optic neuropathy

Table 2. Visual symptoms of cases with uniocular anterior ischemic optic neuropathy

Visual symptoms	No. of Pts. without T.A.	No. of Pts. with T.A.
1. Loss or deterioration of vision usually of sudden onset, reducing vision to:		
a) NPL	—	4
b) PL	—	1
c) HM	2	1
d) CF	—	1
2. Loss of lower field of vision	2	1
3. Loss of central vision	1	—
4. "A shadow over the eye"	1	—
5. "A curtain over the eye"	1	—
6. "As if looking through a lace curtain"	1	—
7. Bumped into people on one side because of defective vision on that side	2	—
8. Sudden onset of blurred vision	2	—
Total number of patients	12	8

Table 3. Initial visual acuity in unilateral anterior ischemic optic neuropathy

Visual acuity	No. of Pts. with T.A.	No. of Pts. without T.A.
6/6–6/12	1	5
6/36–6/60	0	4
CF–HM	2	3
PL in upper nasal quadrant	1	0
NPL	4	0

of non-arteritic type, BONAMOUR [60], and BONA-MOUR et al. [61] mentioned that vision is never lost completely and is usually 6/60 or better. This was not true in the present study; my findings agree with those of FRANÇOIS et al. [185], MILLER et al. [388], and BURDE [73] in that visual acuity can vary from near normal to no perception of light (NPL).

2. In bilateral anterior ischemic optic neuropathy visual loss tends to be somewhat more marked than in unilateral disease. On follow-up, BURDE [73] recorded improvement in visual acuity of more than two lines in 13 out of 39 eyes with impaired vision and no change in visual acuity and/or field defect in 43 eyes with anterior ischemic optic neuropathy of non-arteritic category. In the present series, the final outcome of visual acuity at the end of follow-up was as follows:

a) In Bilateral Anterior Ischemic Optic Neuropathy (Table 4):

Table 4. Final visual acuity in bilateral anterior ischemic optic neuropathy cases as compared to initial visual acuities

Patient number	Initial visual acuity		Final visual acuity	
	right eye	left eye	right eye	left eye
1	NPL	NPL	PL	NPL
2	NPL	HM	NPL	HM
3	NPL	6/18	NPL	NPL
4	NPL	NPL	HM	HM
5	6/12	6/60	6/6	CF

1. There was no change in four eyes (three patients), with no perception of light (NPL) in three and hand motions (HM) in one.

2. Vision deteriorated in two eyes—in one (case 3) from 6/18—to no perception of light on the day after the first consultation. No perception of light developed in the opposite eye three days after the onset of visual symptoms in the right eye, despite treatment with systemic corticosteroids for less than 24 hours. The left eye of patient 5 deteriorated from 6/60 to counting fingers (CF).

3. Vision improved in four eyes (three patients). In case 4 vision improved to hand motion in a small area in both eyes in two weeks; the area of hand motion gradually increased so that the patient had only a central scotoma in one eye and vision in the lower temporal field in the other. In the right eye of patient 1 vision improved in two days to perception of light in the temporal part. The right eye of patient 5 improved from 6/12 to 6/6 in three days with corticosteroids.

b) In Unilateral Anterior Ischemic Optic Neuropathy:

1. No change was seen in 11 cases.

2. Vision deteriorated in three patients—from 6/9 to no perception of light within two days of onset in one; from 6/12 to 6/60 with a central scotoma in the second; and from hand motion to perception of light in the third. This occurred even though patients 1 and 3 were treated with a corticosteroid. The second and third patients deteriorated within 10 to 14 days of the onset. The first patient experienced a constant phenomenon of seeing golden-black geometric figures in the center of vision with no perception of light.

3. Vision improved in six patients; to 6/6 from 6/60 in one and 6/12 in another; to 6/4 from 6/6 in one; to 6/36 from 5/60 in one and to counting fingers from hand motion and perception of light. Usually this improvement took 4 to 6 weeks.

Change in visual acuity during the follow-up was related to the following factors:

Time Interval between the Onset of Visual disturbance and First Consultation (Start of Therapy). This did not seem to alter the visual outcome significantly unless the patient did not seek ophthalmologic care until optic atrophy had already started. Under this circumstance, it is possible that early therapy might have made some difference, as suggested by the data in Table 6. However, it is impossible to be sure.

Presence of Temporal Arteritis as a Cause of Anterior Ischemic Optic Neuropathy. The criterion was a positive temporal artery biopsy for temporal arteritis. Table 5 summarizes the findings.

Table 5. Relationship of visual outcome with presence or absence of temporal arteritis

Temporal arteritis	Number of patients	Visual acuity during follow-up		
		No change	Improvement	Deterioration
Present	11	64%	9%	27%
Absent	14	50%	42%	8%

The data indicate that in anterior ischemic optic neuropathy due to temporal arteritis, the chance that vision will improve is much less than the chances it will deteriorate compared to anterior ischemic optic neuropathy due to no temporal arteritis. Thus, temporal arteritis carries a poorer prognosis for the final outcome of visual acuity than does the arteriosclerotic form.

Relationship of Systemic Corticosteroid Therapy and Presence or Absence of Temporal Arteritis to Final Outcome of Vision. This is summarized in Table 6. The data are interesting and instructive; they indicate that the best outlook for visual acuity in anterior ischemic optic neuropathy is with no temporal arteritis and corticosteroid therapy. Prognosis is worst in patients with temporal arteritis. Systemic corticosteroids have to be given in temporal arteritis patients to prevent the disease from spreading to the second eye and to treat systemic symptoms. Prognosis is also poor in patients with arteriosclerotic anterior ischemic optic neuropathy who do not receive corticosteroid therapy, but it is better than for temporal arteritis.

Fundus Changes

The classic description of the fundus in anterior ischemic optic neuropathy, as found in the literature, is pale edema of the optic disc, usually accompanied by optic disc and peripapillary hemorrhages, and invariable optic atrophy in later stages. These signs are almost invariably considered to be the only fundus findings, although "exsudates" at the posterior pole have been mentioned occasionally. Retinal vessels usually are described as normal.

The main ocular abnormalities in these cases are revealed when the fundus is examined. They can be as follows:

1. Optic Disc Changes

Optic disc changes may vary from a variable swelling of the disc to optic atrophy in all patients, depending upon the time interval after

Table 6. Relationship of systemic corticosteroid therapy and temporal arteritis with final outcome of vision

Group	Systemic steroid therapy and temporal arteritis	Number of patients	Visual acuity during follow-up		
			No change	Improvement[a]	Deterioration[a]
I	With therapy and temporal arteritis	11	64%	9%	27%
II	With therapy and no temporal arteritis	8	12.5%	75%	12.5%
III	No therapy and no temporal arteritis	6	83%	17%	Nil

[a] of two or more lines on Snellen's chart.

the onset of anterior ischemic optic neuropathy in which the patients are seen. When seen within a few days after the onset of visual disturbance, the optic disc is always swollen. If a patient is seen within a few hours after the onset of visual deterioration, the optic disc may show swelling (Fig. 14d). FOULDS [170] mentioned that optic disc swelling may develop a few days before loss of vision; I have not encountered any such instance so far. The optic disc swelling peaks in about 2 to 3 days after the onset of visual deterioration. In the present study, when patients were seen during these early stages of anterior ischemic optic neuropathy, the optic disc showed the following ophthalmoscopic appearances:

a) In Anterior Ischemic Optic Neuropathy Due To Temporal Arteritis

This group included eleven of 25 patients of Category I (p. 25) and only a few of Category II (p. 25). The appearances of the swollen discs could be classified into two distinct types:

1. In about half of the eyes the disc appeared almost chalky-white (Figs. 14a, d, 15a, 16a, 17a, d). Stereoscopic examination revealed a white mass deep to the superficial transparent nerve fiber layer of the optic disc; the mass looked like a white infarct (of the prelaminar region) that had merged with an almost equally white zone around the disc (presumably infarcted pigment epithelium) so that disc margins could not be delineated. The superficial nerve fiber layer of the optic disc was frequently transparent though somewhat edematous. Swelling of the optic disc and infarction in one eye initially involved only a part of the optic disc, even when the patient could not perceive light (Fig. 17a). Later the entire disc became involved (Fig. 17d). This type of change in the optic disc almost always involved ultimately the entire disc. Superficial capillaries in the surface nerve fiber layer of the optic disc were neither congested nor

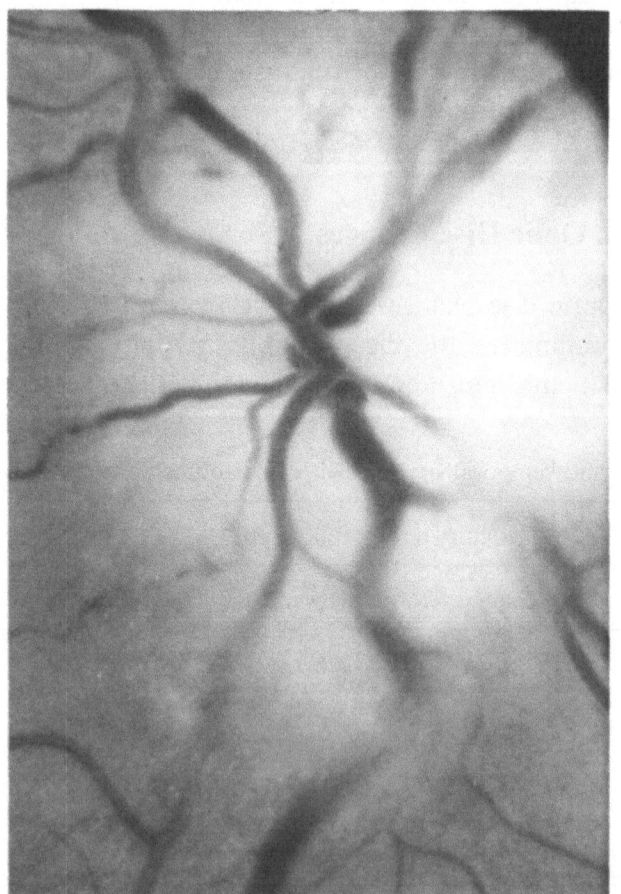

a

Fig. 14a–i. Both eyes of a 65-year-old woman with temporal arteritis, bilateral anterior ischemic optic neuropathy and no perception of light in either eye.

a, b, c) Right fundus on day after onset of blindness.
a) *Fundus photograph* showing chalky-white swelling of the optic disc, with a small superficial retinal hemorrhage above.
b and c) *Fluorescein fundus angiograms*
b) *Retinal arterial phase* showing non-filling of the optic disc, peripapillary choroid and watershed zone inferiorly.
c) *Retinal venous phase* showing non-filling of the optic disc.

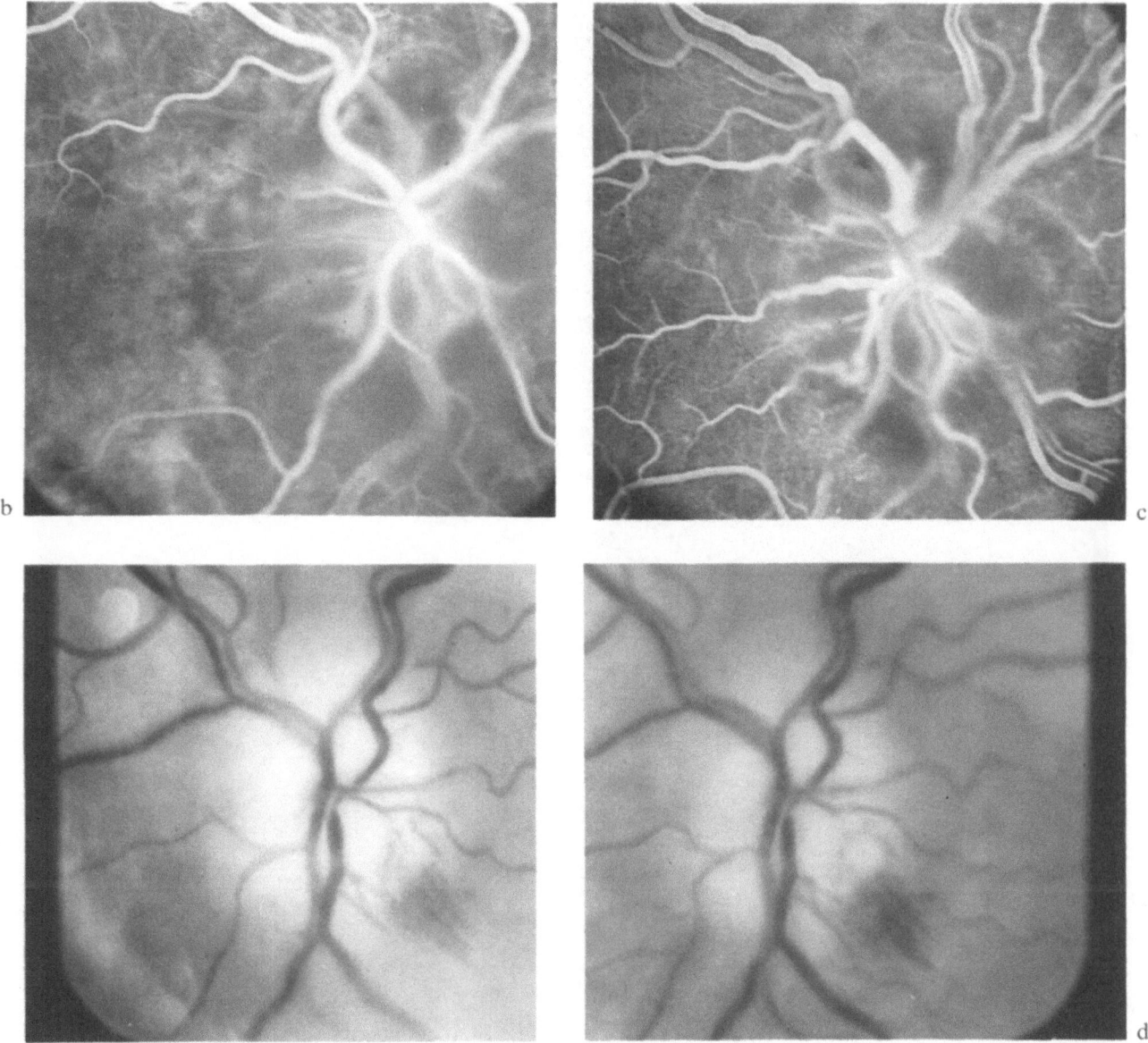

Fig. 14 (continued)

d, e, f) Left fundus on the day of onset of blindness.

d) *Stereoscopic fundus photographs* showing chalky-white swelling of the optic disc, with superficial retinal hemorrhage inferotemporally at the optic disc margin.

e and f) *Fluorescein fundus angiograms*

e) *Retinal arterial phase* showing no filling of the optic disc and choroid.

f) *Retinal venous phase* showing no filling of the optic disc and faint patchy filling of the choroid.

g) *Late phase about 30 minutes after (c)* showing fluorescein staining of the optic disc.

h and i) *Fundus photographs* 3 months after onset of anterior ischemic optic neuropathy showing bilateral cupping and atrophy of the optic discs – (h) right and (i) left fundi

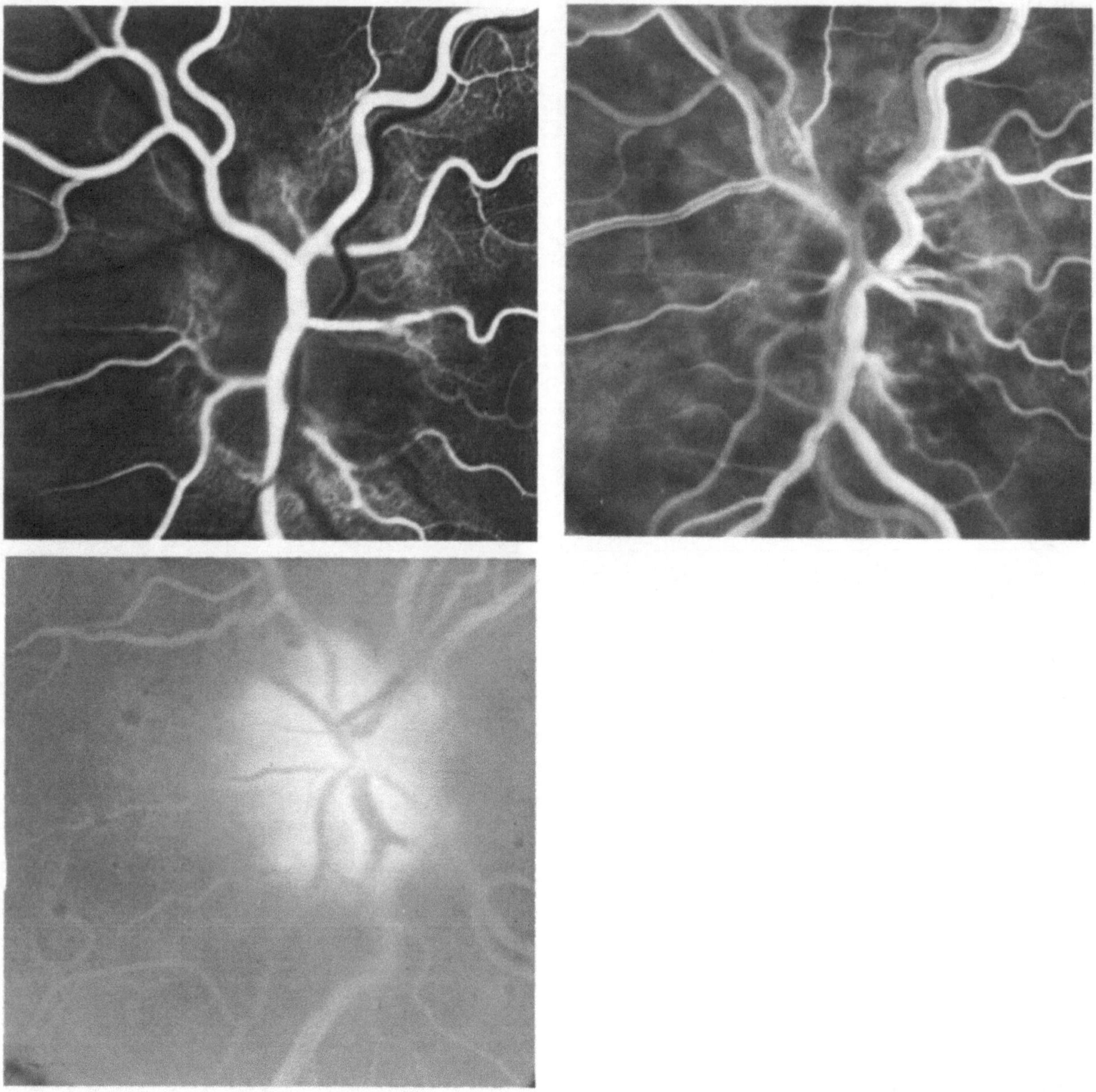

e

f

g

Fig. 14. (continued)

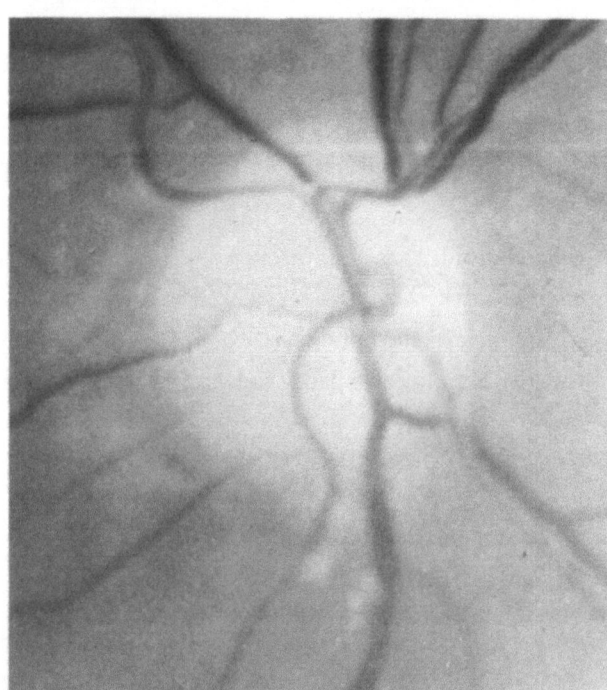

h

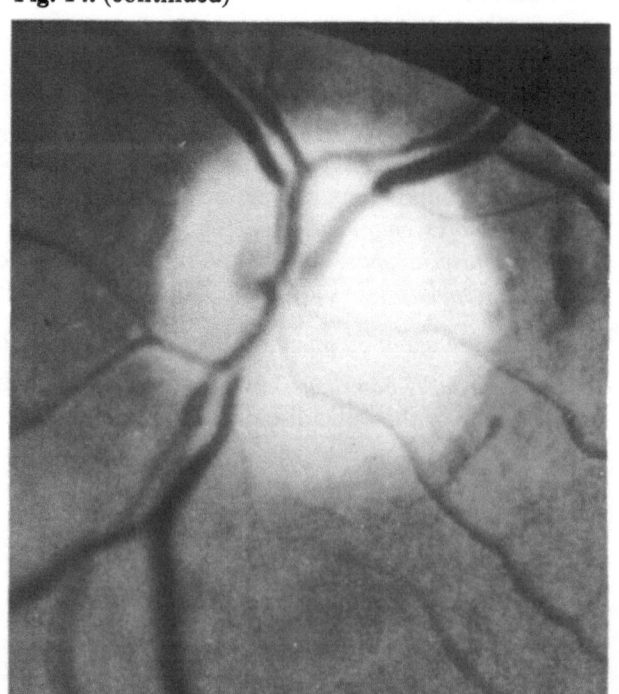

i

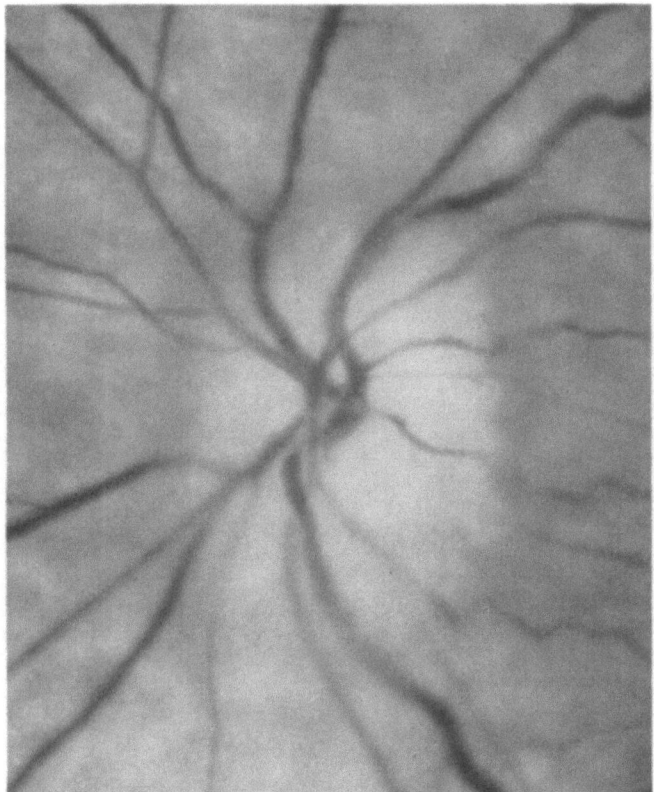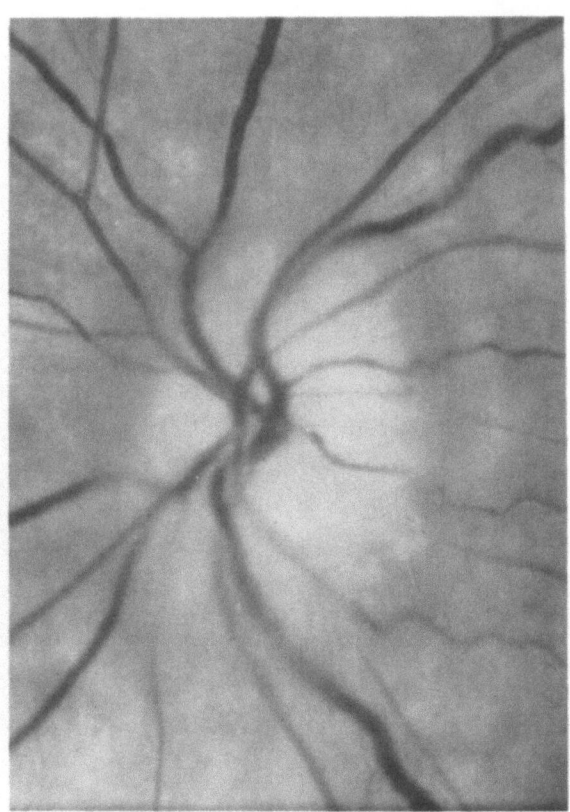

Fig. 15a–f. Left eye of 80-year-old woman with temporal arteritis, left anterior ischemic optic neuropathy and no perception of light in that eye.

a, b, c, d) Two days after onset of anterior ischemic optic neuropathy.

a) *Stereoscopic fundus photographs* showing chalky-white swelling of the optic disc, with no hemorrhages.

b, c, and d) *Fluorescein fundus angiograms.*

b) *Retinal arterial phase* showing non-filling of the optic disc, peripapillary choroid and most of the choroid except in lower temporal sector.

c) *Retinal venous phase* showing non-filling of the optic disc, some of the peripapillary choroid and the watershed zone below.

d) *Late phase* (25 minutes): Showing no staining of the optic disc although a faint staining of the big retinal veins on the disc is seen.

e) *Fluorescein fundus angiogram* during the retinal arteriovenous phase 3 months after the above angiograms showing non-fluorescence of the optic disc, with normal filling of the choroid.

f) *Stereoscopic fundus photographs* 29 $^1/_2$ months after the onset of anterior ischemic optic neuropathy, showing cupping of the optic disc

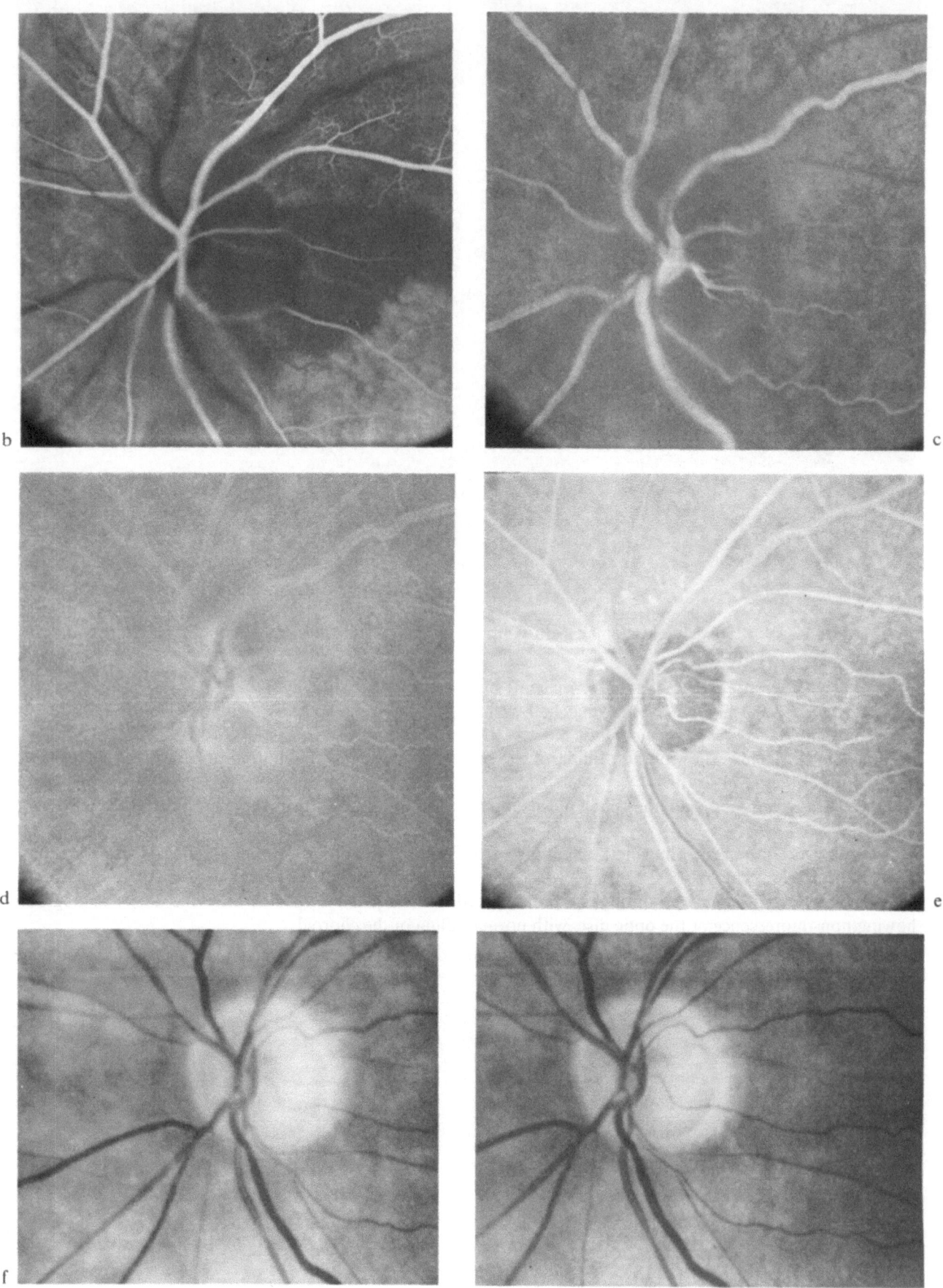

Fig. 15 (continued)

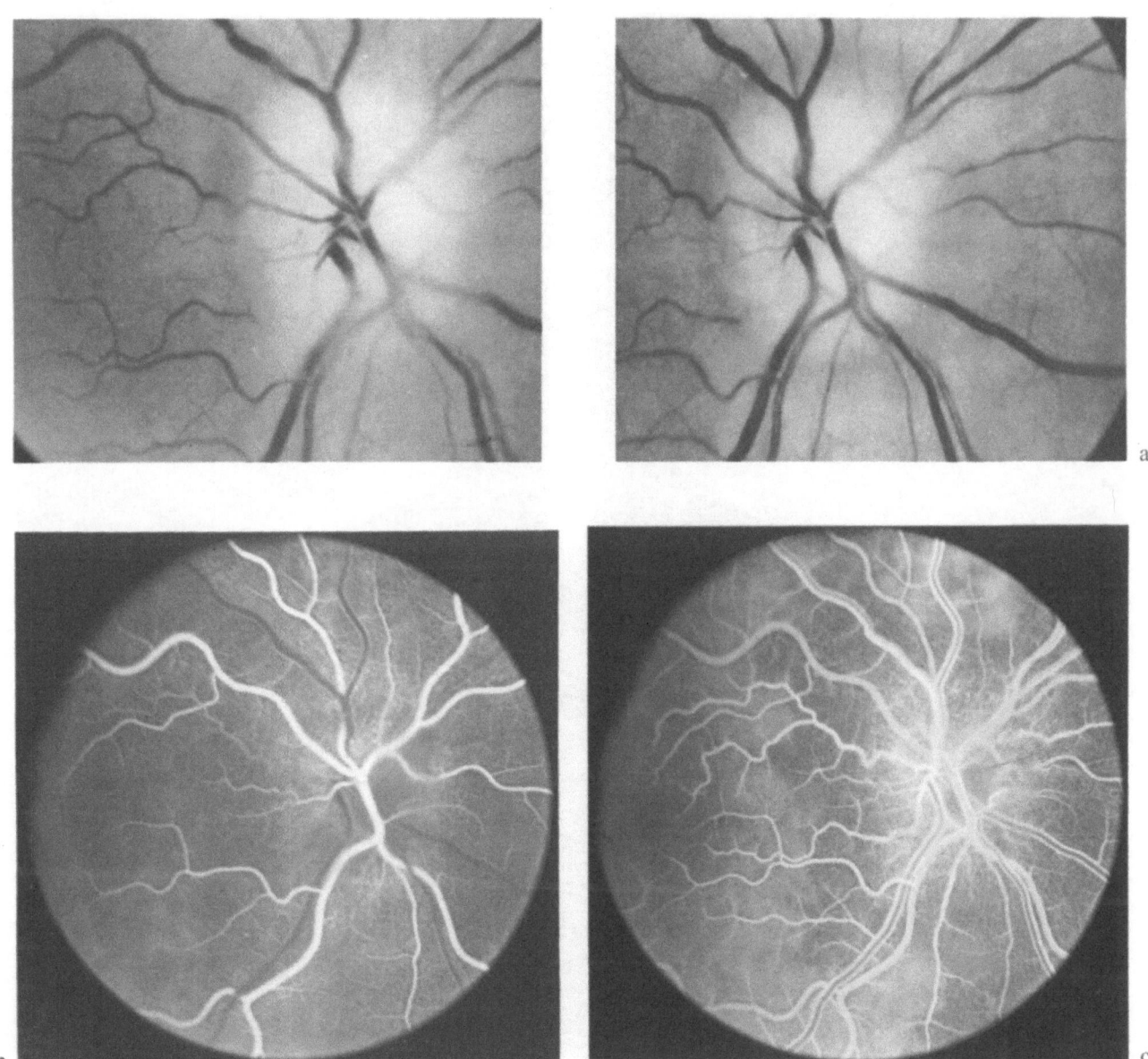

Fig. 16a–j. Right eye of a 72-year-old woman with temporal arteritis, anterior ischemic optic neuropathy and no perception of light in that eye.

Fig. a, b, c, d, e) Three days after onset of anterior ischemic optic neuropathy and on the day of no perception of light.

a) *Stereoscopic fundus photographs* showing chalky-white swelling of the right optic disc, with no hemorrhages.

b, c, d, and e) *Fluorescein fundus angiograms.*

b) *Retinal arterial phase* showing no filling of the choroid and optic disc.

c) *Retinal arteriovenous phase* showing no filling of the optic disc, peripapillary choroid and nasal choroid, with filling of the temporal choroid.

d) *Retinal venous phase* showing no filling of the optic disc and peripapillary choroid, with filling of rest of the choroid except the inferior watershed zone.

e) *Late phase* (15 minutes)—showing no fluorescence of the optic disc. Angiograms five days later showed a similar filling pattern.

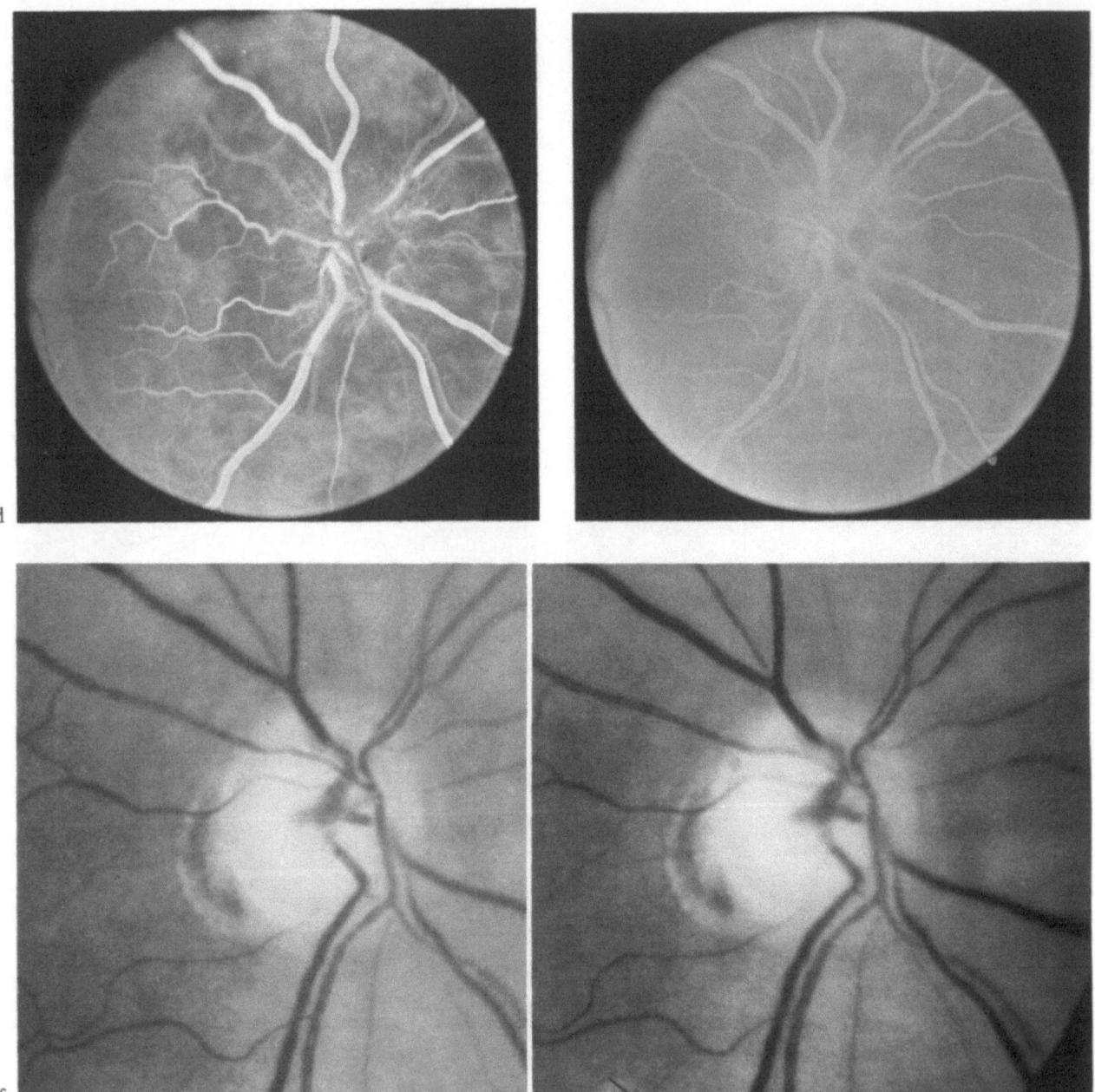

Fig. 16. (continued)

f, g, h, i) 38 days after Fig. a–e.

f) *Stereoscopic fundus photographs* showing cupping of the optic disc and temporal peripapillary chorioretinal degeneration.

g, h and i) *Fluorescein fundus angiograms.*

g) *Retinal arteriovenous phase* showing complete choroidal filling but no filling of the optic disc and degenerated part of the peripapillary region.

h) *Retinal venous phase* showing the same as in Fig. g.

i) *Late phase* (15 minutes) showing no staining of the optic disc but shows fluorescence of the peripapillary region (compare with Fig. e).

j) 13¹⁄₄ months after onset of the anterior ischemic optic neuropathy. *Stereoscopic fundus photographs*—showing cupping of the optic disc which is identical to that seen in Fig. f

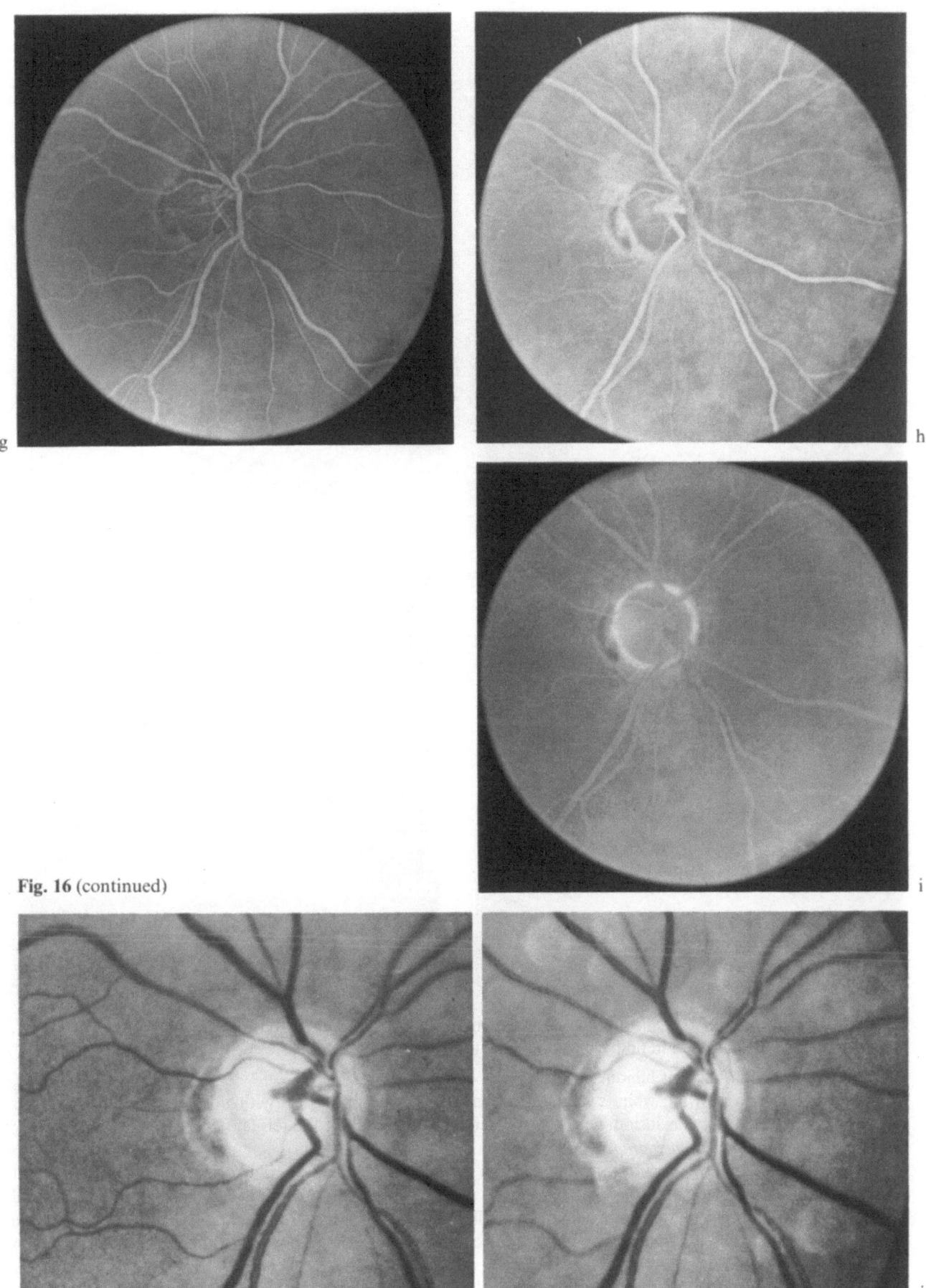

g

h

i

Fig. 16 (continued)

j

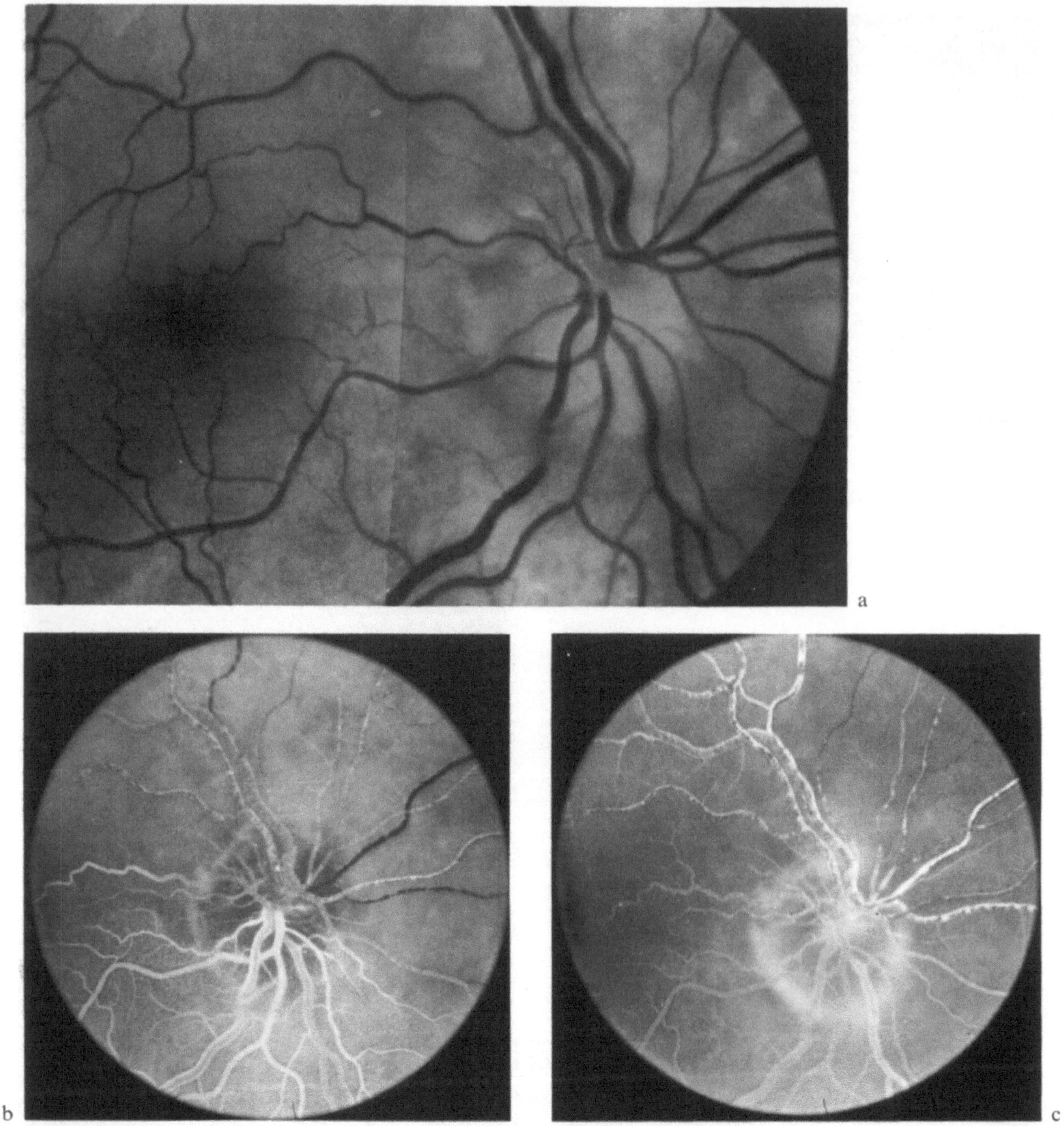

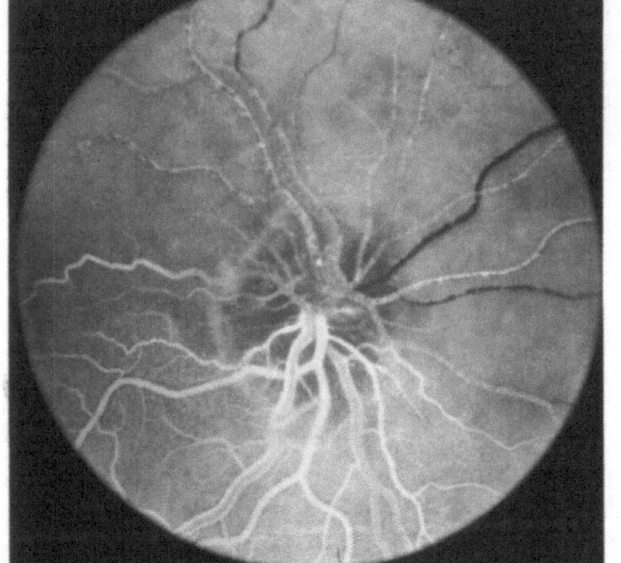

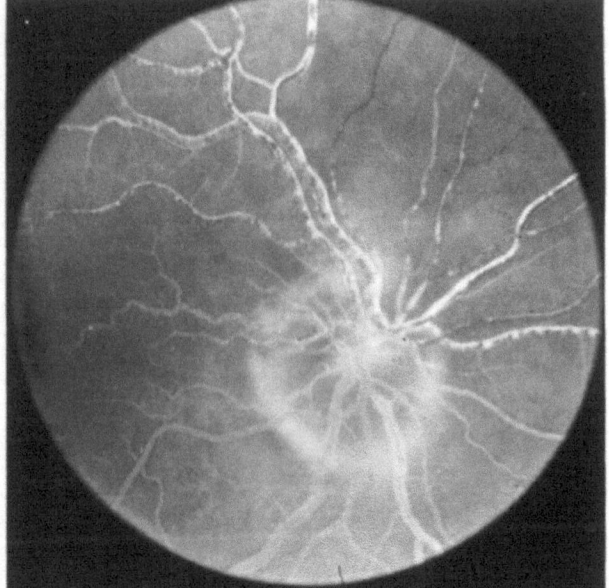

Fig. 17a–l. Right eye of a 71-year-old woman with temporal arteritis, right anterior ischemic optic neuropathy, cilioretinal artery occlusion, and no perception of light in that eye.

a, b, c) Two days after onset of blindness.

a) *Fundus photograph* showing white swelling of lower part of the optic disc with normal color of the upper part, and cilioretinal artery occlusion, with retinal edema of upper half of the retina.

b and c) *Fluorescein fundus angiograms.*

b) *Retinal arteriovenous phase* showing filling of the retinal vessels in lower half of the retina by the patent central retinal artery, with non-filling of the vessels in upper half of the retina supplied by the cilioretinal artery (irregular fluorescein sludging due to an earlier injection of fluorescein), and no filling of the optic disc in spite of this being the second consecutive injection of fluorescein. Choroidal filling is difficult to assess in this second injection.

c) *Late phase:* Showing sludging of fluorescein in the cilioretinal artery and the accompanying retinal vein, no fluorescence of the disc.

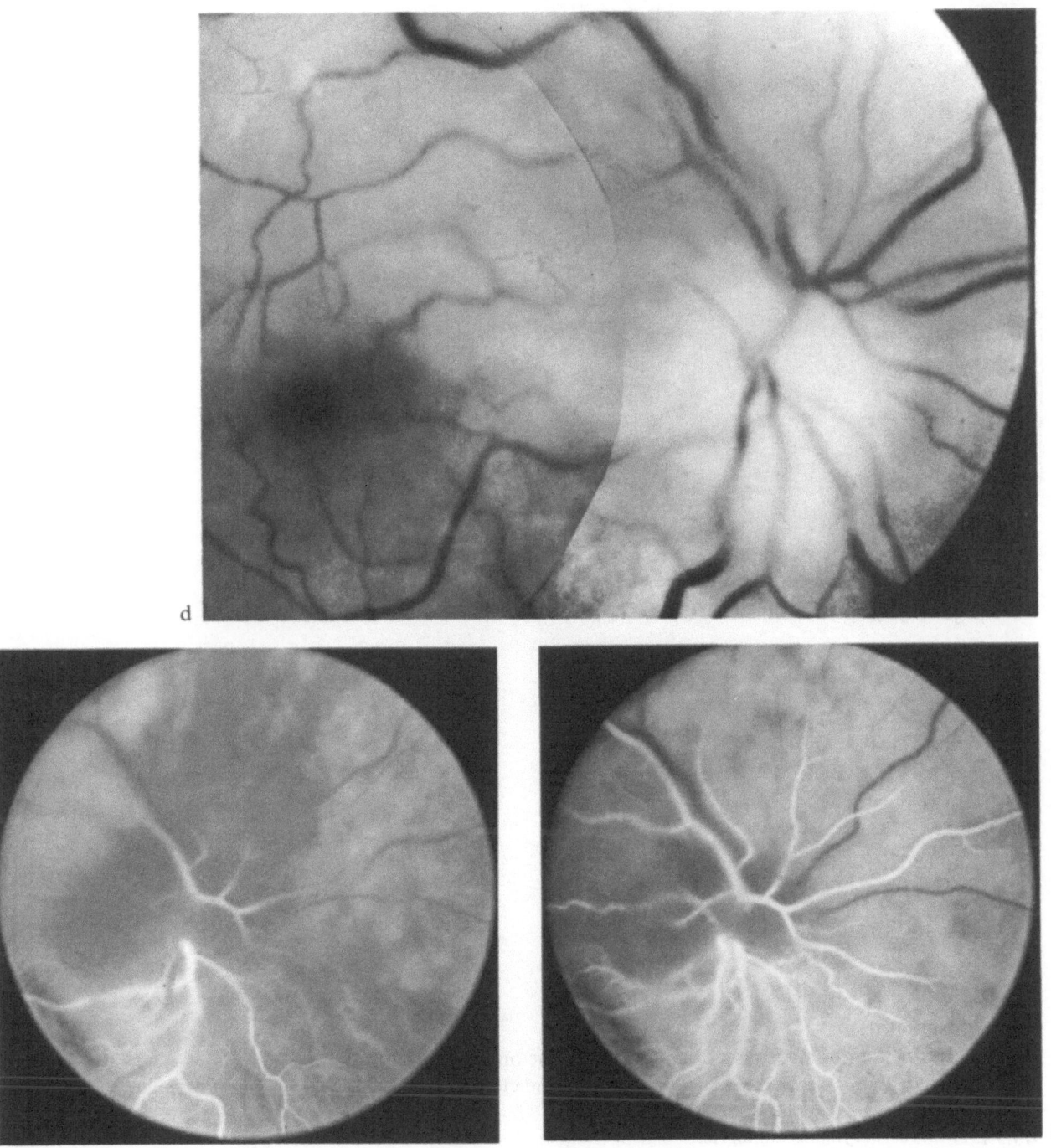

Fig. 17 (continued)

d, e, f, g) Four days after onset of blindness.

d) *Fundus photograph* showing chalky-white swelling of the entire optic disc (compare with Fig. a) with edema of the upper half of the retina.

e, f, g) *Fluorescein fundus angiograms.*

e) *Retinal arterial phase:* Showing filling of the central retinal artery but the cilioretinal artery has just started to fill slowly. No filling of the optic disc, peripapillary choroid and superior watershed zone in the choroid, with faint filling of rest of the choroid.

f) *Retinal arteriovenous phase* showing the cilioretinal artery still in arterial phase. The optic disc shows no filling but the choroid fills completely.

g) *Late phase* showing some staining of the center and lower temporal part of the optic disc.

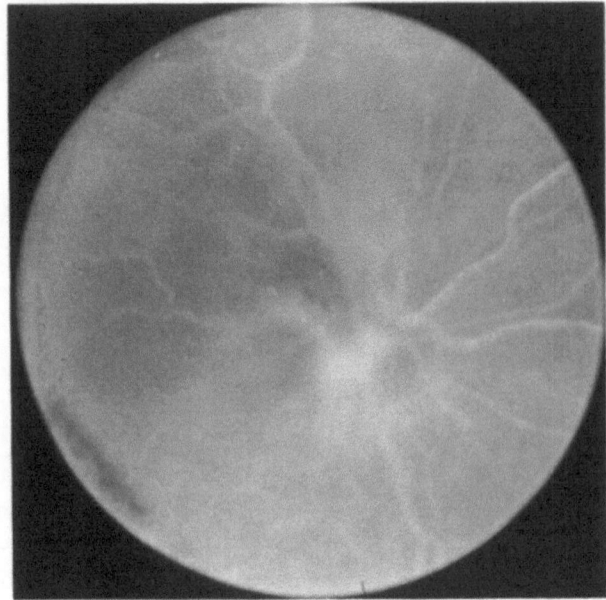

g

Fig. 17 (continued)

h, i, j, k, l) 8$^1/_2$ months after onset of anterior ischemic optic neuropathy.

h) *Stereoscopic fundus photographs* showing atrophy and cupping of the optic disc with peripapillary chorioretinal degeneration.

i, j, k, l) *Fluorescein fundus angiograms*

i) *Pre-retinal arterial phase* showing cilioretinal artery and the choroid fill before the central retinal artery (compare with Fig. b, e), with no filling of the optic disc.

j) *Retinal arteriovenous phase* showing normal filling of retinal and choroidal vasculature with no filling of the optic disc and choriocapillaris in the peripapillary choroid.

k) *Retinal venous phase* showing no filling of the disc and small vessels of the peripapillary choroid.

l) *Late phase* showing well-defined and faintly fluorescent optic disc

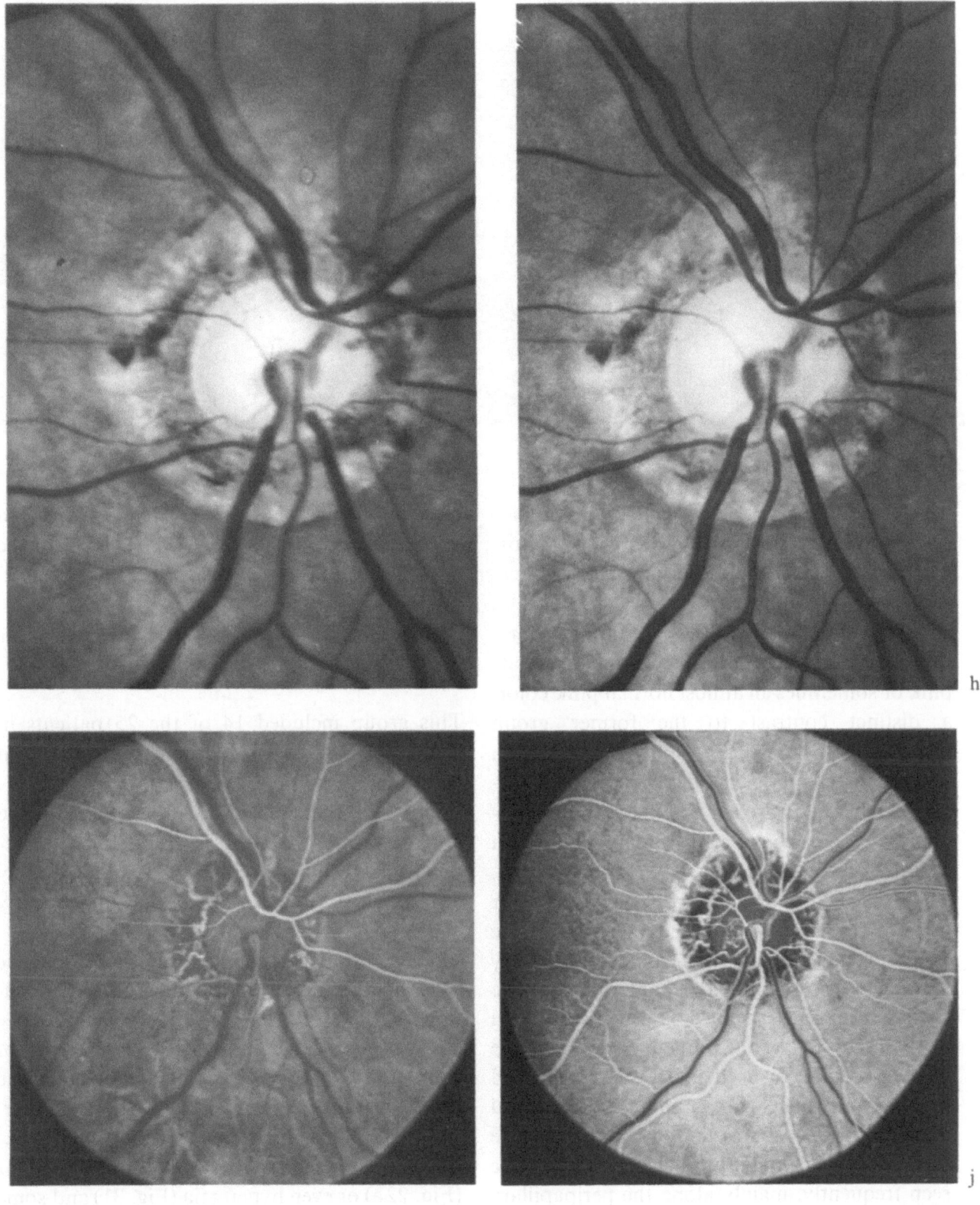

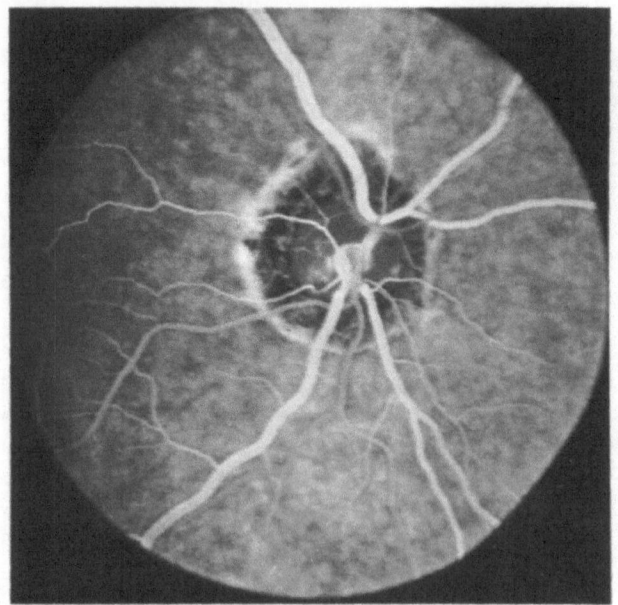 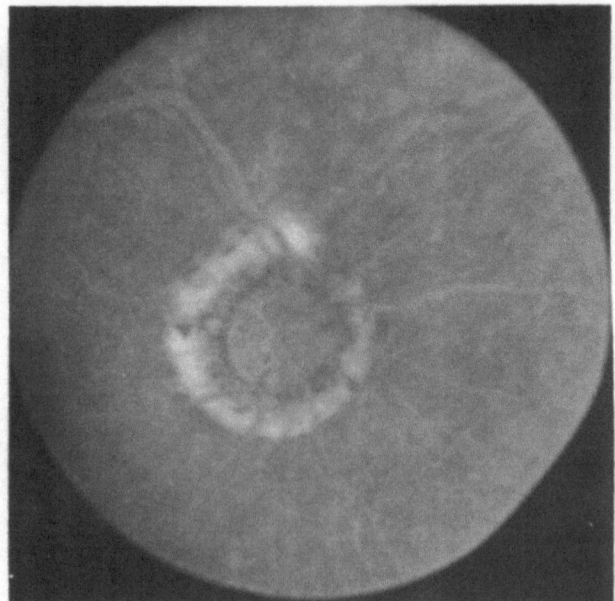

k   l

Fig. 17 (continued)

visible. Hemorrhages on or near the optic disc were rare and, when present, were mostly minor. Central depression of the optic disc was still present.

2. In the other half of the eyes in this group, the optic disc was edematous and had a pale pink or sometimes an almost normal pink color, a distinct contrast to the former group (Fig. 18a). In most however, there was no definite hyperemia of the disc. Stereoscopic examination revealed edema of the disc and frequently a deeper pallor; the prelaminar region appeared to be edematous and somewhat pale. The normal color of the surface nerve fiber layer was superimposed on the prelaminar edema. The edema extended into the immediate peripapillary region. In discs with sectoral anterior ischemic optic neuropathy, edema was usually maximal in the involved part. Although the rest of the disc was not free from edema, it was less marked over the uninvolved part. In some of the sectoral cases edema was almost uniform over the entire disc. Superficial flame-shaped hemorrhages were seen frequently, mainly along the peripapillary capillaries, and usually were minor, although marked hemorrhages on and around the disc (Fig. 18a) were seen in one eye. An edematous disc of this type could be confused with edema of the optic disc due to other causes, although in anterior ischemic optic neuropathy edematous

discs frequently tended to be slightly paler than edematous optic discs of other types. Also, the edema usually is not very marked.

b) In Anterior Ischemic Optic Neuropathy Due To Arteriosclerosis

This group included 14 of the 25 patients in Category I (p. 25), in addition to most eyes in Category II (p. 25).

Most of these discs resembled (a2) above (Figs. 19a, 20a, 21a, 22a, 23b, 24i, 31) frequently with minor or no pallor, and only rarely (a1) (in 2 of 12 eyes examined at a very early stage—Figs. 24a, 25a).

Thus, during early stages of anterior ischemic optic neuropathy, if ophthalmoscopic examination of the optic disc reveals a chalky-white swollen disc with no superficial congestion of capillaries and none or minor hemorrhage, the disease is most probably due to temporal arteritis. When the disc shows edema and a near normal (Fig. 20a) or slightly pale color (Fig. 22a) or even hyperemia (Fig. 31) and some hemorrhages on and around the disc, the pathology probably is not due to temporal arteritis but due to arteriosclerosis. However, no hard-and-fast rules are possible. The chalky-white swollen discs possibly represent massive infarction of the optic nerve head and retrolaminar

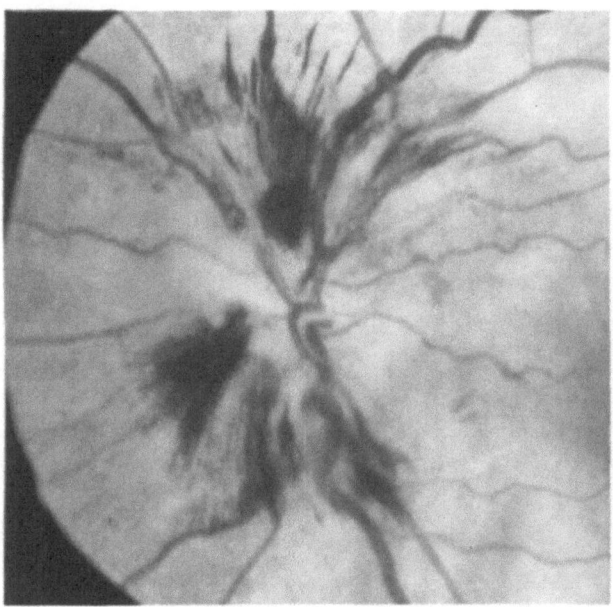
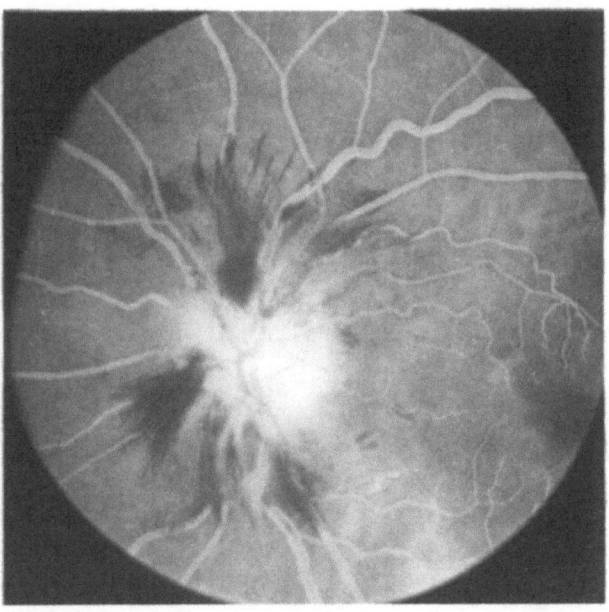

Fig. 18a and b. Left eye of a 75-year-old woman with temporal arteritis, ischemic optic neuropathy and no perception of light in that eye.

a, b) Nine days after onset of anterior ischemic optic neuropathy.

a) *Fundus photograph* showing pale pink edema of the optic disc and multiple superficial hemorrhages.

b) *Fluorescein fundus angiogram:* during the late phase showing diffuse staining of the optic disc

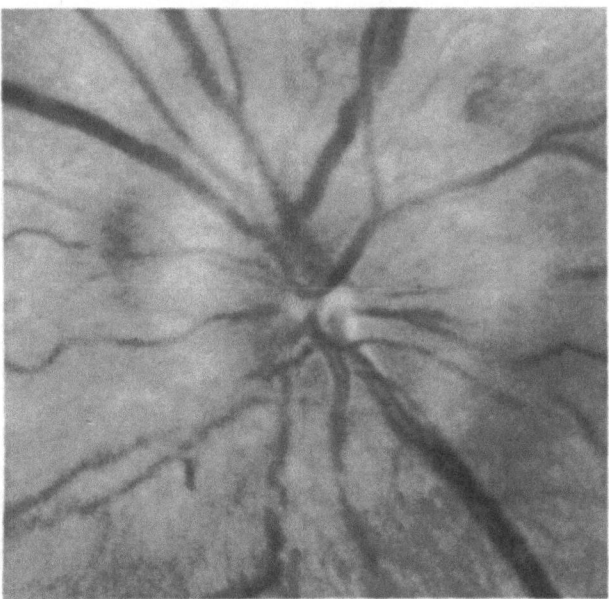
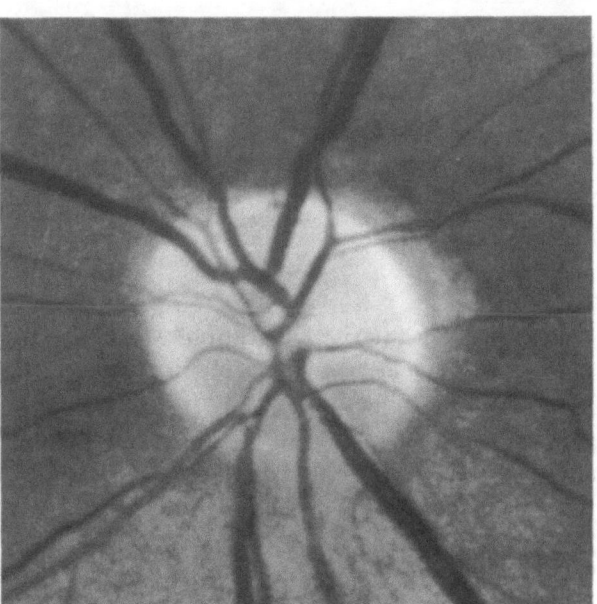

Fig. 19. a and b. Left eye of a 67-year-old man with left inferior altitudinal hemianopia of sudden onset, partial anterior ischemic optic neuropathy, visual acuity of 6/60, and no evidence of temporal arteritis.

a) $2^1/_2$ weeks after onset: *Fundus photograph* showing edema of the optic disc, maximum in upper half of the optic disc.

b) $2^1/_2$ years after onset: *Fundus photograph* showing pallor of upper half of the optic disc with normal lower half.

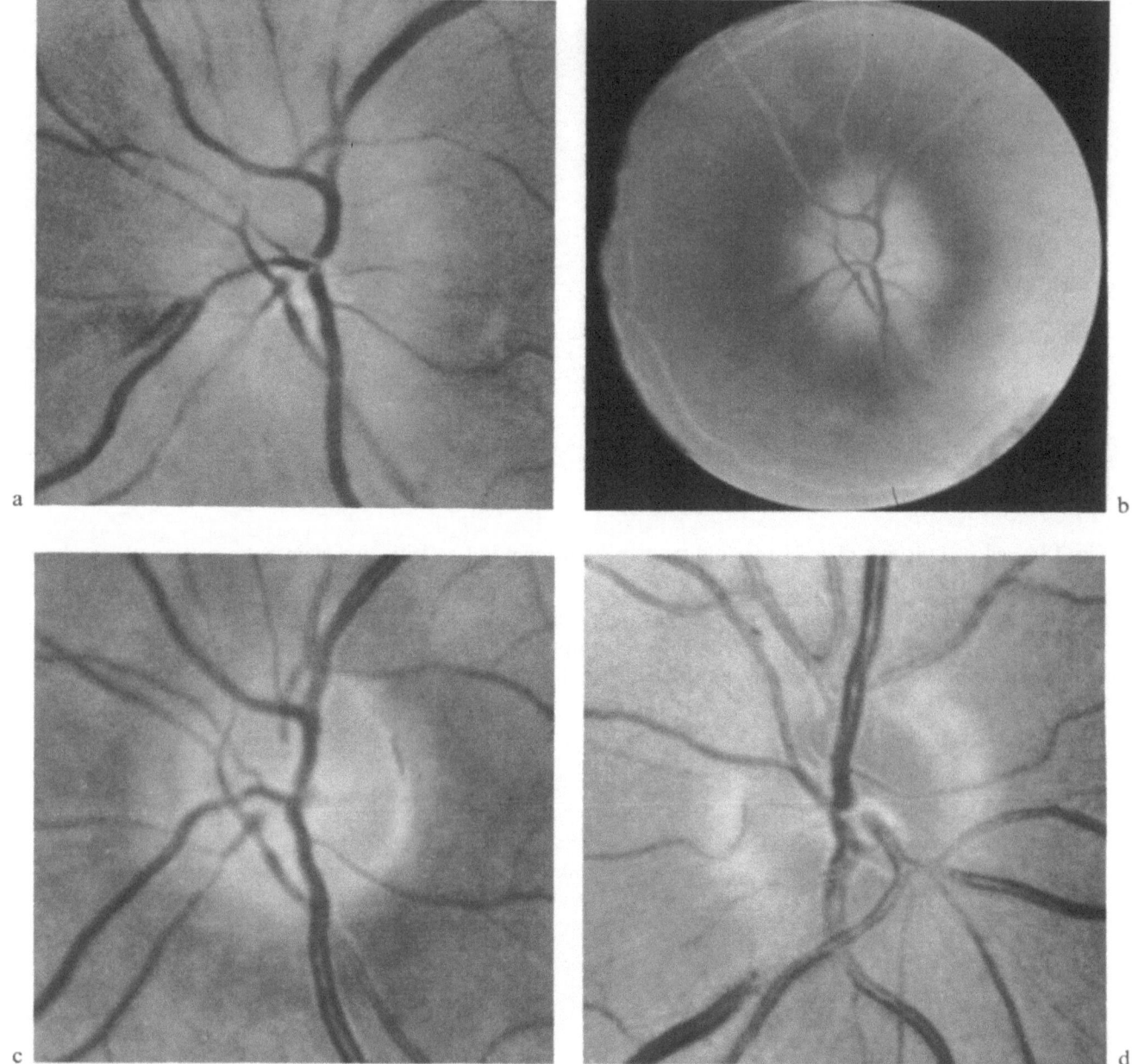

Fig. 20a–d. Left eye of a 70-year-old woman, who noticed suddenly as if seeing through a lace curtain with the left eye (soon after an attack of left ventricular failure).

a, b) About two weeks after onset.

a) *Fundus photograph* showing generalized edema of the optic disc and a superficial retinal hemorrhage inferonasally.

b) *Fluorescein fundus angiogram* during late phase showing fluorescein staining of the optic disc and adjacent region.

c, d) 5 months after onset. Fundus photographs showing pallor of optic disc (c) as compared to right normal optic disc (d)

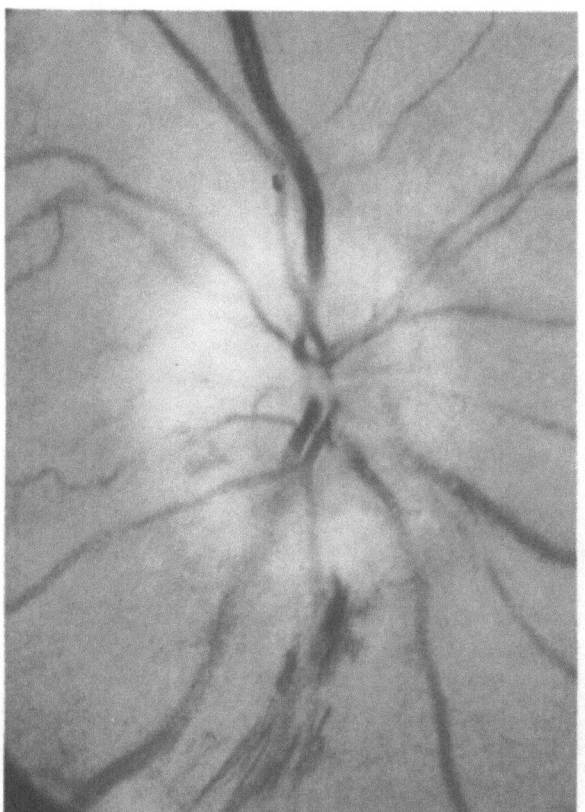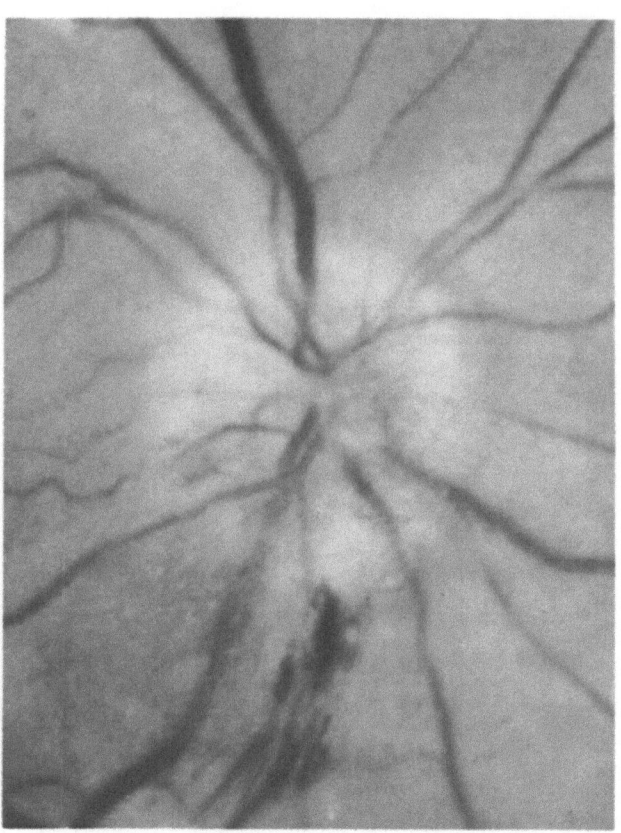

Fig. 21a–e. Right eye of a 61-year-old man with right inferior altitudinal hemianopia of sudden onset 10 days previously, preceded by attacks of transitory blurring of vision in that part for one week; partial anterior ischemic optic neuropathy, visual acuity 6/12 in that eye and no evidence of temporal arteritis.

a) *Stereoscopic fundus photograph* showing swelling of the optic disc with white lesion under the clear but hyperemic superficial layer, and some flameshaped hemorrhages.

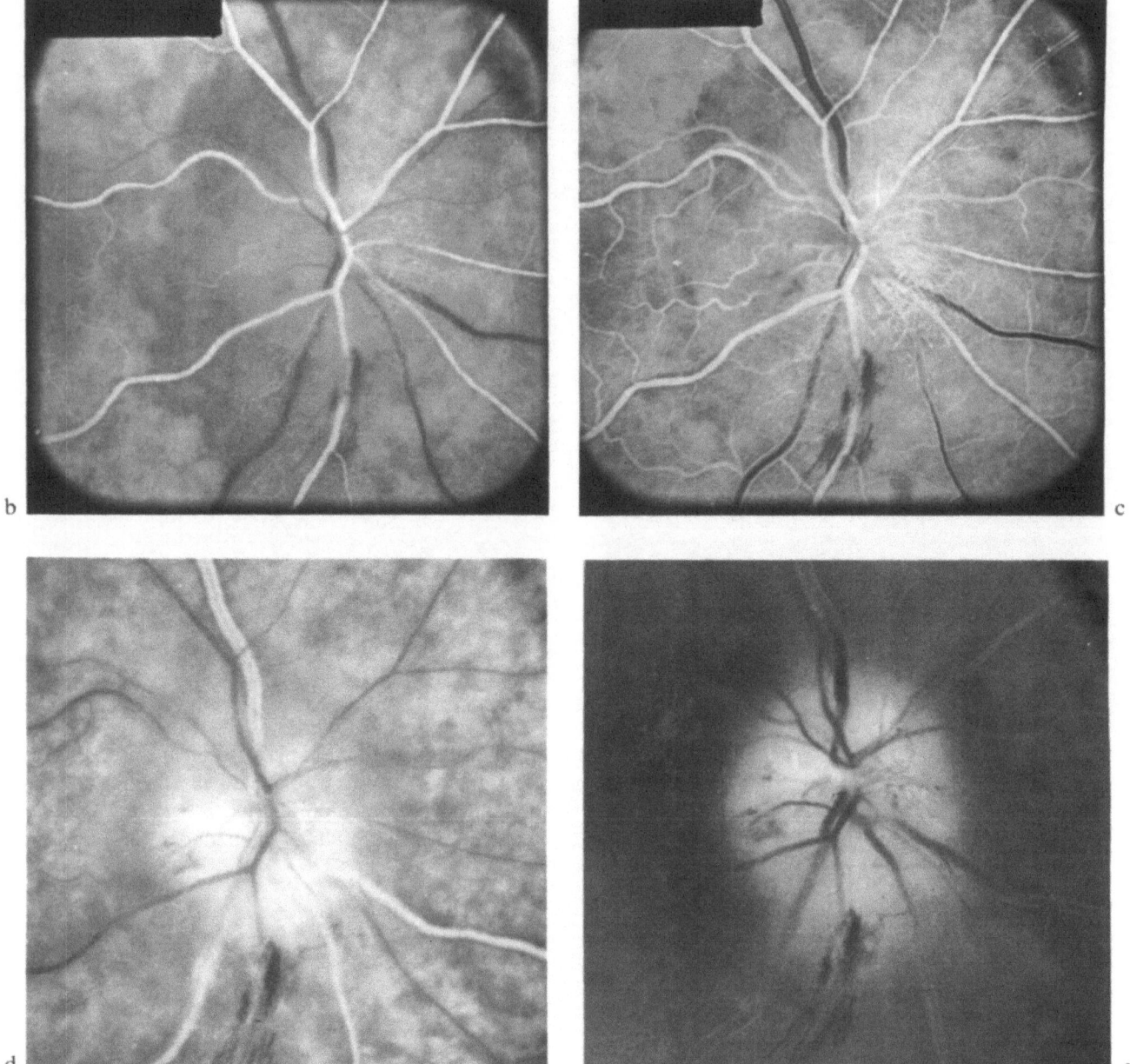

Fig. 21 (continued)

b, c, d, e) *Fluorescein fundus angiograms.*

b) *Retinal arterial phase* showing no filling of the temporal half of the peripapillary choroid and the corresponding part of the optic disc, with patchy filling of the rest of the choroid.

c) *Retinal arteriovenous phase* showing non-filling of superior temporal peripapillary choroid and patchy filling of upper half of the choroid.

d) *Retinal venous phase* showing non-filling of superior temporal peripapillary choroid. Lower half of the optic disc stained with fluorescein and upper half (particularly superior temporal) shows minimal fluorescence.

e) *Late phase* showing diffuse fluorescein staining of the optic disc with blurred margins

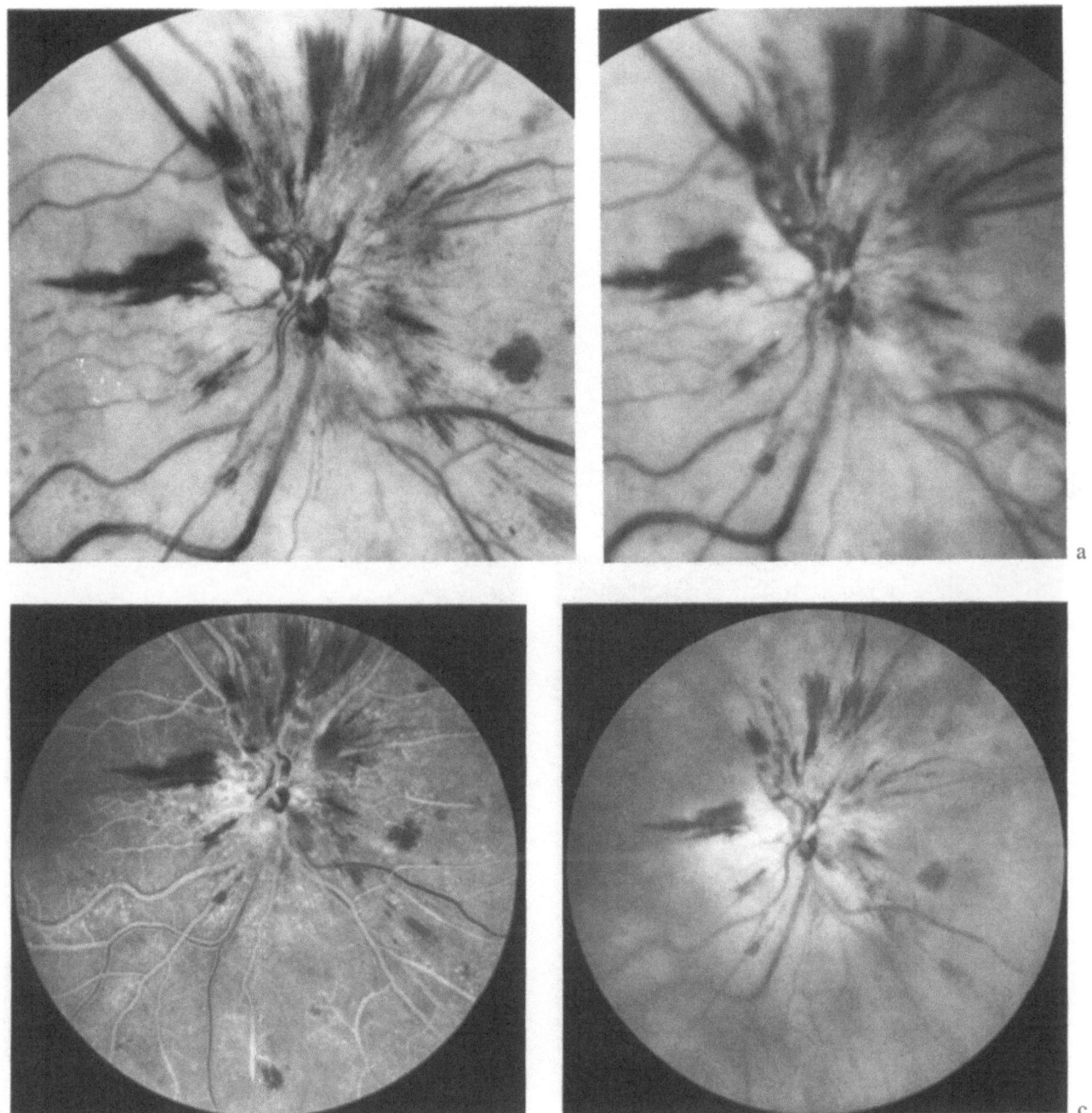

Fig. 22a–f. Right eye of a 60-year-old diabetic woman with sudden onset of blurred vision, visual acuity of 6/12 and inferior altitudinal hemianopia.

a, b, c) 16 days after onset.

a) *Stereoscopic fundus photographs* showing edema of the optic disc which is maximum in the upper nasal half, with superficial retinal hemorrhages and diabetic retinopathy.

b and c) *Fluorescein fundus angiograms.*

b) *Retinal arteriovenous phase* showing normal choroidal filling, masking of upper half of the optic disc by hemorrhages, dilated vessels over the lower part of the optic disc with ill-defined margins, and evidence of diabetic retinopathy.

c) *Late phase* showing fluorescein staining and hyperfluorescence of the optic disc and adjacent region—maximum below and masked above by hemorrhages.

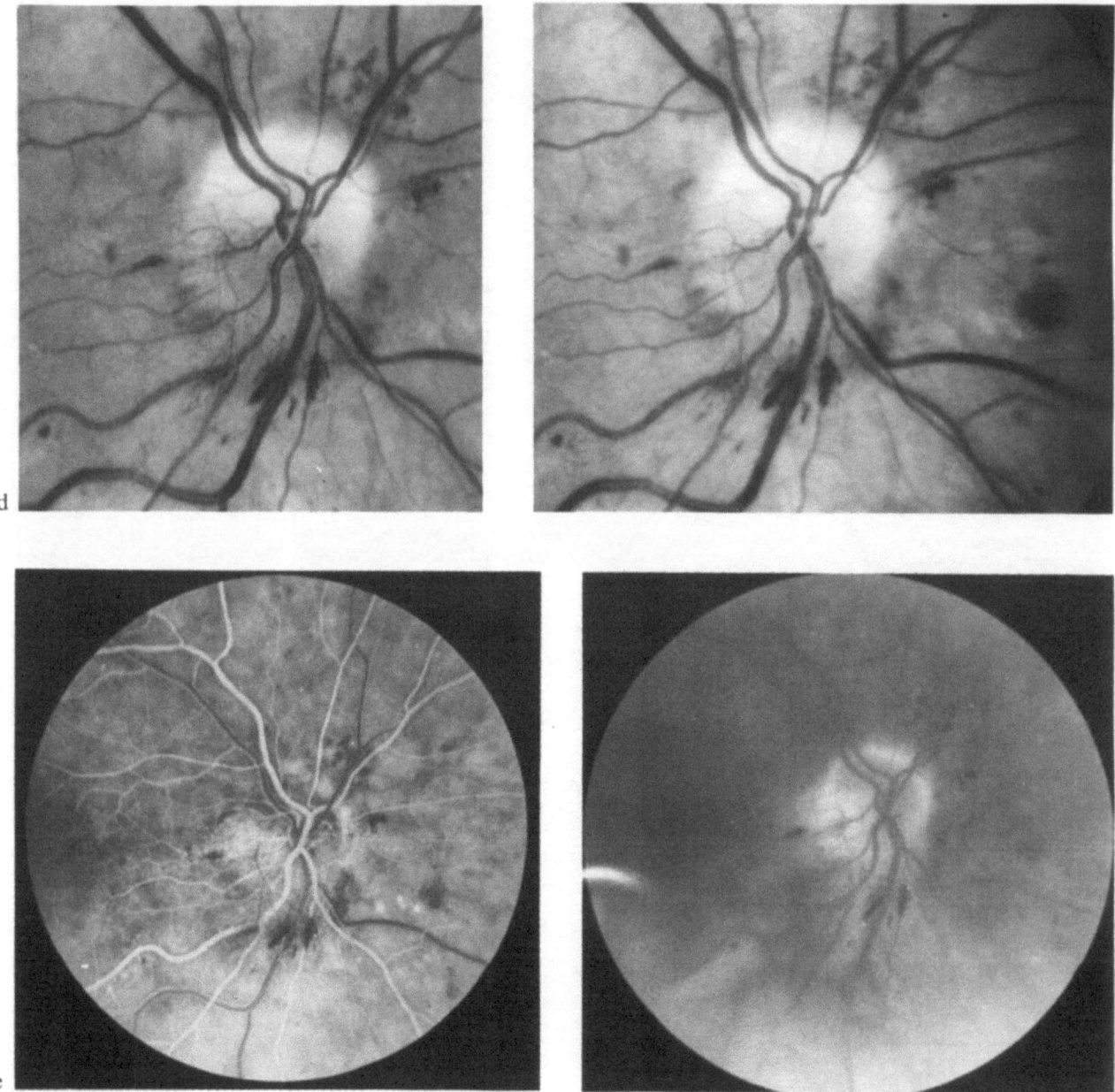

Fig. 22 (continued)

d, e, f) $3^1/_2$ months after onset.

d) *Stereoscopic fundus photographs* showing atrophy of upper half of the optic disc without cupping.

e and f) *Fluorescein fundus angiograms*.

e) *Retinal venous phase* showing non-filling of the atrophic part of the optic disc with dilated vessels and hyperfluorescence of lower temporal part because of diabetic neovascularization. Fluorescein staining of microaneurysms is seen. Superior nasal peripapillary staining is due to absent pigment epithelium in that part.

f) *Late phase* showing non-fluorescence of the atrophic part with staining of the lower temporal part

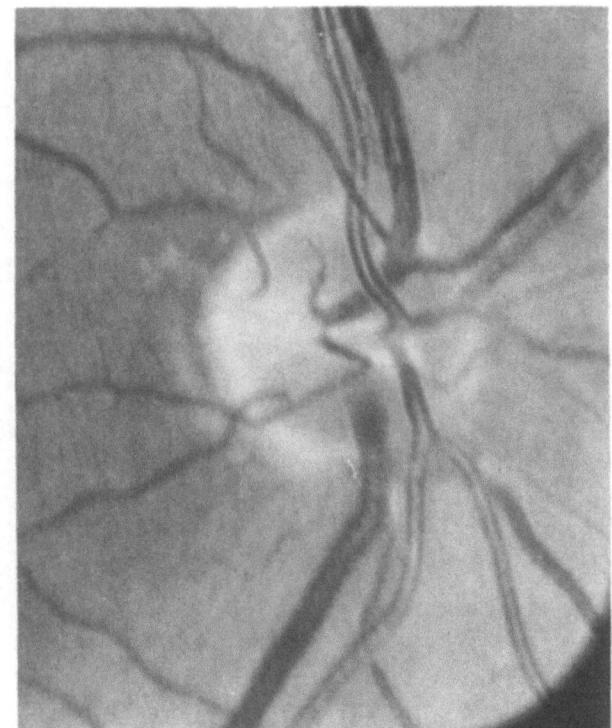

Fig. 23a–f. Right eye of a 59-year-old man with sudden loss of vision in lower field of right eye, visual acuity 6/6-part and superior temporal sectoral anterior ischemic optic neuropathy. He had developed venous stasis retinopathy in left eye 12 years previously.

a) *Fundus photograph* taken 9 months before the onset of above complaint, showing normal optic disc on the right side.

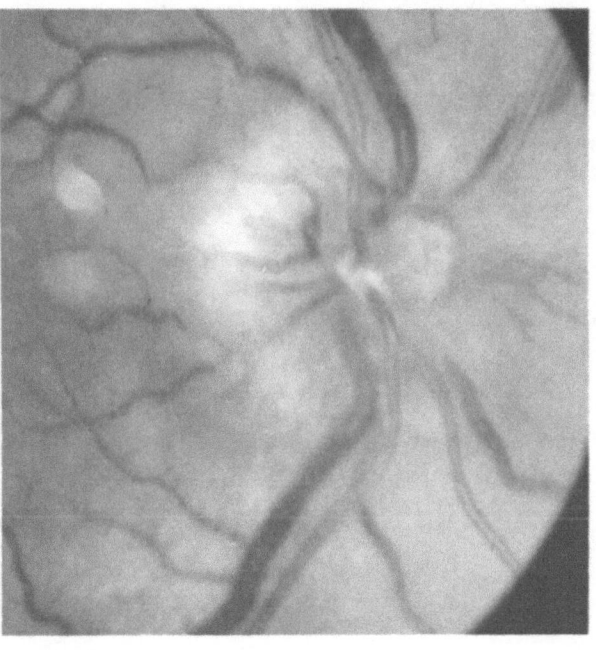

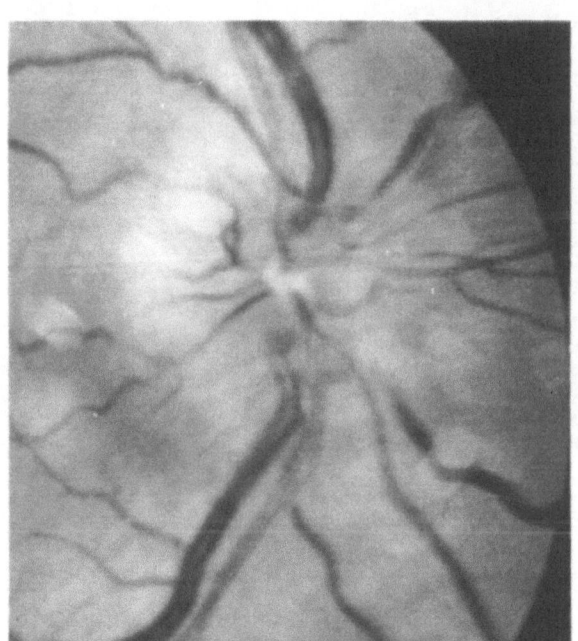

Fig. 23 (continued)

b, c, d, e) 10 days after onset.

b) *Stereoscopic fundus photographs* showing edema of the optic disc, maximum in the superior temporal part.

c, d, e) *Fluorescein fundus angiograms.*

c) *Retinal arterial phase* showing non-filling of the superior temporal part of the optic disc, temporal half of the peripapillary choroid and adjacent choroid in superior temporal part.

d) *Retinal arteriovenous phase* showing complete filling of the choroid. Inferior temporal part of the optic disc shows dilated vessels.

e) *Late phase* showing fluorescein staining of the optic disc, maximum inferotemporally' and blurred margins.

f) *Fundus photograph* two months after onset, showing pallor of the superior temporal part of the optic disc

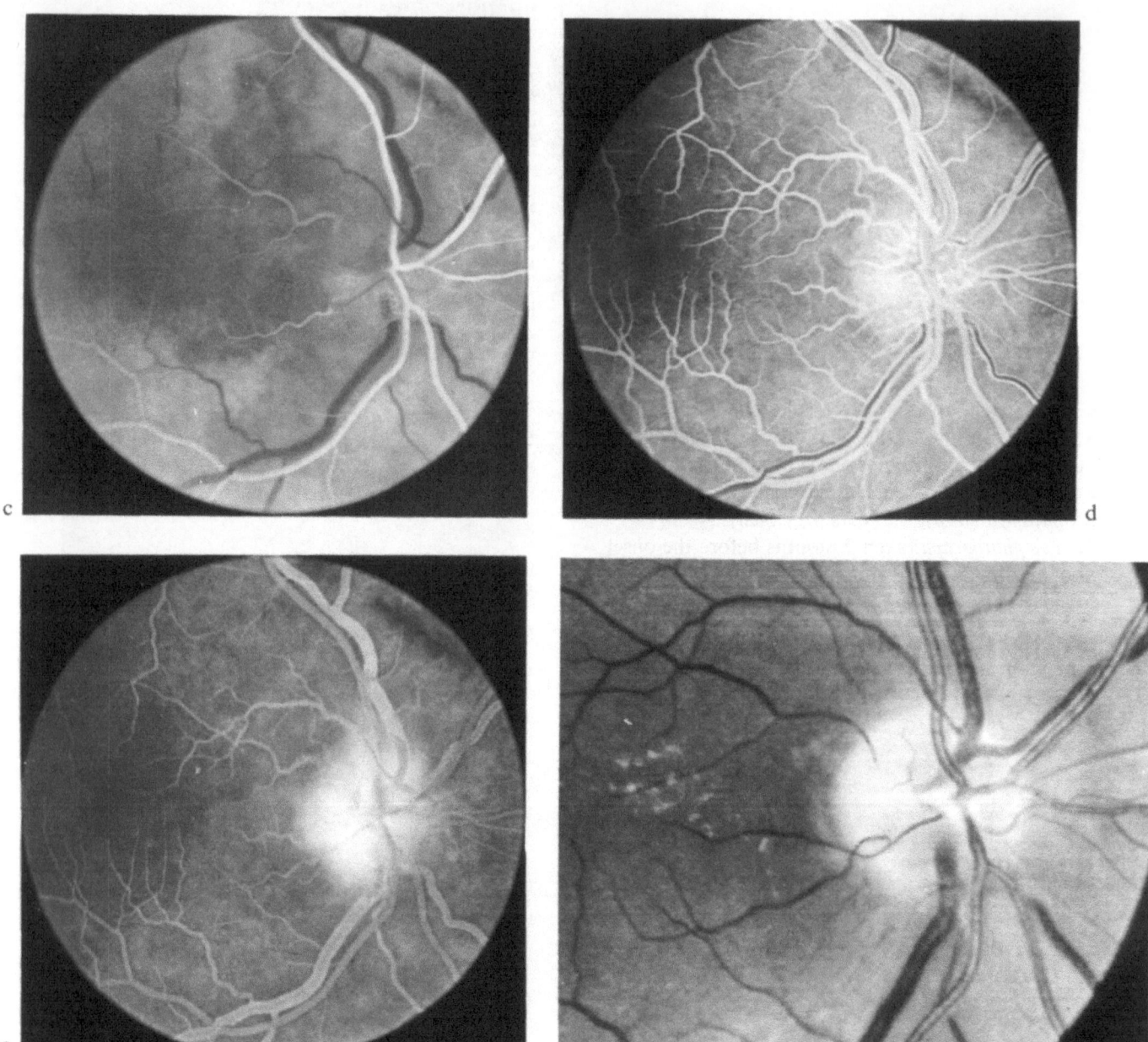

Fig. 23 (continued)

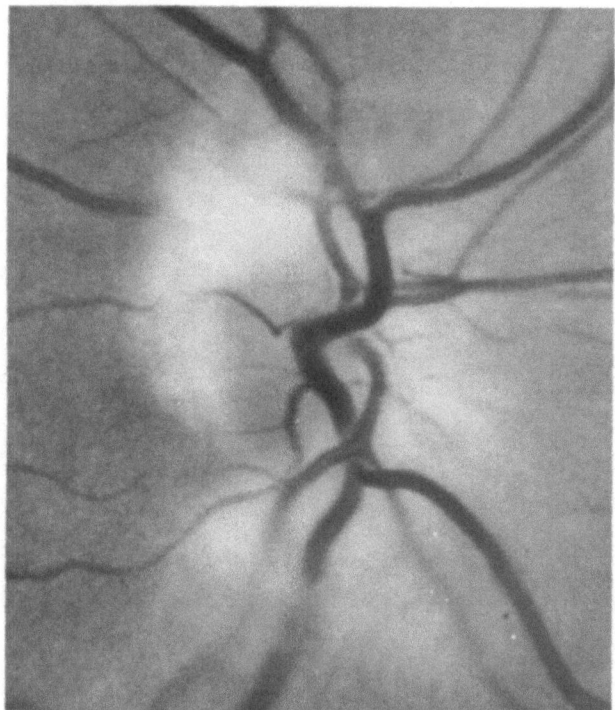
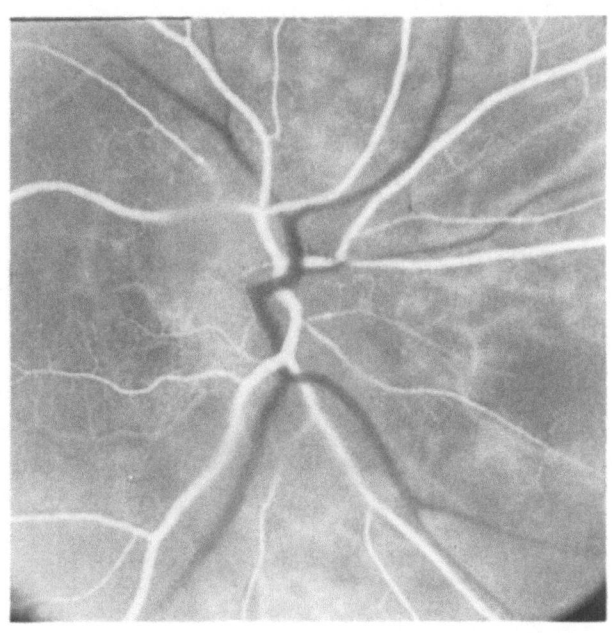

a   b

Fig. 24a–o. Both eyes of a 78-year-old man with bilateral deterioration of vision, visual acuities being 6/12 in the right eye and 6/60 in the left eye and a negative temporal artery biopsy for temporal arteritis.

a, b, c, d, e, f, g, h) Right eye

a, b, c, d, e) 22 days after onset of visual disturbance.

a) *Fundus photograph* showing white edema of the optic disc above, below and nasally with extension on to the adjacent peripapillary region; and normal-looking temporal part. No retinal hemorrhages.

b, c, d and e) *Fluorescein fundus angiograms.*

b) *Retinal arterial phase* showing non-filling of the temporal choroid and optic disc, with filling of a few major choroidal vessels in nasal half.

c) *Retinal arteriovenous phase* showing filling of nasal choroid, temporal peripapillary choroid, and complete filling of the optic disc. No filling of the temporal choroid is seen.

d) *Retinal venous phase* showing better filling of the choroid than seen in (c) although temporal choroid is still empty. Nasal half of the optic disc shows staining with fluorescein. The optic disc margins are not seen except in inferior temporal region.

e) *Late phase* showing diffuse staining of the optic disc with blurred margins except for the inferior temporal margin.

f, g and h) 5 weeks after onset.

f) *Fundus photograph* showing pallor of upper half of the optic disc and fairly pink-looking lower part. The disc margins are well-defined. Retinal vessels have irregular lumen.

g and h) *Fluorescein fundus angiograms.*

g) *Retinal arteriovenous phase* showing filling of whole choroid (compare with c) with temporal part of the optic disc filling better than the nasal part.

h) *Retinal venous phase* showing normal filling of the choroid with nonfluorescence of the optic disc (compare with d). The optic disc was nonfluorescent during the late phase also.

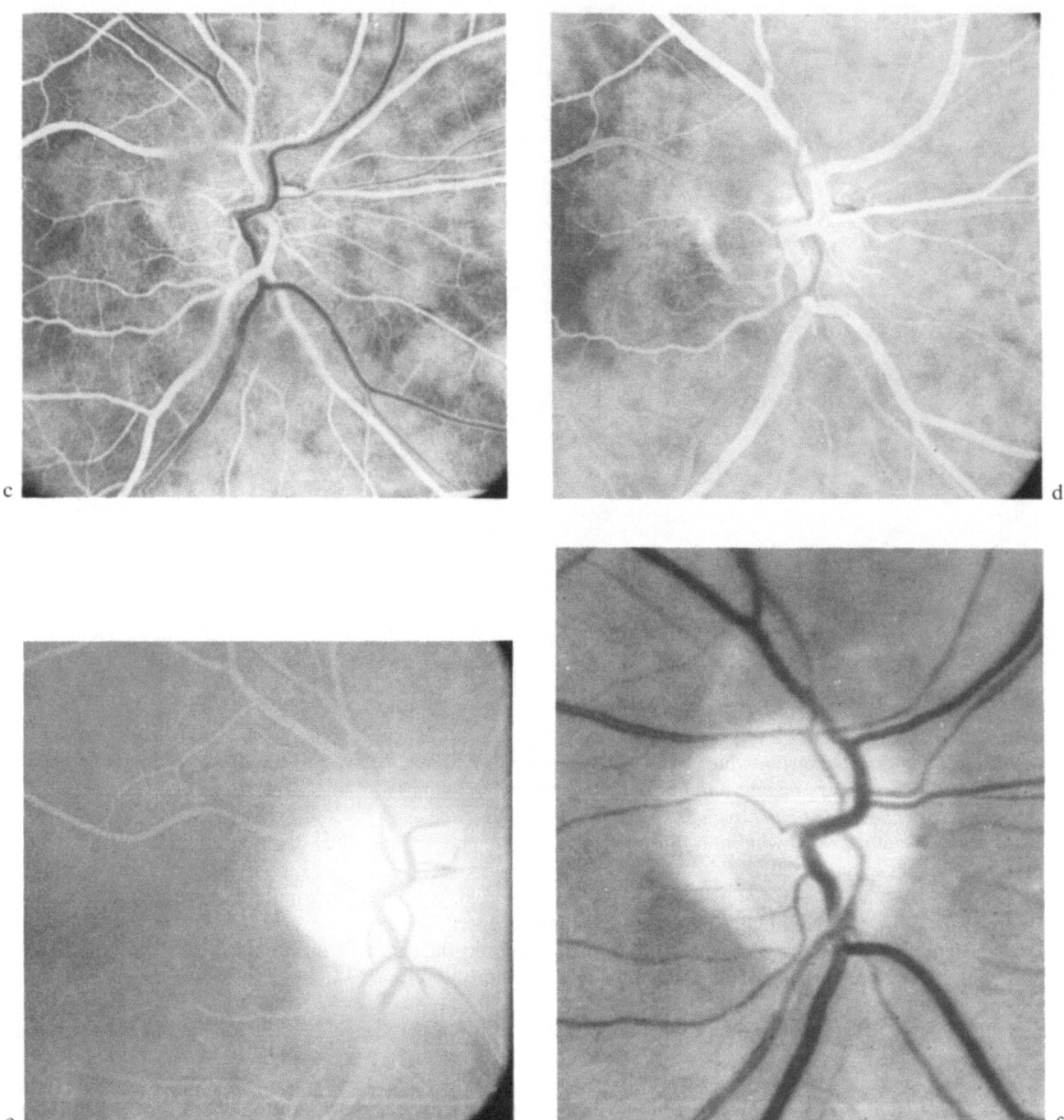

Fig. 24 (continued)

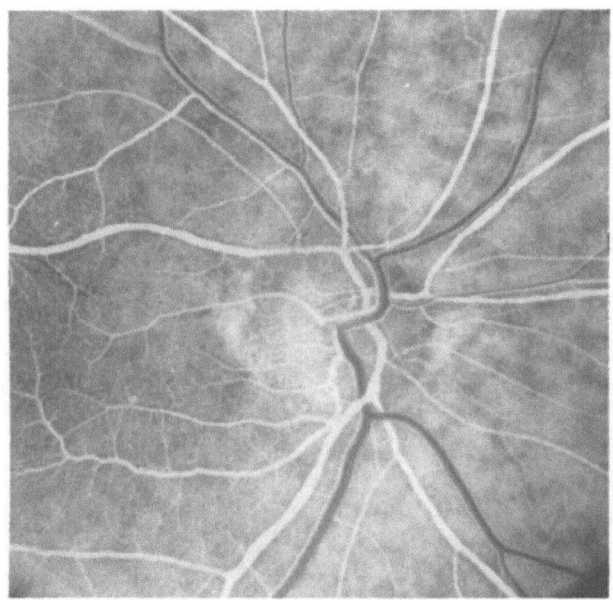
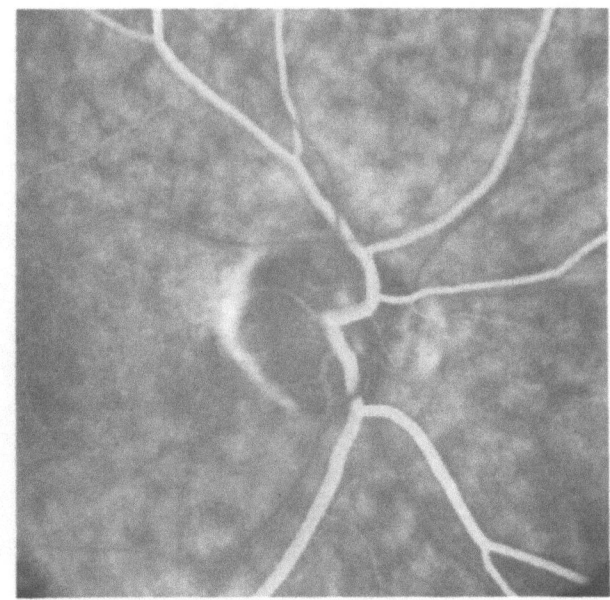

g

h

Fig. 24 (continued)

i, j, k, l, m, n, o) Left eye

i, j, k, l) 23 days after onset of visual disturbance.

i) *Fundus photograph* showing temporal part of the optic disc pale white with a few small punctate hemorrhages and blurred margins. Nasal part of normal color.

j, k, l) *Fluorescein fundus angiograms.*

j) *Retinal arterial phase* showing filling of nasal half of the choroid (supplied by the medial posterior ciliary artery) and optic disc, with temporal part of the choroid (supplied by the lateral posterior ciliary artery) empty. Fluorescence of temporal part of the optic disc due to previous injection of fluorescein for Fig. b–e.

k) *Retinal venous phase* showing filling of the whole choroid, with nasal normal part of the optic disc less fluorescent.

l) *Late phase* showing abnormal fluorescence of the optic disc due to staining—maximum in temporal part.

m, n, o) 5 weeks after onset.

m) *Fundus photograph* showing pallor of temporal part of the optic disc and degeneration of peripapillary region, with normal color of nasal part of the disc.

n, o) *Fluorescein fundus angiograms.*

n) *Retinal arterial phase* showing nasal part of the choroid and optic disc (supplied by the medial posterior ciliary artery) filling with fluorescein while the temporal part of the disc and choroid (supplied by the lateral posterior ciliary artery) empty (Compare with j).

o) *Retinal venous phase* showing filling of the entire choroid but a nonfluorescent optic disc (compare with k). The optic disc was also nonfluorescent during late phase

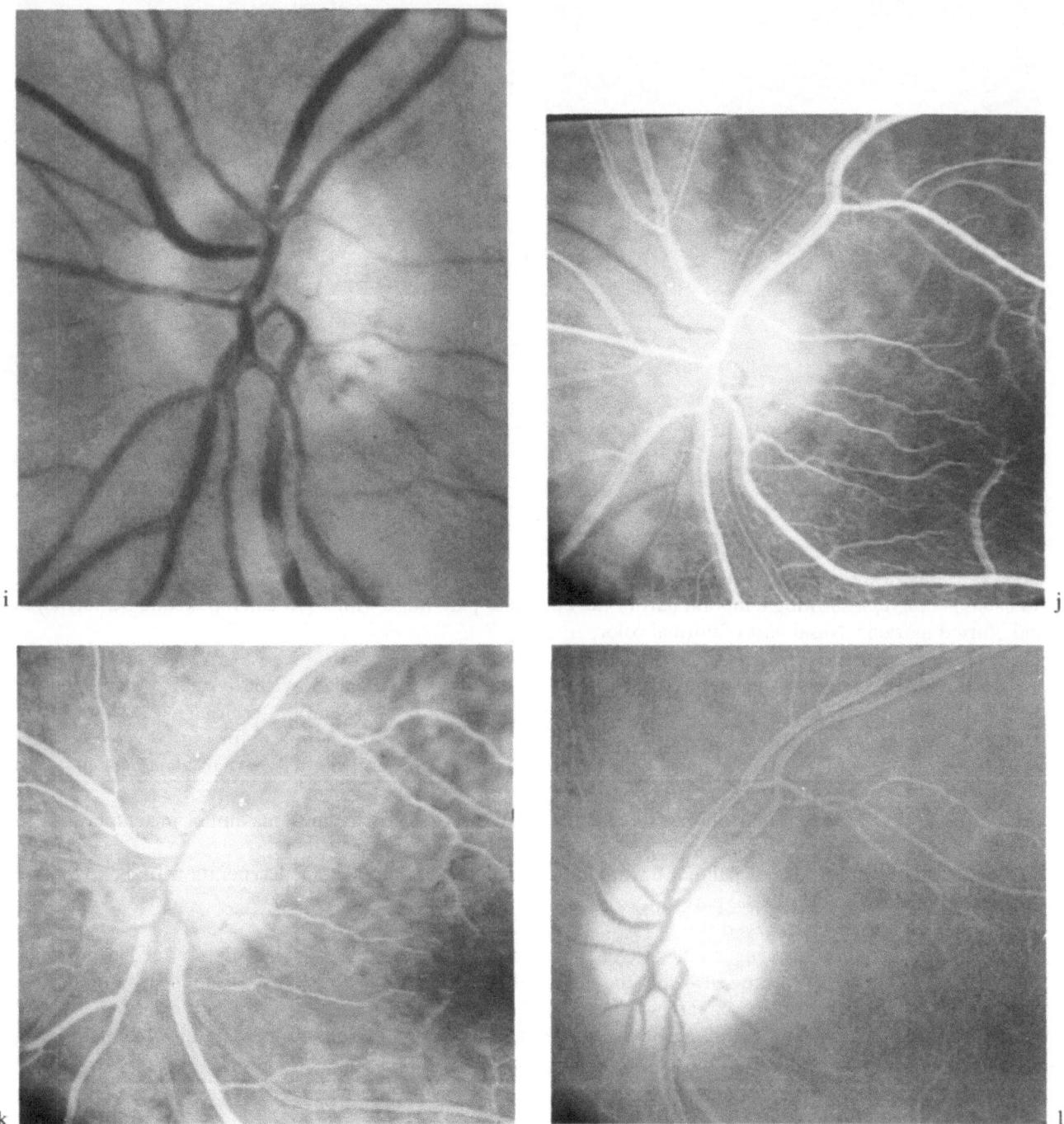

Fig. 24 (continued)

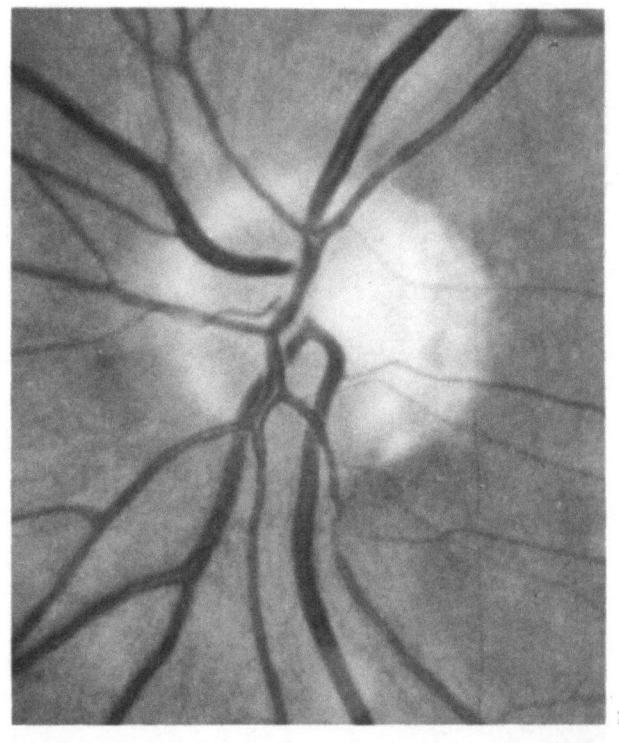

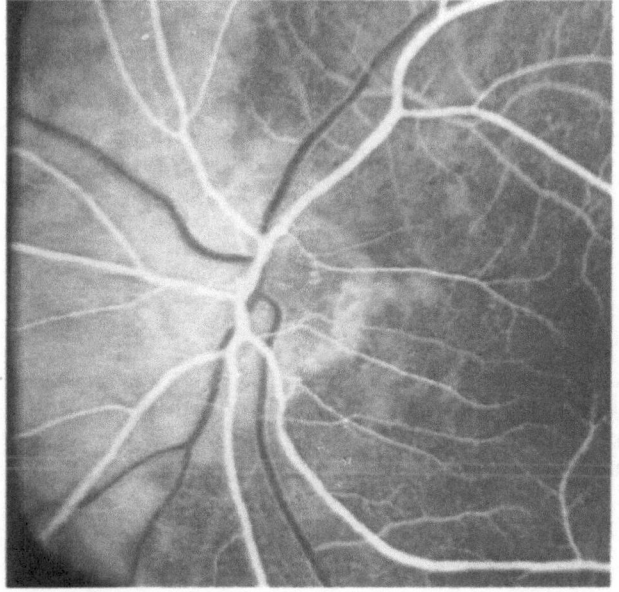

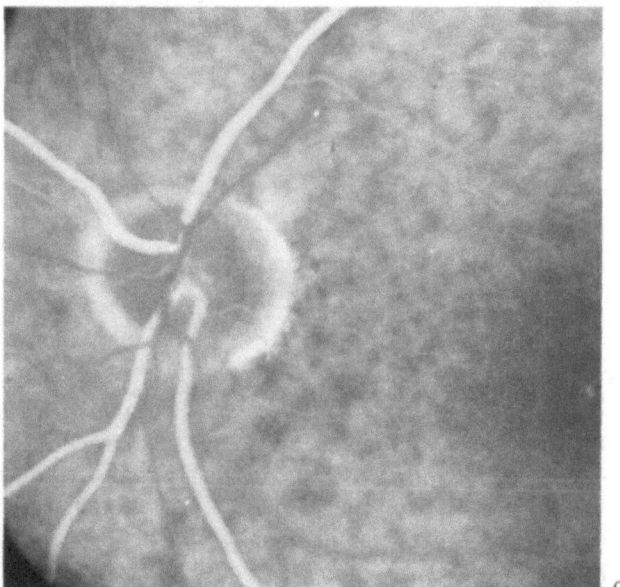

Fig. 24 (continued)

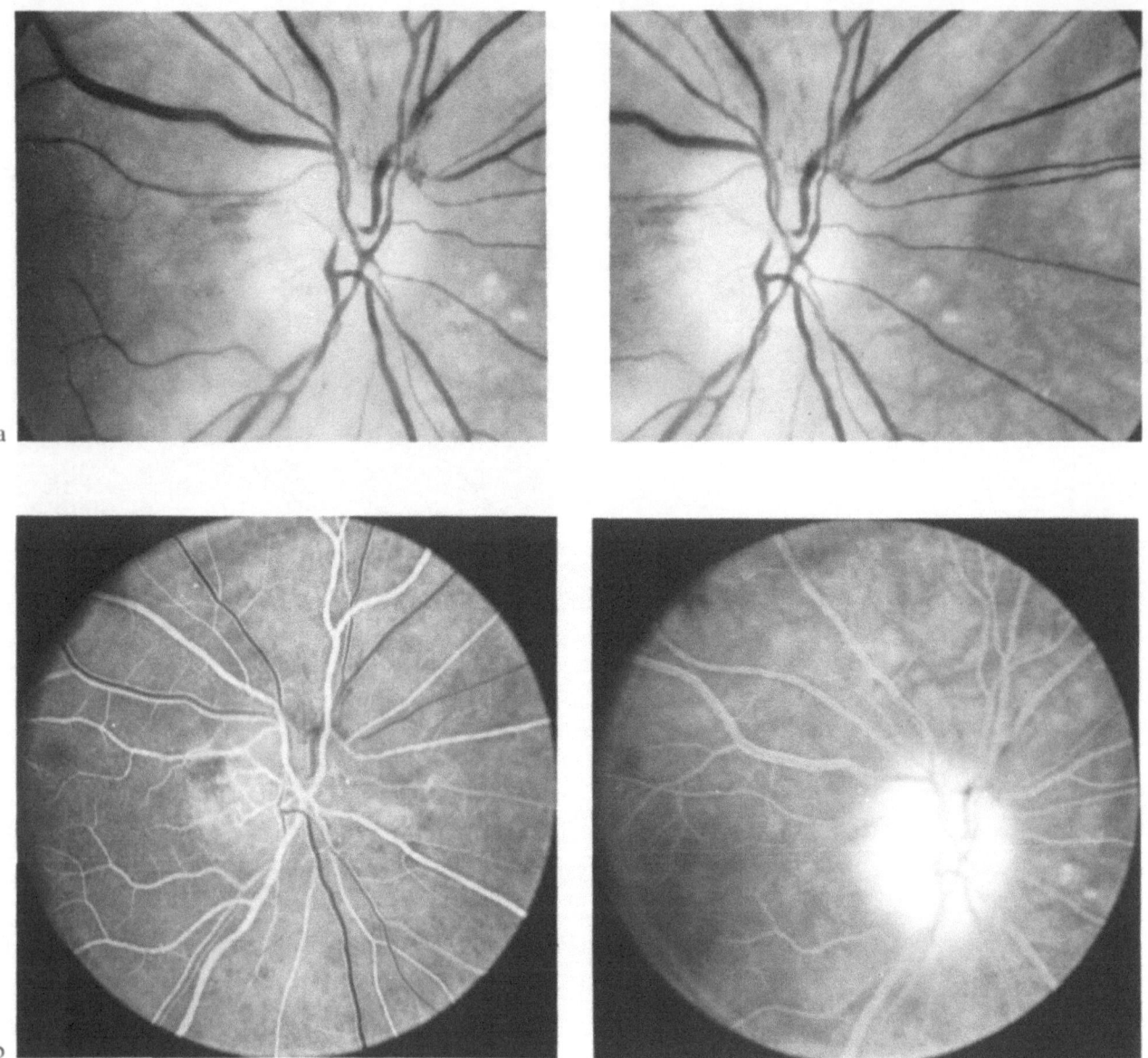

Fig. 25a–c. Right eye of a 61 1/2-year-old woman with sudden deterioration of vision to 5/60 in the right eye, no evidence of temporal arteritis and seen 3 weeks after onset of disturbance of vision.

a) *Stereoscopic fundus photographs* showing swelling of the optic disc with indistinct margins, a white lesion under the superficial transparent retina, superficial striate hemorrhages and arteriosclerotic retinal vessels.

b, c) *Fluorescein fundus angiograms.*
b) *Retinal arteriovenous phase* showing complete filling of the choroid and optic disc.
c) *Late phase* showing staining of the optic disc, particularly of the white lesion

optic nerve, because in all eyes there was marked cupping of the optic disc on resolution, which generally was much more marked than in type (a2). A partial ischemic optic neuropathy may become total after several days (Fig. 17); this finding has also been reported by other authors [185, 474]. SARAUX et al. [474], in arteriosclerotic anterior ischemic optic neuropathy, reported optic disc edema with some hyeremia on the first day, pale optic disc the second day, and several days later the optic disc was pink. I did not observe this pattern.

BONAMOUR et al. [61] reported some cases which, according to them, were anterior ischemic optic neuropathy, but their clinical description is that of optic disc vasculitis type II, as described by me [252].

The optic disc swelling usually starts to subside about 7 to 10 days after it begins. About a month or more later a pale atrophic disc, usually with well-defined margins, is seen (Figs. 14h, i, 15f, 16f, j, 17h, 19b, 20c, 22d, 23f, 24f, m). The time interval between the onset of anterior ischemic optic neuropathy and the development of optic atrophy has been reported to be a few weeks [384], four weeks to four months [342], several weeks [474], 2 to 3 months [60] and from the fifteenth day [61]. In some patients with bilateral disease, if anterior ischemic optic neuropathy develops in an eye when its fellow eye is already atrophic, the condition may be misdiagnosed as the Foster-Kennedy syndrome [338, 474].

At the end of the follow-up period, 21 of the 30 eyes in my series still retained some degree of vision, indicating that a variable number of nerve fibers has survived. Even during the acute phase, though the disc may be swollen diffusely, some degree of vision may still exist. Diffuse edema in the optic disc may make it very difficult to outline an infarcted sector. In my series, when optic atrophy supervened, the distribution of disc pallor and visual acuity was as follows (Table 7):

The patient who could see 6/5 with diffuse optic atrophy in that eye reported that she seemed to be seeing through holes in a lace curtain (Fig. 20); involvement of nerve fibers scattered in patches over the entire optic disc must have been responsible for these symptoms and for the diffuse optic atrophy.

Cupping of the Optic Disc. In the present series the relationship of optic disc cupping to anterior ischemic optic neuropathy was studied to learn more about the mechanism of this phenomenon in general because:

a. Our previous studies indicated that anterior ischemic optic neuropathy, glaucoma, and low-tension glaucoma are manifestations of ischemia of the anterior part of the optic nerve [245, 246, 247, 250, 261, 263, 264], with anterior ischemic optic neuropathy an acute process, the other two chronic. Therefore, optic disc changes in anterior ischemic optic neuropathy should significantly clarify similar changes in glaucoma and low-tension glaucoma.

b. In all previous reports of anterior ischemic optic neuropathy there is hardly any mention of the incidence of optic disc cupping in these

Table 7. Relationship of optic atrophy and visual acuity

Distribution of pallor in optic disc	No. of eyes	Final visual acuity								
		NPL	PL	HM	CF	6/60	6/36	6/12	6/9	6/6 or better
Upper $^1/_2$–$^2/_3$	7	–	–	–	1	–	–	1	2	3
Temporal	3	–	–	–	2	–	1	–	–	–
Inferior temporal	1	–	–	–	1	–	–	–	–	–
Diffuse	19	9	2	3	2	1	1	–	–	1

cases. BEGG *et al.* [31, 32] reported notching of the neuroretinal rim in patients with sectoral anterior ischemic optic neuropathy in chronic simple glaucoma, occurring some 2 to 3 months after the original hemorrhage had disappeared. DRANCE [130] commented that after the usual anterior ischemic optic neuropathy, the optic nerve atrophies but rarely cups. MILLER [390] mentioned cupping of the optic disc without exception in anterior ischemic optic neuropathy due to temporal arteritis, but gave no other details.

In the present series, optic discs were cupped in 13 eyes (Figs. 14h, i, 15f, 16f, j, 17h, 26a, b, 27m). Cupping usually developed about 2 to 3 months after the onset of anterior ischemic neuropathy, sometimes in as little as six weeks. The cupping progressed rapidly so that after 3 to 4 months it was maximum; thereafter it increased only minimally in eyes followed for up to 12 to 20 months (Figs. 16f, i).

Cupping of the optic disc was correlated with:

Intraocular Pressure. In all the eyes, intraocular pressure was within normal limits (less than 20 mm-Hg on applanation tonometry) and was no higher than in those with no cupping.

Temporal Arteritis. When anterior ischemic optic neuropathy was due to temporal arteritis (i.e., positive temporal artery biopsy for temporal arteritis), the optic disc was cupped to a variable degree (Figs. 14h, i, 15f, 16f, j, 17h, 26a, b, 27m) in 80 percent of the eyes; in the remaining 20 percent, optic atrophy was present (visual acuity was no perception of light in two and counting fingers in one) but lens opacities interfered with satisfactory evaluation of the disc. In contrast, when anterior ischemic optic neuropathy was *not* due to temporal arteritis, cupping was seen in only 12.5 percent (Table 8) of the patients and was comparatively milder than in patients with temporal arteritis.

Size of Physiologic Cup in Contralateral Normal Eye. These measurements were undertaken to rule out (a) pre-existing cupping due to so-called burnt-out high pressure glaucoma of a congenital nature, and (b) the possibility that a big physi-

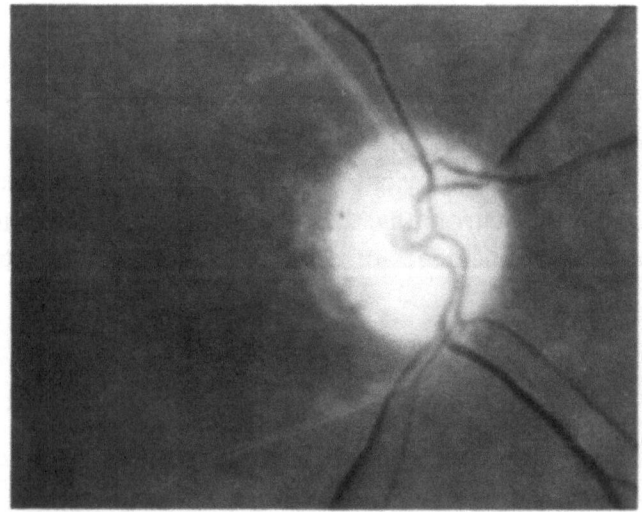
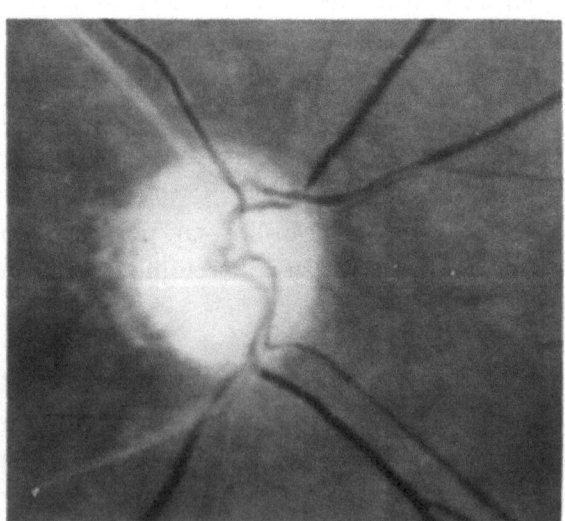

Fig. 26a–c. Both eyes of a 72-year-old woman with bilateral loss of vision (No perception of light in right eye and hand motion in left eye) 9 months previously, with temporal arteritis.

a, b) *Stereoscopic fundus photographs* showing pale, atrophic and cupped optic discs in right (a) and left (b) eyes, with sheathing of right retinal arteries.

c) *Fundus photograph* of right eye showing multiple chorioretinal degenerative patches. These were also seen in the left eye

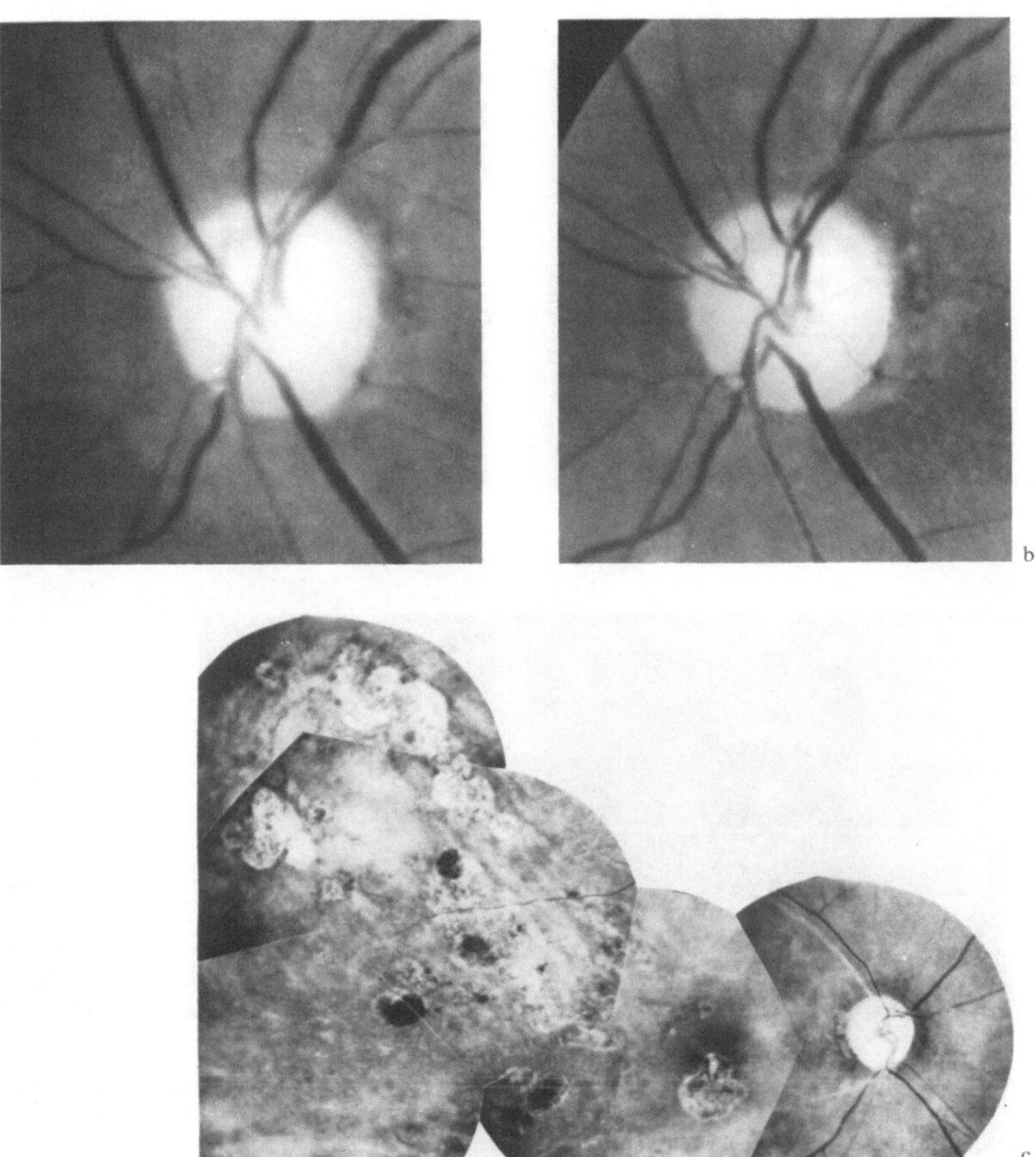

Fig. 26 (continued)

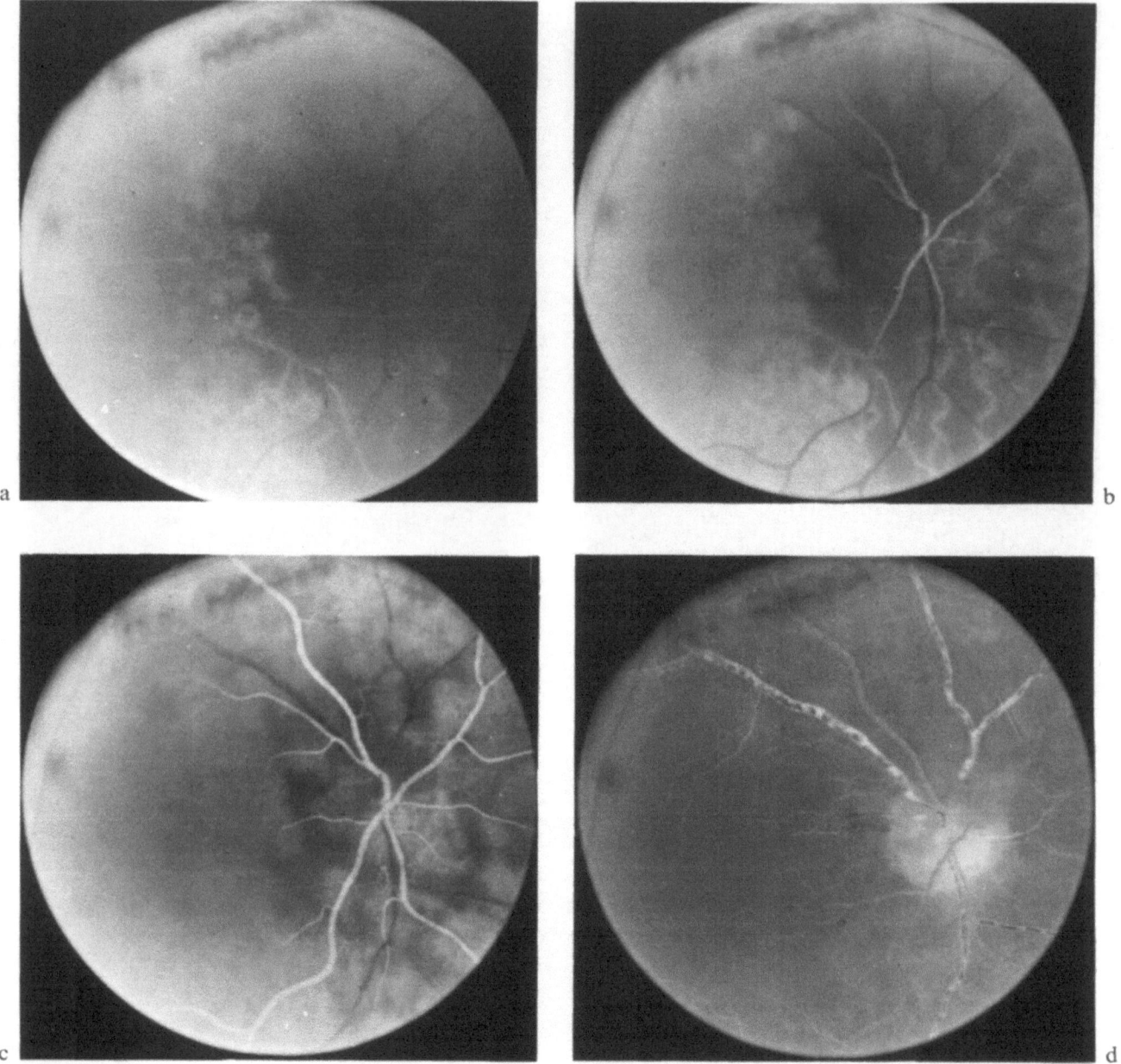

Fig. 27 a–m. Right eye of a 72$^1/_2$-year-old man with temporal arteritis, right partial anterior ischemic optic neuropathy, visual acuity of perception of light in upper nasal part and central retinal artery occlusion.

a, b, c, d) *Fluorescein angiograms:* 3 days after onset of deterioration of vision.

a) shows adequate filling of the temporal choroid (in the region of the lateral posterior ciliary artery distribution) except in the peripapillary choroid. There is no filling of the optic disc, peripapillary choroid, nasal choroid (in the region of the medial posterior ciliary artery distribution) and central retinal artery.

b) Shows start of filling of the central retinal artery and medial posterior ciliary artery almost simultaneously and sluggishly 4–5 seconds after (a).

c) 10 seconds after (b) showing no filling of upper two-thirds of the optic disc and adjacent peripapillary choroid. Rest of the peripapillary choroid shows sparse and patchy filling. Sludging of fluorescein is seen in the retinal arterioles, with no filling of the retinal veins.

d) *Late phase* shows sludging of circulation in the retinal veins and fluorescein staining of lower half of the optic disc.

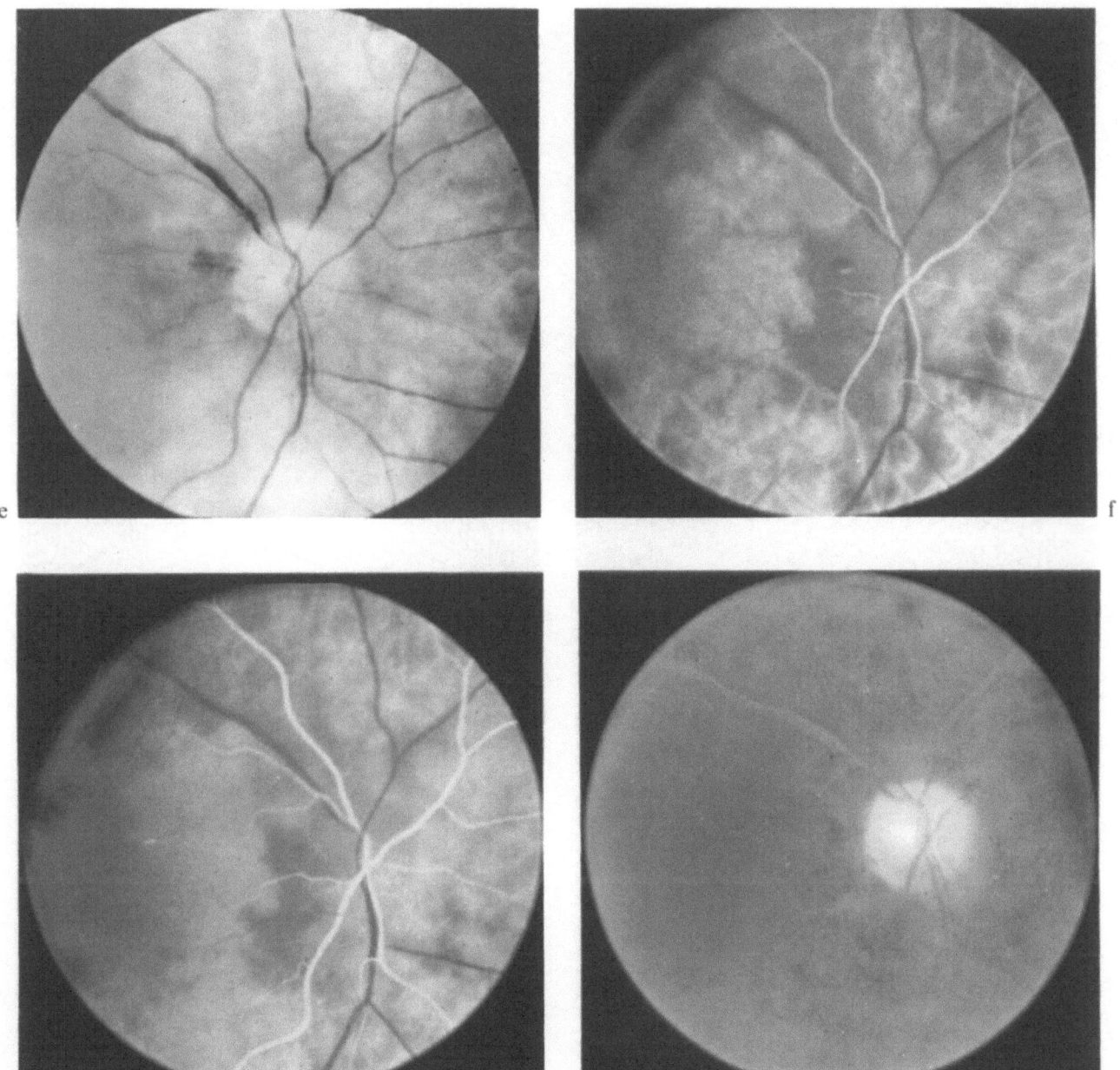

Fig. 27 (continued)

e, f, g, h) Six days after the onset.

e) *Fundus photograph* shows pallor of upper two-thirds of the disc and slight blurring of the upper margin with no significant edema of the disc. Retinal vessels show sludging of blood which is less than seen in (d).

f) Shows filling of the central retinal artery, choroid (temporal choroid better than nasal choroid), and lower third of the optic disc; with no filling of the superior watershed zone in the choroid, temporal and superior peripapillary choroid and upper two-thirds of the disc; and poor filling of the lower watershed zone of the choroid.

g) $3^{1}/_{2}$ seconds after (f), shows filling of the central retinal artery, temporal choroid (supplied by the lateral posterior ciliary artery) except for the temporal peripapillary choroid, slightly patchy filling of the nasal choroid (supplied by the medial posterior ciliary artery); and no filling of the upper two-thirds of the optic disc, superior and temporal peripapillary choroid and superior watershed zone of the choroid. Superior watershed zone and peripapillary choroid took 20 seconds to fill. Retinal circulation still very sluggish.

h) *Late phase* shows fluorescein staining of the optic disc—less in lower third than upper two-thirds, with slightly blurred margins.

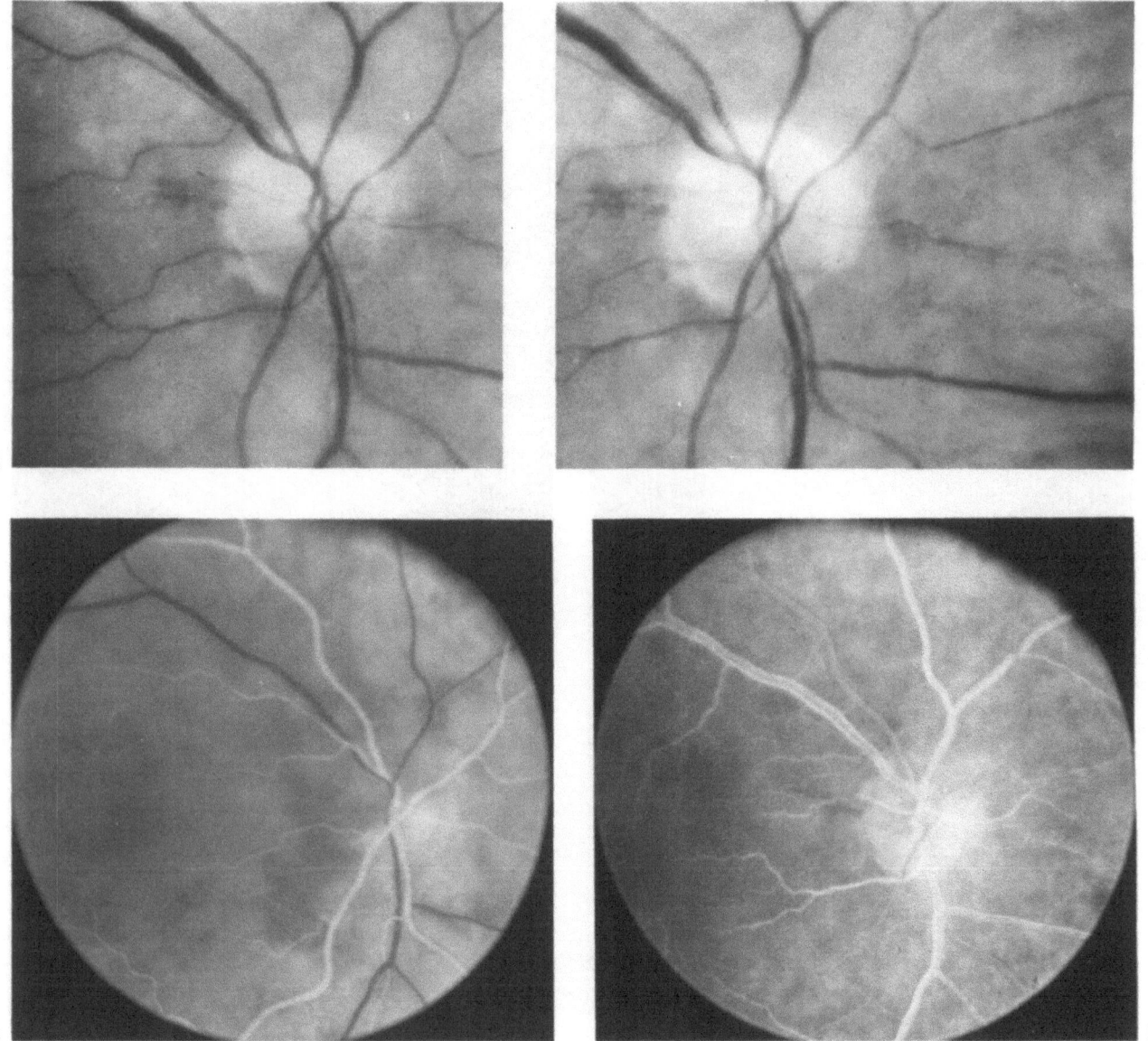

Fig. 27 (continued)

i, j, k) 11 days after onset.

i) *Stereoscopic fundus photographs* show pale upper two-thirds and normal looking lower third of the optic disc, with no sludging of blood in the retinal vessels. A small temporal retinal hemorrhage is seen near the margin of the disc.

j and k) *Fluorescein fundus angiograms* show a much improved retinal, nasal choroidal and optic disc circulation as compared to the above angiograms. However, filling defect in the temporal and superior peripapillary choroid, and superior watershed zone of the choroid still persist till late. Upper two-thirds of the optic disc shows poor filling. Retinal circulation still slow though better than before. (j)—retinal arterial phase and (k) venous phase.

l) 25 days after onset. *Fluorescein fundus angiogram* during late phase shows more staining of the upper two-thirds of the optic disc, i.e., the ischemic part and less of the normal third with well-defined margins (compare with d and h).

m) One year after onset. *Stereoscopic fundus photographs* showing pallor of upper part of the optic disc with cupping, particularly of superior nasal part

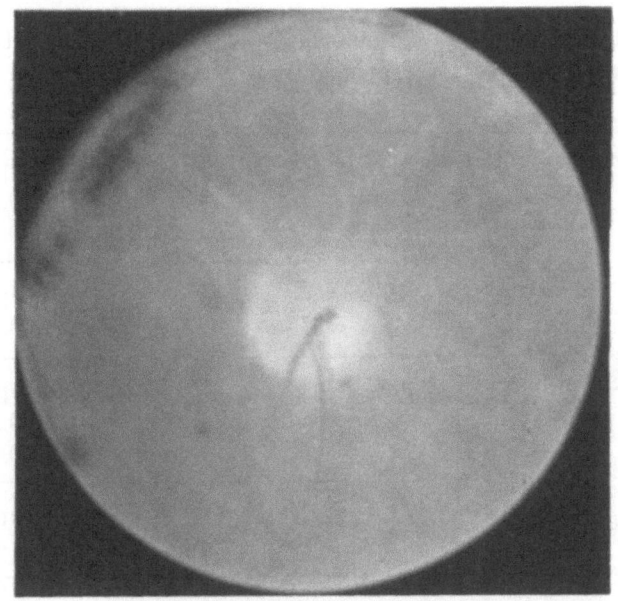

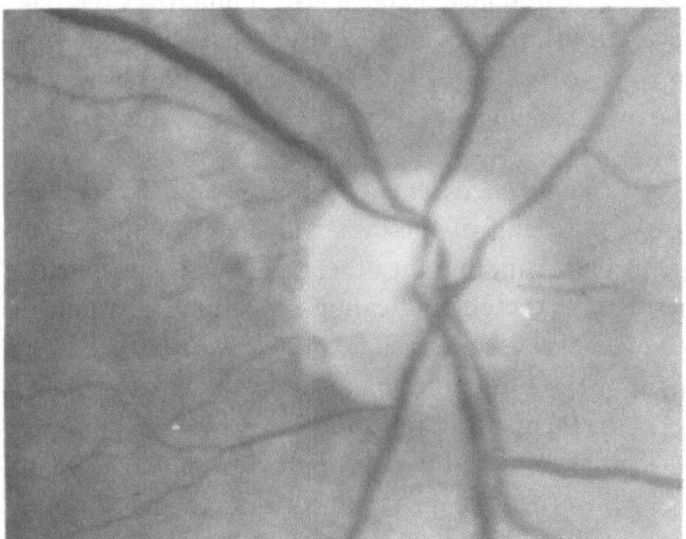

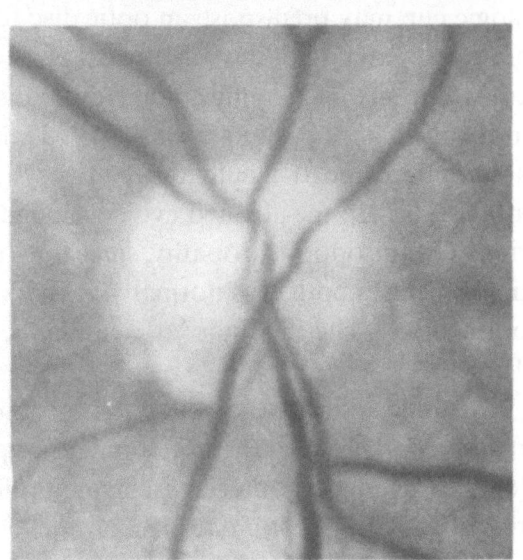

Fig. 27 (continued)

Table 8. Correlation of optic atrophy, cupping of the optic disc, temporal arteritis and final visual acuity

Optic atrophy	No. of eyes	Cupping of optic disc	Temporal arteritis present	Temporal arteritis absent	Final visual acuity								
					NPL	PL	HM	CF	6/60	6/36	6/12	6/9	6/6
Diffuse	10	Present	9	1[a]	8[b]	0	1	0	1	0	0	0	0
	7	Absent	0	7	0	0	2	1	0	2	0	0	2
Sectoral	3	Present[c]	2	1	0	0	0	2[d]	0	0	0	1	0
	7	Absent	0	7	0	0	0	3	0	0	1	0	3

[a] This eye had a very shallow saucer-shaped cupping as compared to the other eyes with cupping.

[b] In one of these, optic atrophy was more marked in the temporal than the nasal part, and so was the cupping.

[c] Atrophy and cupping involved upper $1/2$–$2/3$ of the optic disc in two eyes.

[d] One eye also had central retinal artery occlusion.

Table 9. Correlation of pathological cup size of physiological cup in the contralateral normal eye

Type of optic atrophy	Pathological cupping	No. of eyes	Size of physiological cup in normal fellow eye	Bilateral involvement
Diffuse	Present	10	No cup seen = 3 eyes C/D 0.2 = 2 eyes C/D 0.3 = 1 eye	4 eyes of 2 patients
	Absent	7	No cup seen = 3 eyes C/D 0.5 = 1 eye	3 eyes of 2 patients*
Sectoral	Present	3	No cup seen = 3 eyes C/D 0.2 = 1 eye C/D 0.3 = 1 eye	Nil
	Absent	7	No cup seen = 6 eyes	One eye of patient marked* above

ologic cup may predispose an optic disc to cupping, compared to discs with normal physiologic cups. The size of the physiologic optic disc cup in the normal opposite eye was studied with the assumption that it would reflect the "state of affairs" before the affected eye developed anterior ischemic optic neuropathy, since for all practical purposes both eyes normally have identical optic discs. The findings are summarized in Table 9.

The data indicate that there is no significant relationship between the development of pathologic cupping after anterior ischemic optic neuropathy and the original size of the cup, as judged from the opposite normal eye. In fact, in two eyes with maximum generalized cupping, the normal eye showed no physiologic cup; similarly when the normal eye had the largest cup of the series (i.e., C/D 0.5), the opposite affected eye showed no pathologic cupping. All eyes either did not have a physiologic cup or the size of the cup was within normal limits; in no case was a large cup found in the opposite eye.

Type of Optic Atrophy. Table 8 summarizes the findings. The data indicate that the incidence of optic disc cupping with diffuse optic atrophy is much higher than with sectoral atrophy. This higher incidence may be related to the higher incidence of temporal arteritis in diffuse optic atrophy.

Visual Acuity. Table 8 also summarizes the relationship between final visual acuity and cupping. The data show that visual acuity decreases with increasing cupping.

Hemorrhages on the Optic Disc and near its Margins. Half of the eyes with hemorrhages developed cupping; the other half showed no evidence of it, thereby indicating no definite relationship between hemorrhage and cupping. BEGG *et al.* [31] on the other hand, used these hemorrhages as their sole criterion of the presence of anterior ischemic optic neuropathy in glaucoma and recorded the development of notching of the involved neuroretinal rim.

Pathogenesis of cupping of the optic disc is discussed on p.74.

2. Retinal Changes

In the present study, in about half of the eyes a variable number of small superficial flame-shaped retinal hemorrhages were seen at the margins of the optic disc, sometimes extending to the adjacent retina (Figs. 14d, 18a, 20a, 21a, 22a, 25a, 27e). Congestion of the radial peripapillary capillaries was seen occasionally, but was in no way as frequent or extensive as that seen in optic disc edema of intracranial hypertension. In marked cases, the retina near the margin of the optic disc showed patchy edema and haziness, partially or completely masking the retinal vessels in the localized area (Figs. 14a, 15a, 17d, 21a, 24a). The nerve fiber layer over the optic disc usually was transparent though somewhat edematous. Rarely, a small cotton-wool spot was near the margin of the optic disc. Whenever a cilioretinal artery was present, a localized area of retinal edema (infarction) in the region of supply of the artery was seen (Figs. 10, 17a, d); this has also been found by other authors [111, 185, 498, 500]. Since anterior ischemic neuropathy is due to occlusion of the posterior ciliary arteries, a cilioretinal artery will also be occluded. Such retinal infarcts were described by CULLEN [108] (in his Fig. 1) as "exudates" in anterior ischemic optic neuropathy due to temporal arteritis.

3. Retinal Vascular Changes

Arteriosclerosis, often marked in the retinal arteries, is a common finding in these elderly patients, but is not necessarily indicative of pathologic change. In some cases of the present series it was interesting to observe that arteriosclerotic changes were significantly more advanced in the eye with anterior ischemic optic neuropathy than in the other normal eye. Three patients showed evidence of associated retinal arterial occlusion—a big cilioretinal artery supplying the upper half of the retina (Fig. 17) in one patient, the central retinal artery associated with sectoral involvement of the optic disc by anterior ischemic optic neuropathy (Fig. 27) in a second patient, and an old central retinal artery occlusion was seen in the electroretinogram of the third patient who was seen a few weeks after the onset of anterior ischemic optic neuropathy (Fig. 26a). A localized retinal infarction was seen in the distribution of a small cilioretinal artery in both eyes of another patient (not included in this series) after bilateral anterior ischemic optic neuropathy developed (Fig. 10) [245, 246]. Occlusion of the central retinal artery in temporal arteritis has been reported by other

workers as well [70, 79, 89, 106, 107, 152, 220, 382, 384, 417, 460, 500, 552]. Some authors reported occlusion of a branch of the retinal artery [106, 107, 467] but the description suggested that the vessel involved was most probably a cilioretinal artery and not a branch of the central retinal artery.

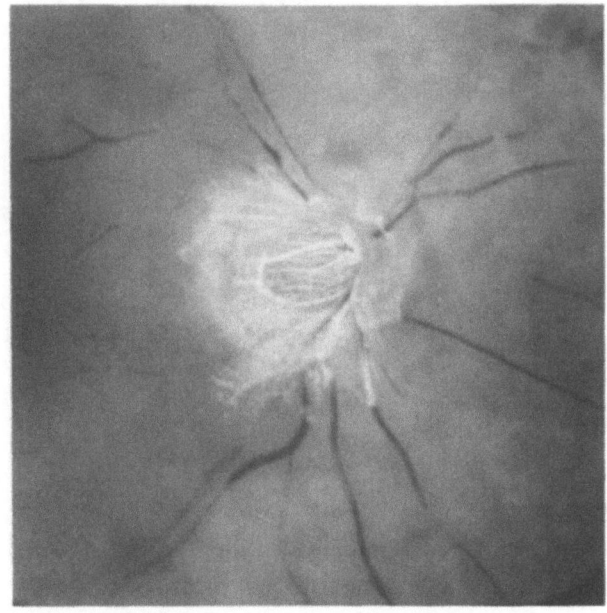

Fig. 28. *Fluorescein fundus angiogram* of a 68-year-old man (with temporal arteritis) two days after onset of central retinal artery occlusion, showing complete filling of the choroid and the blood vessels in the optic disc, without any filling of the central retinal artery

No doubt the central retinal artery can be involved by temporal arteritis independently of anterior ischemic optic neuropathy, and I have seen such cases (Figs. 28, 29). However, occlusion of the central retinal artery in temporal arteritis can be part of the anterior ischemic optic neuropathy process in many cases, and the latter has been missed in the past on simple ophthalmoscopic examination. Central retinal artery occlusion with anterior ischemic optic neuropathy can be explained if one considers the origins of the central retinal artery.

In my studies [502] I found that the central artery of the retina and the medial posterior ciliary artery arise by one common trunk from the ophthalmic artery in 40.4 percent, and divide into the central retinal artery and medial posteri-

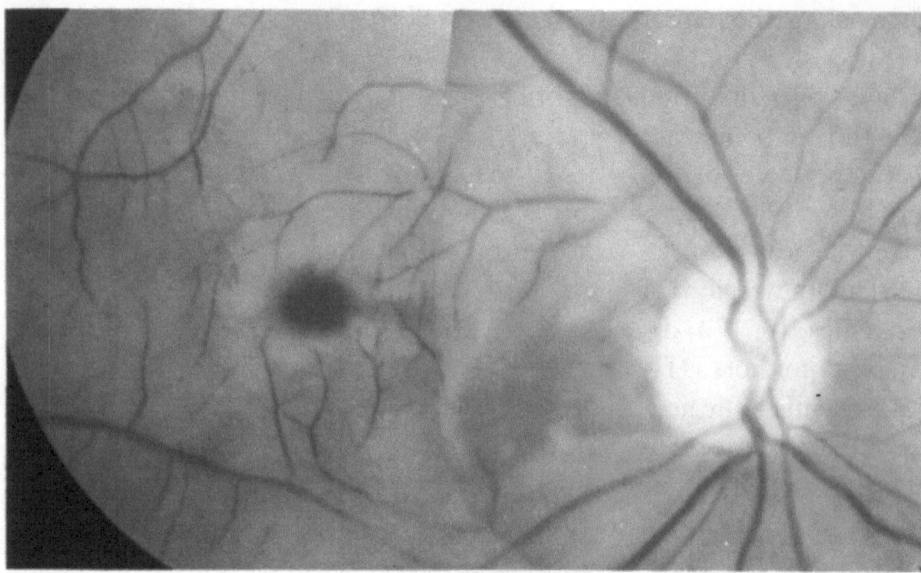

Fig. 29. *Fundus photograph* of left eye of a 68-year-old woman (with temporal arteritis and bilateral central retinal artery occlusion) showing retinal edema except in the area of a patent cilioretinal artery, and cherry-red spot at the fovea

or ciliary artery at some distance from the ophthalmic artery (Fig. 7). Similarly, the central retinal artery may arise in common with the lateral posterior ciliary artery (in 12.5 percent) or with the medial posterior ciliary artery + the lateral posterior ciliary artery (in 6.7 percent). If the occlusion takes place in the common trunk near its origin from the ophthalmic artery, it will occlude both the central retinal artery and one or both posterior ciliary arteries. Thus, central retinal artery occlusion can be seen in anterior ischemic optic neuropathy. The fact that anterior ischemic optic neuropathy is not as commonly associated with central retinal artery occlusion, as suggested by the origin of these arteries, would indicate:

1. The lesion occluding the posterior ciliary arteries involves the arteries at some distance from their origin and is not an extension of the process from the ophthalmic artery. Thus, the posterior ciliary arteries may be selectively vulnerable to involvement in temporal arteritis and in the arteriosclerotic process, factors not shared to the same extent by the central retinal artery. That arteriosclerotic changes may be more marked in the eye with anterior ischemic optic neuropathy than in the opposite eye (as men-

tioned above), would indicate that the central retinal artery is also equally or only slightly less involved by these changes than the posterior ciliary artery.

2. The other important factor that may be responsible for the more frequent occlusion of the circulation in the distribution of the posterior ciliary arteries (and hence the production of anterior ischemic optic neuropathy) compared to the central retinal artery is as follows: when the perfusion pressure in the intraocular arteries falls and an imbalance occurs between intraocular and perfusion pressures, the intraocular distribution of the posterior ciliary arteries, particularly that to the optic nerve head and peripapillary choroid, is much more susceptible to obliteration than is the central retinal artery [250, 264]. This finding has been well demonstrated in patients with anterior ischemic optic neuropathy (p. 72) and indicates that complete occlusion of the posterior ciliary arteries is not essential to the production of anterior ischemic optic neuropathy (as discussed on p. 21). With partial occlusion of the parent trunk of both the posterior ciliary artery and central retinal artery and a fall in diastolic perfusion pressure to below intraocular pressure, anterior ischemic optic neuropathy can

be produced while the retinal circulation may still be intact. Thus, elderly patients with central retinal artery occlusion and pale-looking optic discs should be investigated for temporal arteritis (by erythrocyte sedimentation rate and by intravenous fluorescein angiography). Angiography will show normal filling of small vessels in the optic disc in patients with central retinal artery occlusion unassociated with posterior ciliary artery occlusion (Fig. 28), and no filling of the disc, peripapillary choroid and central retinal artery in anterior ischemic optic neuropathy with central retinal artery occlusion (Fig. 27a). This precaution will prevent anterior ischemic optic neuropathy from developing in the other eye if temporal arteritis is detected early and treated with corticosteroids. Even if central retinal artery occlusion is not associated with anterior ischemic optic neuropathy and is due to temporal arteritis, detecting the arteritis (so that intensive corticosteroid therapy is started early) can prevent involvement of the other eye. For instance, the patient (not included in the present series) whose eye is seen in Fig. 29 (with central retinal artery occlusion), had lost the sight of her right eye four weeks previously due to occlusion of the central retinal artery and possible anterior ischemic optic neuropathy, but temporal arteritis was not suspected until both eyes were blind. Such tragedies can be avoided by investigating every patient over 60 years of age, who is suffering from central retinal artery occlusion, for temporal arteritis.

4. Macular and Peripapillary Changes

Eyes with anterior ischemic optic neuropathy frequently show a variable degree of senile macular degenerative change compatible with age. Similarly, a variable degree of peripapillary degenerative halo—complete or partial—is not rare. During the first 2 to 3 weeks after the onset of acute anterior ischemic optic neuropathy, a whitish lesion continuous with the infarct of the optic nerve head is seen to involve the peripapillary region for a variable distance (Figs. 14a, d, 15a, 16a, 17a, d, 18a, 19a, 24a, i, 25a). In

all probability, this is infarcted pigment epithelium caused by ischemia of underlying peripapillary choroid. Ophthalmoscopically and histopathologically, we have demonstrated similar whitish lesions, caused by ischemic necrosis of the pigment epithelium and outer layers of the overlying retina, in other parts of the fundus in rhesus monkeys when the posterior ciliary arteries were occluded experimentally [253, 260]. Like these experimental lesions, the peripapillary whitish lesion later resolves, leaving a variable amount of chorioretinal degeneration of the involved area (Figs. 16f, j, 17h).

5. Peripheral Chorioretinal Degenerative Patches

In patients with ischemic optic neuropathy, the peripheral part of the fundus may show patches of chorioretinal degeneration. These were seen in 30 percent of the eyes in this series, and the most extensive example is shown in Fig. 26c. The size, shape, and distribution of the patches varied considerably.

Of nine eyes with such patches, 5 could not perceive light, there was nasal hemianopia, with the border passing through the blind spot in one (Fig. 30b) (the patches were only on the temporal part of the fundus, i.e., the region with lateral posterior ciliary artery occlusion), visual acuity was limited to hand motion to counting fingers in two, and in one to $6/12$. We have demonstrated development and evolution of such patches ophthalmoscopically and histopathologically in experimental posterior ciliary artery occlusion in rhesus monkeys [204, 207]. If occlusion of the posterior ciliary artery produces chorioretinal degenerative patches, the question must be asked: Why are these seen in only 30 percent of the eyes with anterior ischemic optic neuropathy when anterior ischemic optic neuropathy is due to occlusion of the posterior ciliary arteries? The rarity of chorioretinal lesions can be explained by the fact that in almost all patients with anterior ischemic optic neuropathy intravenous fluorescein angiography showed some choroidal circulation from posteri-

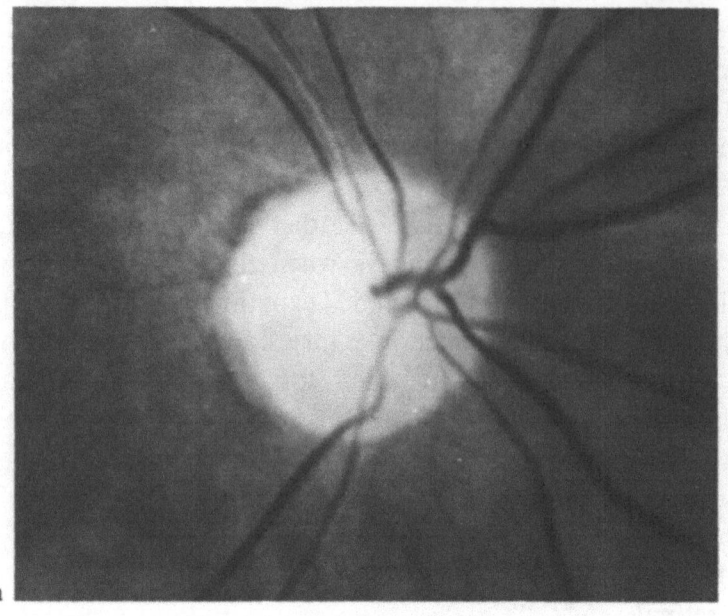

a

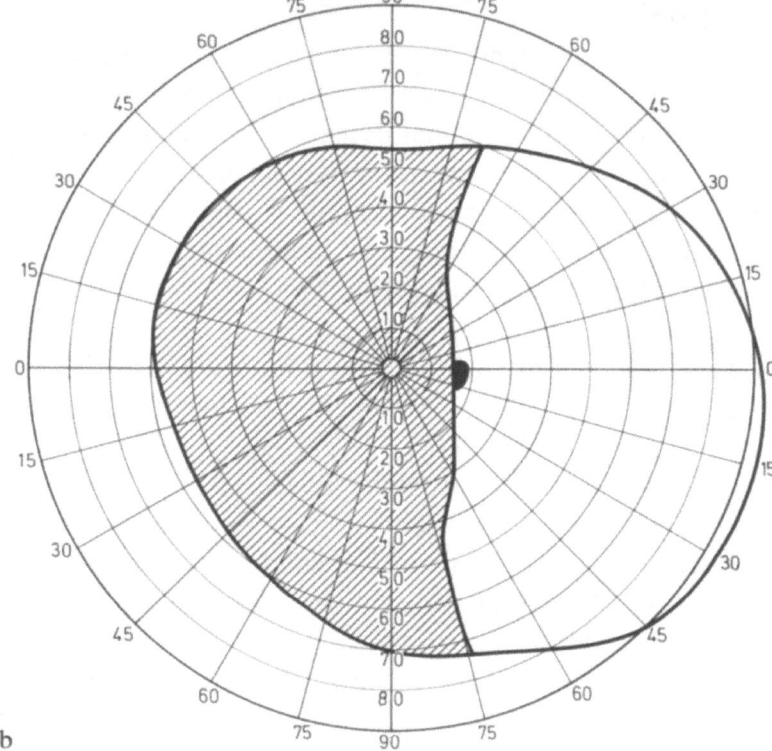

b

Fig. 30a and b. A 67-year-old woman had developed a sudden loss of central vision in the right eye one afternoon 18 months before, which had since remained unaltered. Visual acuity in that eye now counting fingers, in the temporal field; (a) the right optic disc shows atrophy of the temporal half with a normal nasal half and the retinal vessels show a generalized narrowing. (b) The visual fields showed a nasal hemianopia with the border of the hemianopic defect passing through the blind spot. The patient was unaware of this right nasal hemianopia. The left eye was normal

or ciliary arteries by the venous phase of the retinal circulation (e.g., Fig. 16d) even though the peripapillary choroid and optic disc did not fill with dye (Figs. 16b, c, d). Thus, in these cases, the optic disc suffers most, while the poor and delayed circulation in the rest of the choroid is sufficient to prevent the classic fundus lesions seen during experimental complete occlusion of the posterior ciliary arteries. In our studies we found that the pigment epithelium survived, even

in the presence of poor choroidal circulation [253, 260]. In almost all anterior ischemic optic neuropathies, the presence of some choroidal circulation, however poor and delayed, seems to suggest that (a) the main posterior ciliary arteries are markedly narrowed but not completely occluded, or (b) circulation in the occluded posterior ciliary arteries reestablishes itself very quickly. That such rapid restoration can occur is demonstrated by intravenous fluorescein angiography in these patients (p. 73) and in those with central retinal artery occlusion [248]. I think factor (a) is the more important and would be operative even in the presence of factor (b) because perfusion pressure in the posterior ciliary artery circulation would be significantly reduced, producing an imbalance between perfusion and intraocular pressure. Such an imbalance leads to defective perfusion and/or obliteration of vessels in the choroid and peripapillary choroid and depletes the posterior ciliary artery supply to the optic nerve head [264]. Susceptibility to obliteration of the vessels, un-

optic neuropathy and, consequently, the higher susceptibility to ischemia of the optic nerve head and retrolaminar part of the optic nerve compared with the choroid other than the peripapillary can be explained. Therefore complete obliteration of the posterior ciliary arteries is not necessary for the production of anterior ischemic optic neuropathy. This disorder can be produced by any sudden and prolonged reduction in perfusion pressure of the posterior ciliary arteries, to a level below intraocular pressure.

Thus, anterior ischemic optic neuropathy can exist in man without chorioretinal lesions of the type seen in our experimental occlusive studies of the posterior ciliary arteries [253, 260] because—

1. As discussed above, the choroidal circulation is much less susceptible to obliteration than is the peripapillary choroid and posterior ciliary circulation in the optic nerve head.

2. Neural tissue of the optic nerve is far more sensitive to anoxia than pigment epithelium; the latter can survive despite very poor circulation (suggested by our experimental studies [260]). No other fundus abnormality was detected.

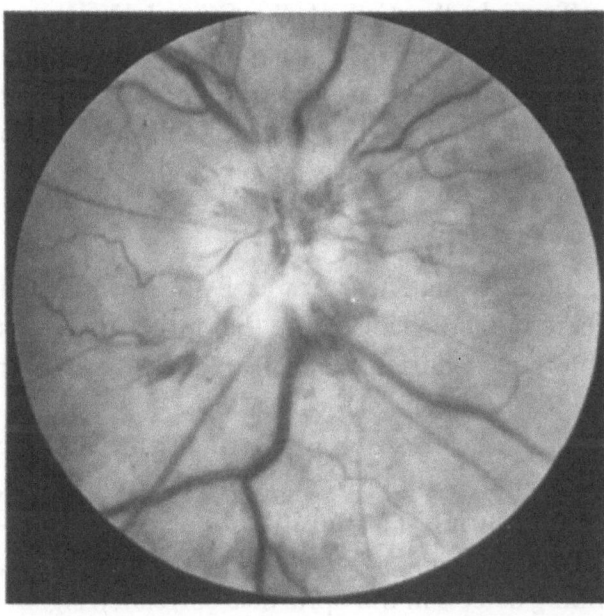

Fig. 31. Right eye of a 74-year-old man with sudden onset of inferior altitudinal hemianopia, superior sector anterior ischemic optic neuropathy, no temporal arteritis, and visual acuity 6/7.5. He had similar trouble in left eye 10 years previously and had residual left inferior altitudinal hemianopia and optic atrophy of upper half of the left disc. *Fundus photograph* of right eye 10 days after onset showing edema of the optic disc with hyperemia and superficial hemorrhages

Intravenous Fluorescein Fundus Angiography

So far, no detailed intravenous fluorescein study on anterior ischemic optic neuropathy is available. FOULDS [170] mentioned that intravenous fluorescein angiography showed incomplete filling of the capillaries in that part of the optic nerve head that corresponds to the visual field defect and may show capillary dilatation and abnormal permeability of disc vessels, with widespread leakage. BEGG et al. [30] showed filling defects or delayed filling in atrophic sectors of the optic disc after sectoral anterior ischemic optic neuropathy and slightly larger filling in the lamina cribrosa. SANDERS [471] described late choroidal filling of the peripapillary region and

der these circumstances is maximal in the optic disc, slightly less in the peripapillary choroid, and least in the rest of the choroid. Thus, nonfilling of the peripapillary choroid and optic disc, with poor and delayed filling of the choroid (Figs. 16b, c, d), in eyes with anterior ischemic disc or filling defects at the disc corresponding with the field defect, dilatation of the peripapillary plexus, and hyperfluorescence of the disc.

In the present study a detailed intravenous fluorescein angiographic study of eyes with anterior ischemic optic neuropathy was conducted. This revealed findings which have either not been mentioned previously or received scant attention in the literature. They not only add considerably to our knowledge of the pathogenesis and management of anterior ischemic optic neuropathy but also aid in its diagnosis.

The angiographic pattern varied not only in eyes in which anterior ischemic optic neuropathy involved the entire optic disc, as compared to those with only sectoral involvement of the disc, but with the time interval between the onset of anterior ischemic optic neuropathy and angiographic examination.

Angiography showed the following:

1. Optic Disc Changes

a) In Anterior Ischemic Optic Neuropathy Involving the Entire Optic Disc

During the First Week after the Onset of Anterior Ischemic Optic Neuropathy. Fluorescence of the optic disc was not seen during transit of the dye or during the late phases (Figs. 14b, c, e, f, 15b–d, 16b–e, 17b, c, e–g), although very occasionally very late staining may be seen (Fig. 14g).

During the Second Week. Although the optic disc did not fluoresce during transit of the dye, it usually stained with fluorescein during the late phases (Fig. 18b).

From the Third Week Onwards. The optic disc showed fluorescence during either the retinal-arterial or the arteriovenous phase and later showed staining with blurred margins (Fig. 20b).

After about Two Months. When the optic disc swelling subsided and optic atrophy was established, the optic disc usually showed no or very

faint fluorescence during the transit of dye and the late phases (Figs. 15e, 16g–i, 17i–l).

b) Sectoral Anterior Ischemic Optic Neuropathy

The normal part of the optic disc filled normally while the ischemic part either did not fill (Figs. 27a–d, f, g) or filled very late during the transit of dye (Figs. 21b–d, 23c, d, 24b–d, 25b, 27i, k), depending upon the age of the lesion. During the late phases, the pattern was as follows:

During the First Week. Usually only the normal part stained with fluorescein (Fig. 27d).

Towards the End of the Second Week and Thereafter. The ischemic part started to stain more than the normal part (Fig. 27h) and had a blurred border, with a transitional period when the whole disc stained equally well (Figs. 21e, 22c, 23e, 24e, l).

When Optic Atrophy was Established. When there was no edema, only the normal part was fluorescent during the transit of dye and later on (Figs. 22e, f, 24n, o) [251].

In eyes with sectoral anterior ischemic optic neuropathy, filling defects in the optic disc, shown during the transit of fluorescein, correlated significantly with visual field defects. Also, filling defects in the optic disc correlated significantly with those in the peripapillary choroid during the transit of dye, when seen during the first couple of weeks after onset; after that period, once choroidal circulation was restored, such correlation usually was not seen.

2. Choroidal Circulation

a) In Anterior Ischemic Optic Neuropathy Involving the Entire Optic Disc

During the First Week after the Onset of Anterior Ischemic Optic Neuropathy. There was markedly delayed and poor filling of the choroid by the posterior ciliary arteries (Figs. 14b, c, e, f, 15b, c, 16b–d). The earlier a patient was seen, the more marked the filling defect was; within a few hours after the onset of anterior ischemic optic neuropathy, practically no choroidal filling was detected during the retinal transit of dye (Figs. 14e, f). One posterior ciliary artery might fill before the other (Figs. 15b, 16c, 17e), but all filled slowly. The choroid filled either in the retinal venous phase or more commonly afterwards; only rarely did the posterior ciliary arteries start to fill during the retinal arteriovenous phase. Filling of the peripapillary choroid was delayed much more than the rest of the choroid—in fact, during the first three days it frequently did not show filling (Figs. 14e, f, 16a–d) or did not fill till the late retinal venous phase or even later (Figs. 14b, c, 15b, c, 17e, f). Filling of the choroid and peripapillary choroid, particularly of the latter, was frequently patchy; complete filling occurred very slowly. In some eyes filling of the choroid deteriorated towards the second half of the week, before it improved.

During the Second Week. The posterior ciliary artery circulation started to improve, usually slowly, so that choroidal and peripapillary filling could be seen in the late retinal arteriovenous phase. The improvement was slower in the peripapillary choroid than in the rest of the choroid; the filling there might not be completed until the retinal venous phase. This filling gradually improved with time, although the choroidal circulation might still not fill until the retinal arteriovenous phase (by the end of the third week).

Watershed areas between the lateral and medial posterior ciliary arteries were usually the last to fill. The superior watershed zone generally showed the filling defect more frequently and longer than did the inferior watershed zone (Fig. 17e).

b) In Sectoral Anterior Ischemic Optic Neuropathy

Angiography in some of these eyes showed a filling defect in the choroid and peripapillary choroid, which was localized to the sector corresponding to the location of the anterior ischemic optic neuropathy or which was more extensive. However, this was noticed in only a few of the eyes (Figs. 21b, c, 24b–d, j, n, 27a–c, f, g, j). After about 2 to 3 months choroidal circulation usually was restored to normal (Figs. 15e, 16h, 17i–k, 22e). Delayed filling persisted slightly longer in the peripapillary than in the rest of the choroid.

A choroidal filling defect during the transit of dye, when angiography was performed soon after the onset of anterior ischemic optic neuropathy, correlated significantly with ischemia of the optic disc. Once the choroidal circulation improved, this correlation disappeared. Choroidal circulation improved significantly within a week or even less, so that occlusion might escape detection if angiography were not performed within the first few days after onset. Optic disc ischemia and peripapillary choroid filling defects during the transit of dye correlated significantly during the initial stages of ischemic optic neuropathy. As peripapillary choroid filling improved, this correlation also disappeared. The peripapillary choroid filling defects lasted longer than did those in the choroid.

3. Retinal Circulation

Retinal circulation generally was perfectly normal on angiography but was involved in the following two eyes—

a) Cilioretinal Artery Occlusion

In a patient with right anterior ischemic optic neuropathy, the big cilioretinal artery, supplying the upper half of the retina was occluded; circulation in the central retinal artery supplying the lower half of the retina was normal (Figs. 17b, c). Filling of the cilioretinal artery and choroid had improved significantly by the fourth day (Figs. 17e, f) and was perfectly normal when the patient was seen 8 $1/2$ months later (Figs. 17i, j).

I have recently seen another similar patient

(not included in this series), in whom the cilioretinal artery supplied blood to the lower half of the retina. This patient developed anterior ischemic optic neuropathy of the lower half of the optic nerve head and retinal infarction of the lower half of the retina associated with a superior altitudinal field defect. The choroidal and cilioretinal artery circulation was normal when he was seen 27 days after the onset of anterior ischemic optic neuropathy. However "hibernation of the blood in the retina" [248] in the distribution of the cilioretinal artery was seen, i.e., the retinal arteriovenous phase was missing. In this patient, the anterior ischemic optic neuropathy was of an arteriosclerotic nature, while in the first patient it was due to temporal arteritis.

These studies indicate that the so-called *branch retinal arterial occlusion* described with anterior ischemic optic neuropathy by various authors is, in all probability, an occlusion of a cilioretinal artery.

b) Central Retinal Artery Occlusion

Anterior ischemic optic neuropathy involved the upper half of the right optic disc in a patient with temporal arteritis and was associated with central retinal artery occlusion (Fig. 27). Angiography on the third day after the onset of visual disorders showed normal filling of the lateral posterior ciliary artery in this eye (Fig. 27a). However, the onset of filling in both the medial posterior ciliary and central retinal artery was delayed by five seconds (Fig. 27b). Complete filling took more than one minute, with a retinal arteriovenous gap of 23 seconds (in the normal left eye of this patient the central retinal artery filled in 12 seconds, with a retinal arteriovenous gap of three seconds; Figs. 27c, d). With the passage of time circulation in both the central retinal and medial posterior ciliary artery improved (Figs. 27f, g, j, k). The mechanism of the involvement of the central retinal with the medial posterior ciliary artery in occlusive disorders has already been discussed (p. 68).

Within the first few days after the onset of ischemic optic neuropathy, the retinal venules

over the swollen optic disc sometimes showed fluorescein leakage (Figs. 15d, 16e, 17g) and some engorgement of the radial peripapillary capillaries.

These intravenous fluorescein angiography findings of the optic disc, choroid, and retina in anterior ischemic optic neuropathy do not bear any significant resemblance to the true edema of the optic disc as seen in intracranial hypertension and other conditions. Thus intravenous fluorescein angiography can help to differentiate anterior ischemic optic neuropathy from other types of optic disc swelling. As has been shown, the intravenous fluorescein angiographic pattern keeps changing as the time interval between onset of anterior ischemic optic neuropathy and examination changes. This finding should be borne in mind when interpreting these angiograms so as to prevent unnecessary confusion.

4. Chorioretinal Degenerative Lesion in Anterior Ischemic Optic Neuropathy

Fluorescein fundus angiography of the lesions shown in Fig. 26c revealed unmasking and masking of the choroidal fluorescence in the depigmented areas and pigmented spots respectively, without late staining of the lesion. In anterior ischemic optic neuropathy, I have not seen, so far, an acute chorioretinal ischemic lesion of the type we produced experimentally and studied by fluorescein fundus angiography [260].

Pathogenesis of Cupping of the Optic Disc

Optic disc cupping is a classic feature of chronic simple glaucoma. It was discovered on ophthalmoscopic examination over 120 years ago [214, 302, 304, 443] and was soon confirmed histopathologically by MÜLLER [402]. Cavernous degeneration of the optic nerve in glaucoma was noted by SCHNABEL [480]. In attempts to explain the pathogenesis of optic disc cupping, a very large volume of literature has since accumulated, but the mechanism is still far from clear. The presence of optic disc cupping with no rise in intraocular pressure, first described by VON GRAEFE [215], has further contributed to the confusion. A very high incidence of optic disc cupping has been seen in anterior ischemic optic neuropathy due to temporal arteritis (p. 59). The cupping is identical in all aspects to that seen in glaucoma and low-tension glaucoma. Thus, identical pathologic optic disc cupping occurs in glaucoma, low-tension glaucoma (pseudoglaucoma), and anterior ischemic optic neuropathy. Since anterior ischemic optic neuropathy is an acute process (with a much-telescoped natural history that results in marked cupping within 4 to 5 months after its onset), it has been possible to follow its entire natural history in patients with modern techniques (e.g., stereoscopic ophthalmoscopy, fluorescein fundus angiography and histopathology). Based on these clinical and experimental studies, I have tried to explain the pathogenesis of optic disc cupping in anterior ischemic optic neuropathy and, also presumably, in glaucoma and low-tension glaucoma. The three conditions represent an ischemic disorder of the anterior part of the optic nerve—anterior ischemic optic neuropathy being an acute process while the other two are chronic.

1. Review of Literature

It is impossible to review fully the colossal amount of literature on this subject. Hence an extremely brief review of some of the important views on the subject is given below.

The basic pathologic changes in optic disc cupping are atrophy of the nerve fibers and glial cells and ectasia of the optic disc. Various theories have been postulated to explain the pathogenesis of changes in the optic disc. These can be divided into the following three main groups:

The mechanical theory
The vascular theory
The cavernous degeneration theories.

a) The Mechanical Theory

Since raised intraocular pressure is the cardinal feature of ordinary glaucoma, it is natural that a mechanical explanation should have been the first to be advanced. This theory was first suggested by MÜLLER [402, 403] and subsequently supported by a large number of workers [45, 192, 311, 516, 517]. According to them, raised intraocular pressure produces herniation of the walls of the eyeball at its weakest spot (presumed to be the lamina cribrosa), causing ectasia of the optic disc. Atrophy of the nerve fibers represents pressure atrophy due to direct pressure on nerve fibers as well as on ganglion cells in the retina. The most important factor is considered to be loss of the normal plane of the lamina cribrosa, producing sharp kinking and compression of nerve fibers [509]. LAKER [333] and BIRNBACHER et al. [45] claimed to have produced optic disc cupping in dead eyes by raising intraocular pressure. NEUMANN et al. [408] reported repeated transient optic disc cupping by elevated intraocular pressure, which returned to normal when the pressure was lowered. Similar reversible cupping that returns to normal when intraocular pressure is reduced has been reported by VON GRAEFE [217], LANGE [337], SHAFFER et al. [492] and others. SHAFFER [491] and SHAFFER et al. [492] suggested that the cupping is due to atrophy of the astroglial tissue of the prelaminar region. SZYMANSKI et al. [522] reported the production of optic disc cupping by a sudden lowering of intracranial pressure. FUCHS [191, 192], based on histopathologic studies, postulated that the anterior glial fibers disappear first, and then the fibers in the lamina cribrosa. The connective tissue layers of the latter fibers bow backwards under the influence of raised intraocular pressure and become sclerosed at first, then thin and atrophic, and finally fragmented. He also stated that the nerve fibers undergo pressure atrophy at the same time.

b) The Vascular Theory

LAGRANGE et al. [332] considered optic disc cupping to be due to vascular interference in the optic disc secondary to raised intraocular pressure, the latter causing vascular obliteration and sclerosis, which produce neural atrophy. Reduction of the capillary network in the optic nerve head and resultant ischemia were considered responsible for cupping by ELSCHNIG [156], CHRISTINI [101, 102], FRANCOIS et al. [178, 179] and KALVIN et al. [310]. A large numer of workers, based on their clinical and/or experimental studies, have considered that visual field defects and changes in the optic nerve head in glaucoma are vasogenic in origin [9, 25, 41, 53–55, 101, 102, 128–130, 133–137, 139–143, 145, 156, 159, 160, 162, 171, 178, 179, 187, 194, 230, 234–236, 245, 246, 250, 262–264, 268, 310, 331, 346, 355, 365, 379, 380, 394, 409, 410, 452, 453, 455, 472, 504, 521, 537, 538, 559, 582].

Optic disc cupping without any rise in intraocular pressure has been observed commonly, since its first description by VON GRAEFE in 1857 [215]. This has naturally caused some workers to question the role played by raised intraocular pressure in the production of cupping. Hence some have postulated that optic disc cupping and associated changes are due to a vascular lesion within the nerve, and that raised intraocular pressure is coincidental [100, 101, 366, 367, 372, 452]. DALSGAARD-NIELSEN [114], SJÖGREN [504] and VAIL [545] described atherosclerotic occlusion of small nutrient arteries supplying the lamina cribrosa, as a cause of ischemic degeneration and disintegration of the nerve fibers without proliferative gliosis. This is said to lead to backward displacement of the lamina cribrosa, with pallor and optic disc cupping. NIEDERMEIER [409] believed the vascular changes in the lamina cribrosa were trophic in origin. DEWECKER [558] stated that nutritional disturbances of the disc decrease its resistance to normal intraocular pressure so that it yields to the pressure. DUKE-ELDER [139–143, 145] considered that the changes in the optic nerve head and visual fields depend upon a relative vascular insufficiency that varies with the ratio between intraocular and capillary pressure. DUKE-ELDER's view has been supported by recent studies as a valid explanation of changes in the optic disc and visual fields in glaucoma and low-tension glaucoma [30, 32, 130, 133, 134, 171, 250, 264, 268, 331].

GAFNER and GOLDMANN [194], GOLDMANN [205], NORDMANN [411] and BECKER and SHAFFER [27] postulated that raised intraocular pressure shunted blood away from the optic nerve head, leading to degeneration of neural tissue.

The vascular basis for involvement of the retrolaminar optic nerve is discussed with cavernous degeneration below.

Recent studies have helped to localize the vascular disturbance in these cases primarily to the posterior ciliary artery circulation [41, 53–55, 159, 245–247, 250, 262–264, 331, 521].

c) The Cavernous Degeneration Theories

Cavernous degeneration of the optic nerve in glaucoma was first described by SCHNABEL [480–482], who considered cupping to be secondary to degeneration of nerve fibers resulting from cavernous degeneration, which, he claimed, preceded cupping. Proliferation of interstitial connective tissue and its contraction pulls back the lamina cribrosa. SCHNABEL mentioned that cavernous degeneration in the lamina cribrosa region produces spaces that coalesce to form one large cavity, exposing the lamina cribrosa itself and resulting in glaucomatous cupping. This view was supported by ELSCHNIG [154, 156], HÜMMELSTEIN et al. [292], SCHNAUDIGEL [483], EVANS [162], WOLFF [572] and a host of others. ELSCHNIG [155], like SCHNABEL, attributed cavernous degeneration in glaucoma to solution of the nerve fibers and optic nerve framework by the abnormal lytic action of intraocular fluid as it passes backwards through the optic nerve. TENG [525] postulated that glaucomatous optic disc cupping is due mainly to degeneration and the disappearance of collagen and optic nerve fibers, produced by the action of vitreous on these tissues. The vitreous enters the optic nerve through congenital or acquired breaks in the surface of the optic disc. TENG stated that raised intraocular pressure did not play a role in optic disc cupping and cavernous degeneration.

LOEWENSTEIN [359] disagreed with the views of ELSCHNIG [155], because cavernous degeneration is located some distance from the lamina cribrosa. He also ruled out the view that degeneration was due to ascending degeneration of the optic nerve, caused by glaucoma, for the same reasons.

Circulatory disturbances as the possible cause of cavernous degeneration have been suggested by a large number of workers [19, 142, 168, 202, 245, 246, 278, 332, 359, 365, 371, 394, 451, 545, 559, 572]. BAILLIART [19] concluded that incomplete occlusion of the central retinal artery causes ischemia and cavernous degeneration. LOEWENSTEIN et al. [360] described cavernous degeneration as due to vascular damage rather than to raised intraocular pressure. PICKARD [434] thought cavernous degeneration was a distinct entity, with only a casual association with glaucoma. He postulated [435] that cavernous degeneration is the result of changes in the circle of Zinn and Haller, because the optic nerve head is supplied only by this structure. WOLFF [572] pointed out that cavernous degeneration classically occurs in any organ in which the blood supply is gradually cut off. Highly differentiated tissue degenerates and disappears before supporting tissue because its requirement for blood is high. Similarly, in the optic nerve empty spaces are formed by the disappearance of nerve fibers, while the glial network and septa remain unchanged. There is no reactionary gliosis or scar tissue formation because of ischemia. Similar views had been expressed by GRADLE [213]. WOLFF [572] was of the opinion that chronic glaucoma cannot produce such a picture. The presence of cavernous degeneration also has been observed in high myopia [17, 413, 516].

Various locations have been cited in the literature for cavernous degeneration: Most marked in the region of the lamina cribrosa (SCHNABEL); some distance from the lamina cribrosa [359]; between and behind the connective tissue layers of the lamina cribrosa [572]; the pre- and retrolaminar regions of the optic nerve, even extending into the brain along the nerve [156]; in the optic nerve head and retrolaminar region [213], and in that part of the optic nerve containing central retinal vessels [155, 202, 213].

ZIMMERMAN [581], in histopathologic examinations of eyes with continuously elevated intraocular pressure, found after six days marked edema of the optic disc, which started to subside one week after onset, with hydropic degeneration in the nerve fibers anterior to the lamina cribrosa and demyelination posterior to the lamina cribrosa. Two weeks after onset, deep optic disc cupping was seen with cavernous degeneration. Spaces were filled with acid mucopolysaccharide, a finding that was more marked two months after onset. These findings were confirmed in experimental studies of raised intraocular pressure in owl monkeys by the same group [230, 310, 334, 582]. They considered the changes to result from ischemic necrosis secondary to raised intraocular pressure. In their India-ink injection studies, HAMASAKI et al. [230] showed nonfilling of vessels in the optic nerve head and in the optic nerve 3 to 4 mm behind the lamina cribrosa. ZIMMERMAN et al. [582] and LAMPERT et al. [334] mentioned that in cavernous degeneration due to ischemic infarct no hyaluronic acid was found in the spaces*, whereas these spaces contained hyaluronic acid in cavernous degeneration of experimental glaucoma. They postulated that the cavernous degeneration in acute glaucoma was a special type, presumably with hyaluronic acid forced from the vitreous into the ischemic infarct in the optic nerve.

2. Recent Studies

In our understanding of the pathogenesis of optic disc cupping, particularly in anterior ischemic optic neuropathy, also in glaucoma and low-tension glaucoma, the following have provided important information:

---

* Presence of acid mucopolysaccharide in cavernous degeneration spaces in anterior ischemic optic neuropathy has recently been demonstrated (HINZPETER, E.N.—European Ophthalmic Pathology Society Meeting 1974, Toulouse, France—Figs. 13d, e, f).

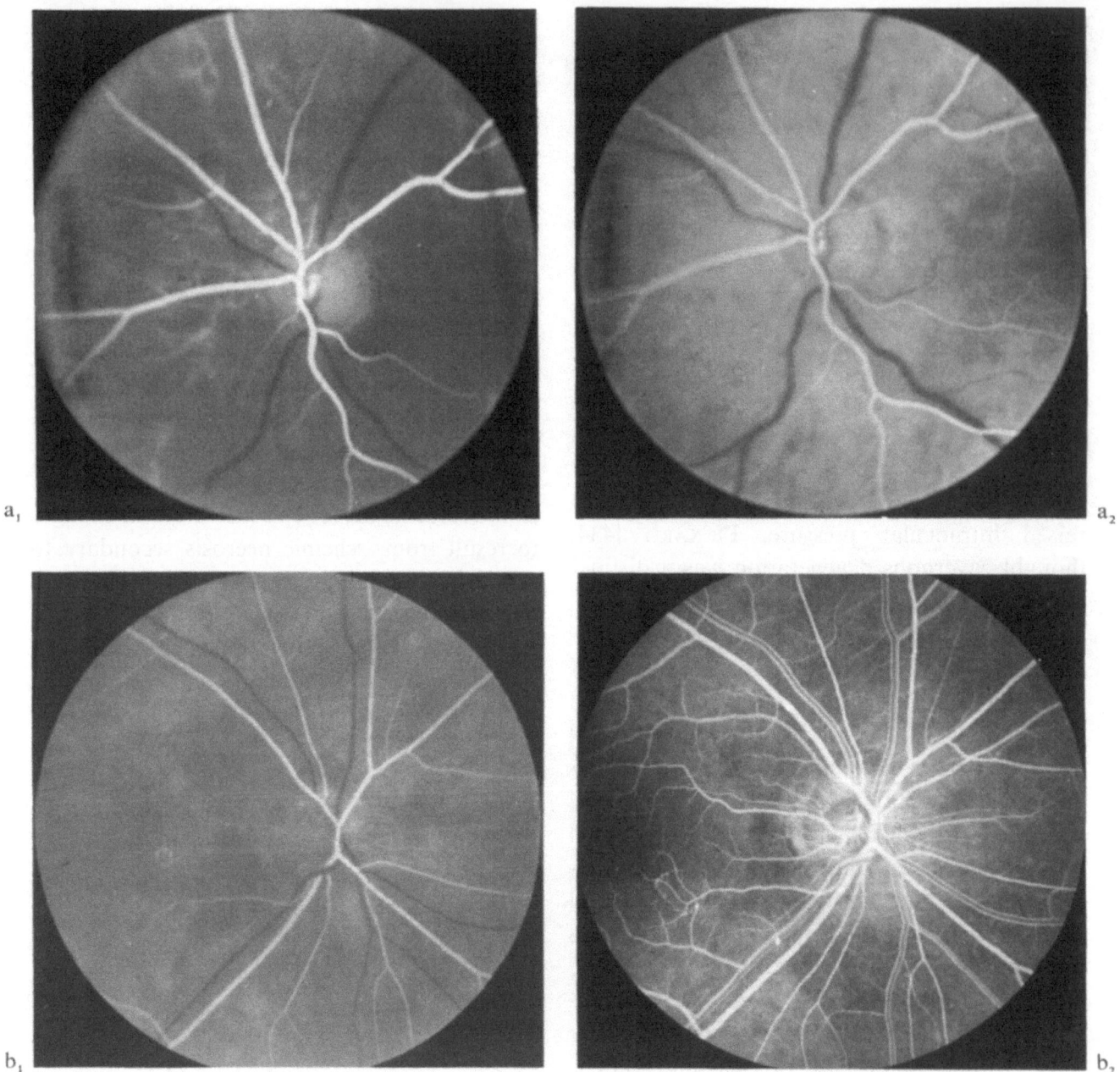

Fig. 32

a) Fluorescein fundus angiograms of left eye of a 47-year-old woman with chronic simple glaucoma and deeply cupped optic disc.

1) *At 60 mm Hg intra-ocular pressure:* Retinal arteries fill without choroidal filling except for a few big choroidal arteries.

2) *At 20 mm Hg intra-ocular pressure 2 days later:* Retinal arterial and choroidal filling normal.

The disc fluorescence seen in 1) and 2) is due to a preliminary test dose of fluorescein and not to disc filling.

b) Fluorescein fundus angiograms of right eye of a 59-year-old woman with visual field defects but normal intra-ocular pressure (20 mm Hg) in both eyes.

1) *During retinal arterial phase:* Shows faint filling of temporal choroid (supplied by lateral posterior ciliary artery) except for the peripapillary choroid and optic disc.

2) *During retinal arteriovenous phase:* Filling of the choroid as in 1)

a. Pattern of arterial supply to the anterior part of the optic nerve (p. 6) (Fig. 2).

b. Fluorescein fundus angiographic findings in patients with anterior ischemic optic neuropathy (p. 71), glaucoma (Fig. 32a), and low-tension glaucoma (Fig. 32 b) [250, 256, 261].

c. Fluorescein fundus angiographic findings in experimental ocular hypertension (Fig. 33) and systemic arterial hypotension [250, 264].

d. Experimental anterior ischemic optic neuropathy in rhesus monkeys produced by occluding the posterior ciliary arteries, with consequent histopathologic changes in the optic nerve (Fig. 12) [261].

e. Histopathologic changes in the optic nerve of patients with anterior ischemic optic neuropathy (p. 13) (Fig. 13).

f. Pathogenesis of anterior ischemic optic neuropathy (p. 14) [255].

As has been mentioned above (p. 13), the area of greatest involvement by infarction in the optic nerve is the optic nerve head and the retrolaminar part. The infarction evolves through liquefaction necrosis (Fig. 13 a) [364] and finally to retrolaminar fibrosis in four months (Fig. 13 c) [272]; these areas are supplied by the posterior ciliary arteries, which are vessels involved in the production of anterior ischemic optic neuropathy (p. 14). Infarction destroys maximally all the neural tissue and to some extent the fibrous connective tissue. Since the entire optic nerve head, except for the superficial nerve fiber layer, is supplied by the posterior ciliary arteries, occlu-

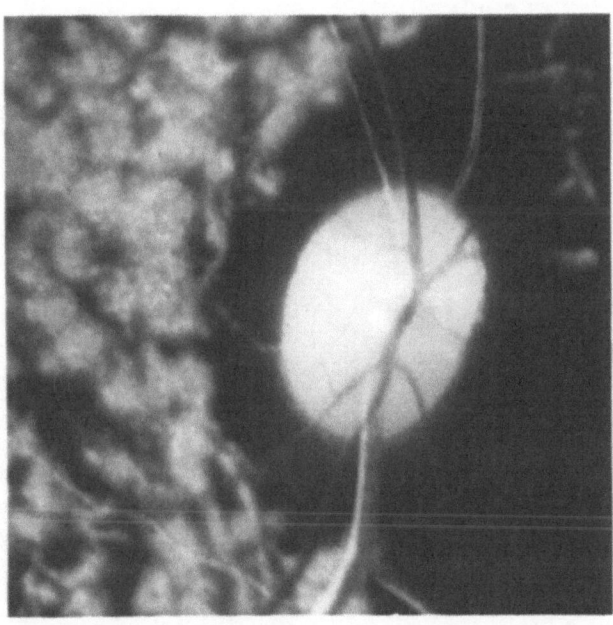 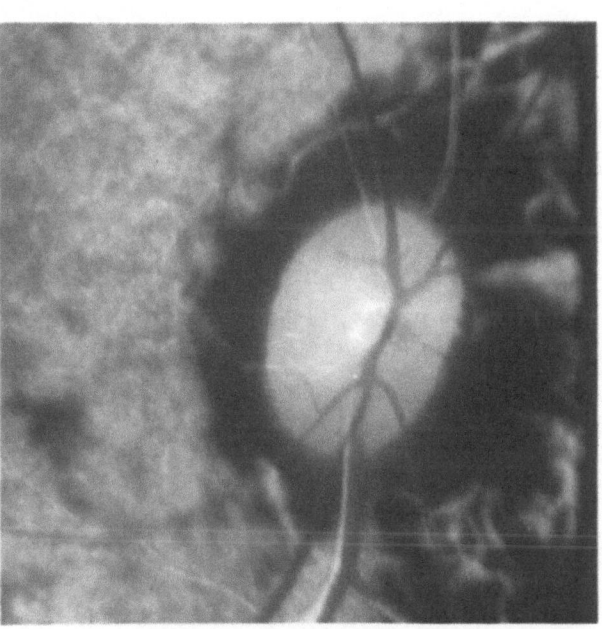

a   b

Fig. 33a and b. Fluorescein fundus angiograms of right eye of cynomolgus monkey (after experimental central retinal artery occlusion, at 70 mm Hg intra-ocular pressure.)
a) Early phase of choroidal filling—showing very slow and patchy filling of the choroid in the temporal half (supplied by the lateral posterior ciliary artery) with only a very early localized filling in the superior nasal choroid but no filling of the peripapillary choroid, superior choroidal watershed zone, inferior nasal choroid and optic disc.
b) 12 seconds after (a) shows complete filling of the choroid, though less than normal, and no filling of the peripapillary choroid and optic disc and patchy filling of the choroid watershed zones above and below (compare with Fig. 16 d).
Fluorescence of the optic disc in (a) and (b) is due to previous fluorescein angiography done a few minutes before these pictures to determine the filling pattern at normal intraocular pressure when the entire choroid and optic disc filled normally.

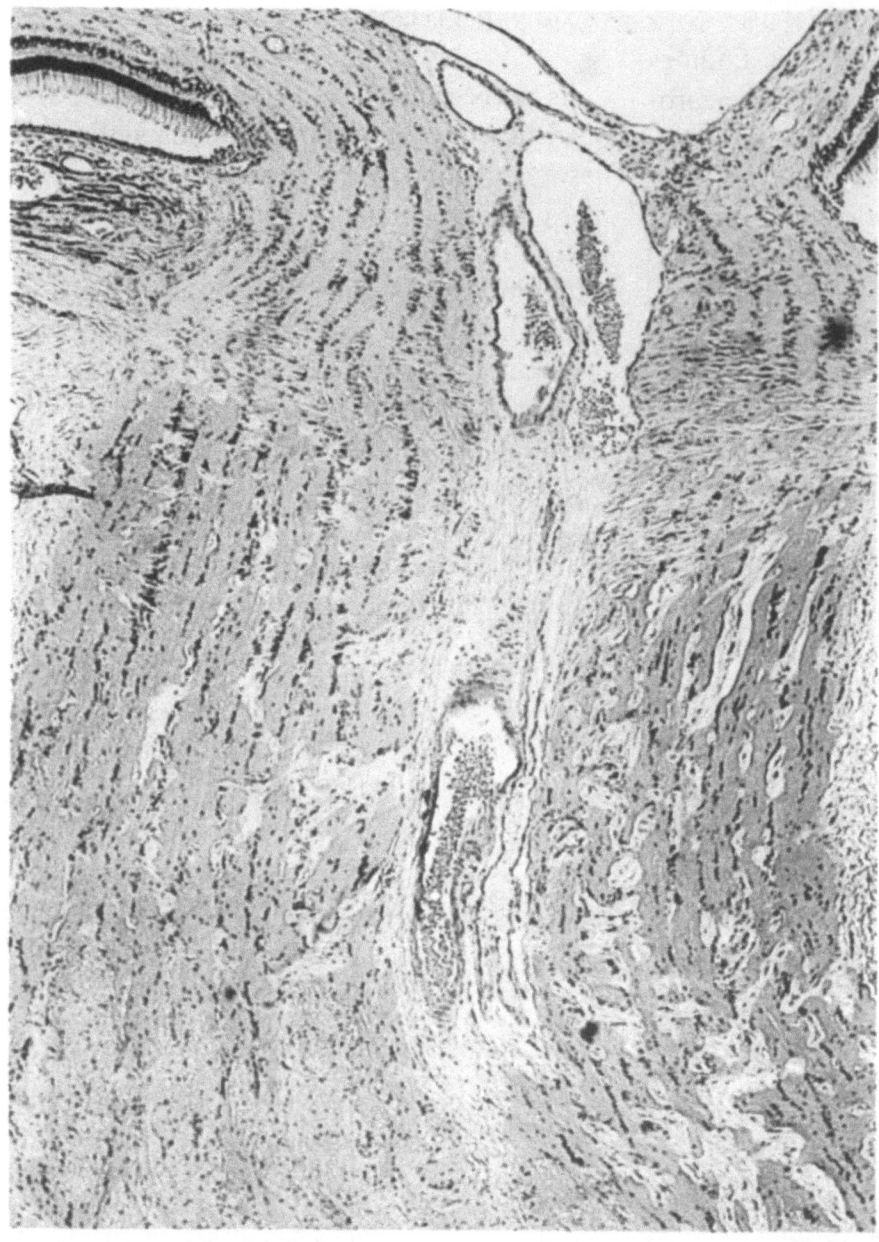

Fig. 34. Longitudinal section of a normal human optic nerve showing normal pattern of the various parts of the optic nerve head and retrolaminar optic nerve. (b) is a higher power of the optic nerve head to show the normal thickness of the neural prelaminar region

sion of the posterior ciliary arteries produces massive infarction of the optic nerve head. Capillaries in the surface nerve fiber layer of the optic disc, though derived from the retinal arterioles, may also become obliterated due to secondary associated edema of the nerve fiber layer. The neural tissue of the prelaminar part of the optic nerve head forms the main part of this structure in front of the lamina cribrosa (Fig. 34). An idea

of the normal thickness of this region can be gained easily from the depth of the normal physiologic cups in cases where the lamina cribrosa forms their floor. Complete destruction of this neural part of the optic nerve head (Fig. 35) will result in a significant amount of cupping. GREEN-FIELD [221] showed a well-developed disc cupping in histological sections of an eye with anterior ischemic optic neuropathy due to temporal

Fig. 34 (continued)

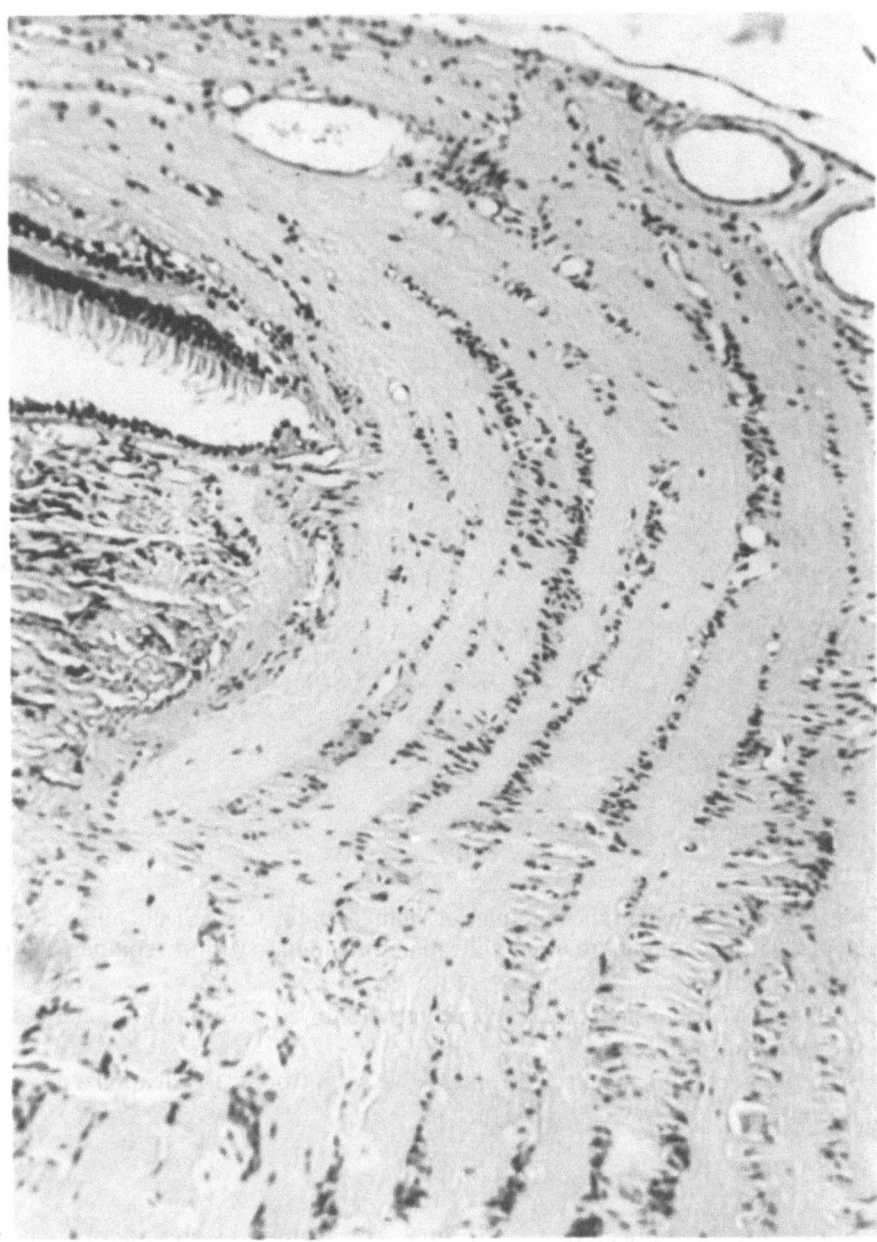

Fig. 34b

arteritis. Central retinal artery occlusion with patent posterior ciliary arteries would not produce as much destruction of the neural tissue in the optic nerve head because:

1. The retinal arterioles supply only a thin superficial nerve fiber layer and not the main part of the optic nerve head.

2. It has been noticed in most cases of central retinal artery occlusion that capillaries in the surface nerve fiber layer, which are of retinal arterial origin, fill profusely through their deep communications with the posterior ciliary prelaminar vessels (Fig. 28) so that the surface layer

does not suffer significant ischemia, unlike the marked ischemia seen in the prelaminar region in anterior ischemic optic neuropathy.

In central retinal artery occlusion, infarction of the inner layers of the retina and retinal nerve fiber layer would produce ascending degeneration of the nerve fibers, so that in the optic nerve head degeneration ultimately involves the optic nerve fibers only, without involvement of glial tissue. Similarly, other conditions involving degeneration of the optic nerve fibers alone in the optic nerve head, e.g., after ascending or descending degeneration of the optic nerve,

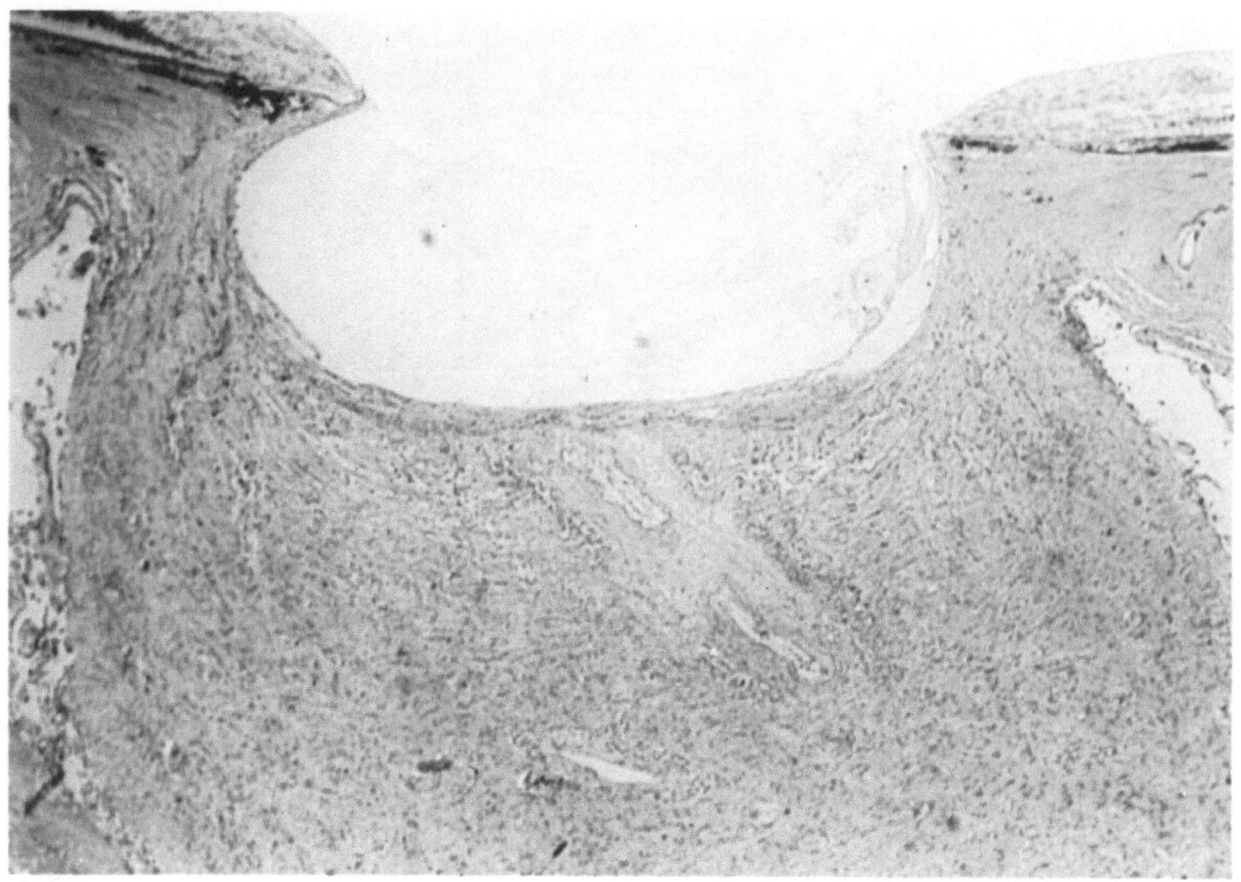

Fig. 35a and b. Microphotographs of human optic nerve head and retrolaminar optic nerve showing deep glaucomatous cupping, markedly atrophic prelaminar region (compare with Fig. 34b) and bowing backward of lamina cribrosa.

a) In a 63-year-old patient: The optic nerve showed cavernous degeneration in the part posterior to the area shown in this picture.

b). In a 65-year-old patient: The optic nerve was atrophic and hyalinized

could not be expected to produce the same amount of prelaminar neural tissue destruction as in anterior ischemic optic neuropathy.

The other important factor in the pathogenesis of optic disc cupping in anterior ischemic optic neuropathy is the change in the retrolaminar part of the optic nerve, which at first undergoes infarction (Figs. 12, 13) and ultimately fibrosis develops (Fig. 13c). Since all the retrolaminar fibrous septa are firmly attached to the posterior surface of the lamina cribrosa (Fig. 1a), fibrosis of the retrolaminar optic nerve would pull the lamina cribrosa backwards by contraction of fibrous tissue. Histopathologic studies demonstrated fully developed retrolaminar fibrosis by about four months after the onset of anterior

ischemic optic neuropathy [272]. Similarly maximum cupping of the optic disc in the present study was seen by about four months (p. 60). Moreover, normal neural tissue occupying the big spaces between the fibrous septa of the optic nerve (Fig. 1d) undergoes liquefaction necrosis and the spaces collapse. In turn the posterior support to the lamina cribrosa collapses. Thus, a combination of these two factors would result in a bowing backwards of the lamina cribrosa, which is seen on histopathology in these eyes (Fig. 35). The other factor that may further play a part in the backward bowing of the lamina cribrosa could be the effect of marked ischemia on the lamina cribrosa itself. The lamina cribrosa is composed partly of connective tissue and

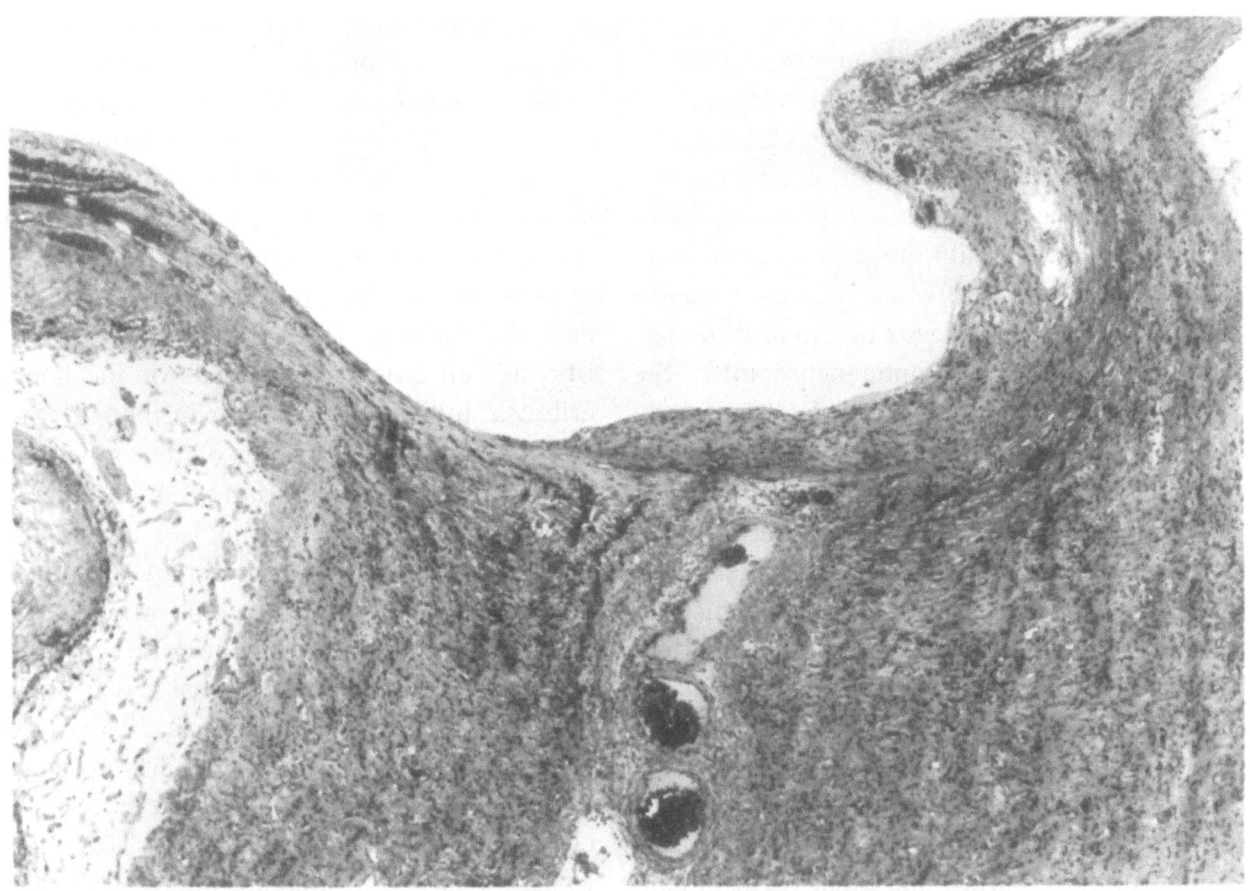

b

partly of neural tissue (p. 5) and could be weakened and thinned by ischemia.

Thus, a combination of the following three factors may be responsible for optic disc cupping in anterior ischemic optic neuropathy:

a) Destruction of the neural tissue in the prelaminar region of the optic nerve head. As mentioned above, it is a thick tissue composed almost entirely of neural tissue.

b) Bowing backwards of the lamina cribrosa due to retrolaminar fibrosis, and absence of normal support of the lamina cribrosa posteriorly by the disappearance of normally large amounts of neural tissue in the retrolaminar optic nerve.

c) Destruction of the neural tissue in the lamina cribrosa and possible weakness of its connective tissue part (as a part of infarction) would further aggravate the bowing backwards of the lamina cribrosa.

I do not feel the intraocular pressure in itself has any significant role to play in cupping in anterior ischemic optic neuropathy, as there is no evidence in this study to suggest that.

MILLER [390] postulated that for optic disc cupping in anterior ischemic optic neuropathy it is essential that both the retinal and posterior ciliary arteries be occluded. All the studies, as discussed in pathogenesis of anterior ischemic optic neuropathy (p. 14), clearly show that anterior ischemic optic neuropathy is due to occlusion of the posterior ciliary arteries, with no involvement of the central retinal artery. In fact, according to the basic definition of anterior ischemic optic neuropathy the central retinal artery is not involved. Similarly in the cases of my series, intravenous fluorescein angiography demonstrated no evidence of central retinal artery occlusion in all except two (Figs. 26, 27); the rest had only occlusion of the posterior ciliary arteries. In the two eyes with associated central retinal artery occlusion, the retinal artery was arising in common with the posterior ciliary arteries (p. 67). Moreover, MILLER tried to differentiate anterior ischemic optic neuropathy from ischemic papillopathy, but it is not clear from his description exactly what his concept of the latter was; his colleague Michael SANDERS [471] had, in fact, used the term *"ischemic papillopathy"* synonymously with anterior ischemic optic neuropathy in an earlier publication.

A comparatively low incidence of optic disc cupping was seen in anterior ischemic optic neuropathy due to arteriosclerosis in the present series. It is not possible to give a satisfactory explanation for this difference. All the evidence in the present study suggests that in arteriosclerotic anterior ischemic optic neuropathy, the ischemic process is not as marked or as massive as in temporal arteritis. It is possible that in arteriosclerotic anterior ischemic optic neuropathy, the ischemic neuropathy is the result of a single transitory hemodynamic crisis in the posterior ciliary arteries, unlike the complete or marked occlusion of the posterior ciliary artery by arteritis in temporal arteritis. Since in the cases due to arteriosclerosis the ischemia is in all probability temporary and transient with a single vascular insult, ischemic changes in the optic nerve head and retrolaminar part are presumably not as marked and extensive as in temporal arteritis. This would explain the better visual acuity, better prognosis, and lower incidence of optic disc cupping in arteriosclerotic anterior ischemic optic neuropathy, compared to temporal arteritic anterior ischemic optic neuropathy. This fact has also been pointed out by DRANCE et al. [133].

Since in glaucoma and low-tension glaucoma, the primary defect is interference with the posterior ciliary artery circulation to the optic nerve head and retrolaminar optic nerve [41, 53, 54, 159, 230, 245, 246, 250, 262, 263, 264] either due to a rise of intraocular pressure (glaucoma) or a fall in perfusion pressure in the posterior ciliary arteries (low-tension glaucoma), the above-mentioned mechanism of optic disc cupping in anterior ischemic optic neuropathy would also apply to glaucoma and low-tension glaucoma. In glaucoma and low-tension glaucoma the factors responsible for the ischemia are ongoing and, unlike those of arteriosclerotic anterior ischemic optic neuropathy, are not transitory in nature. Therefore they would develop far more ischemic changes (and associated

changes) than in arteriosclerotic anterior ischemic optic neuropathy. This factor was well illustrated by studies of DRANCE et al. [133].

Thus it seems optic disc cupping in anterior ischemic optic neuropathy due to temporal arteritis, glaucoma, and low-tension glaucoma is due to combined ischemic degenerative changes in the neural tissue of the prelaminar region of the optic nerve head, the retrolaminar optic nerve, and the lamina cribrosa, with retrolaminar fibrosis and bowing backwards of the lamina cribrosa. Individual variations in the pattern of blood supply of this region of the optic nerve may be responsible for variations in the response to ischemia (acute or chronic) of the anterior part of the optic nerve in different individuals. For example, the central retinal artery during its intraneural course within the optic nerve gives no branch in 25 percent of cases, one branch in 26.6 percent, two branches in 20.3 percent, three branches in 10.9 percent, four branches in 10.9 percent, six branches in 1.6 percent, and eight branches in 1.6 percent [243, 503]. These branches may be located anywhere between the point where the artery enters the optic nerve and the retrolaminar region; their size varies greatly. Branches of the central retinal artery, when and where present, constitute an axial centrifugal vascular system in this part of the optic nerve (Fig. 2). The major blood supply to the optic nerve comes from the centripetal branches of the pial plexus. The latter is formed by recurrent pial branches from the peripapillary choroid and branches of the short posterior ciliary arteries as well as collateral branches from the ophthalmic artery and its branches [241], with marked variations in the amount contributed from different sources (Fig. 2). From this brief account of the blood supply of the intraorbital part of the optic nerve, it is evident that there is tremendous variation in the blood supply of the retrolaminar and intraorbital optic nerve. In some cases the retrolaminar part of the optic nerve may derive its major blood supply from the central retinal artery and only a minor contribution from the posterior ciliary arteries to its peripheral part (via the recurrent pial branches from the peripapillary choroid); such an optic nerve would suffer only minor peripheral ischemia in anterior ischemic optic neuropathy. In contrast to this, in 25 percent of eyes, the central retinal artery gives out no branches within the nerve, and the entire blood supply to the anterior part of the optic nerve comes from the posterior ciliary arteries—such a nerve would suffer massive retrolaminar destruction in the event of anterior ischemic optic neuropathy. Between these two extremes lies a whole spectrum of variations in blood supply to the anterior part of the optic nerve. Moreover, the contribution by the peripapillary choroid to the pial plexus also varies considerably. Indeed, the pattern in the two eyes of the same individual may vary widely. Thus an ischemic disorder of the posterior ciliary artery would show all sorts of variations in the distribution of degenerative lesions in the optic nerve. I feel this variation in the pattern of blood supply is an important factor in determining the dissimilar development of optic disc cupping in different eyes in response to identical posterior ciliary artery ischemia. The involvement of the retrolaminar part of the optic nerve in glaucoma, low-tension glaucoma, and anterior ischemic optic neuropathy has always intrigued workers in the field because it has been difficult to explain how raised intraocular pressure could influence the extraocular part of the optic nerve. Various mechanisms have been postulated to explain this, including the forcing of vitreous or toxic intraocular fluid from the eye into the retrolaminar part of the optic nerve (p. 76), and the existence of a special artery ("the central artery of the optic nerve" [174, 175, 176]) supplying this region. From this description of the arterial supply of the anterior part of the optic nerve (p. 6), we now know that for the retrolaminar part the peripapillary choroid is usually the main, if not the only, source of blood: the peripapillary choroid in turn is not only subjected to intraocular pressure and any imbalance between intraocular and perfusion pressures in the posterior ciliary arteries, but also shows a higher vulnerability to obliteration under these circumstances than the rest of the choroid (Figs. 16d, 32, 33). Thus,

although the retrolaminar part of the optic nerve is not directly subjected to the intraocular pressure, its blood supply is very much influenced by it.

In glaucoma and low-tension glaucoma, cavernous degeneration in the retrolaminar optic nerve, which is again the result of ischemia, is well-established [250]. SPENCER et al. [511] pointed out that the changes in the retrolaminar optic nerve seen by them in their histopathologic study of anterior ischemic optic neuropathy due to temporal arteritis resembled cavernous degeneration. Figure 12b shows experimentally produced cavernous degeneration after posterior ciliary artery occlusion in rhesus monkey and Figs. 13d, e, f show cavernous degeneration in a patient with anterior ischemic optic neuropathy. Various locations for cavernous degeneration in the optic nerve are given in the literature (p. 77). In my study of the distribution of cavernous degeneration on histopathology in patients, I have seen all these variations (Fig. 36). In view of the above-mentioned variations in the contribution by the posterior ciliary artery to the retrolaminar optic nerve, these variations are no surprise. Ischemia of the optic nerve in the region of blood supply by the recurrent pial branches of the peripapillary choroid would produce cavernous degeneration. I agree with WOLFF [572] as to the mechanism of neural degeneration, although he could not explain the factors responsible for such an ischemia.

These findings lead us to believe that optic disc cupping, cavernous degeneration, and visual field defects in anterior ischemic optic neuropathy, glaucoma, and low-tension glaucoma are vasogenic in origin. In the production of vascular disturbances, not only is intraocular pressure important but perfusion pressure in the posterior ciliary arteries is even more important. In fact, it is the balance between the two pressures that is crucial. This helps towards clearing some of the age-old mysteries concerning optic disc cupping and cavernous degeneration without a rise in intraocular pressure.

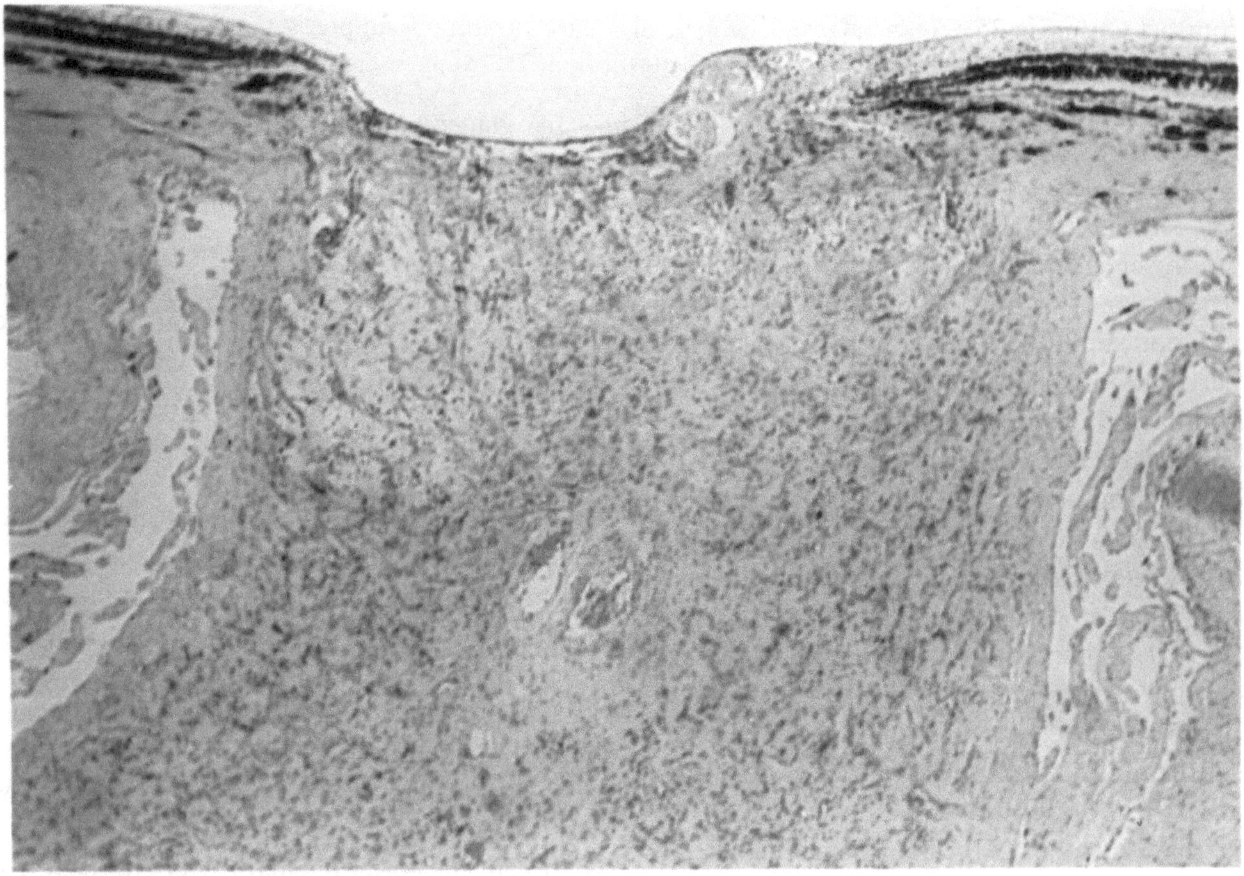

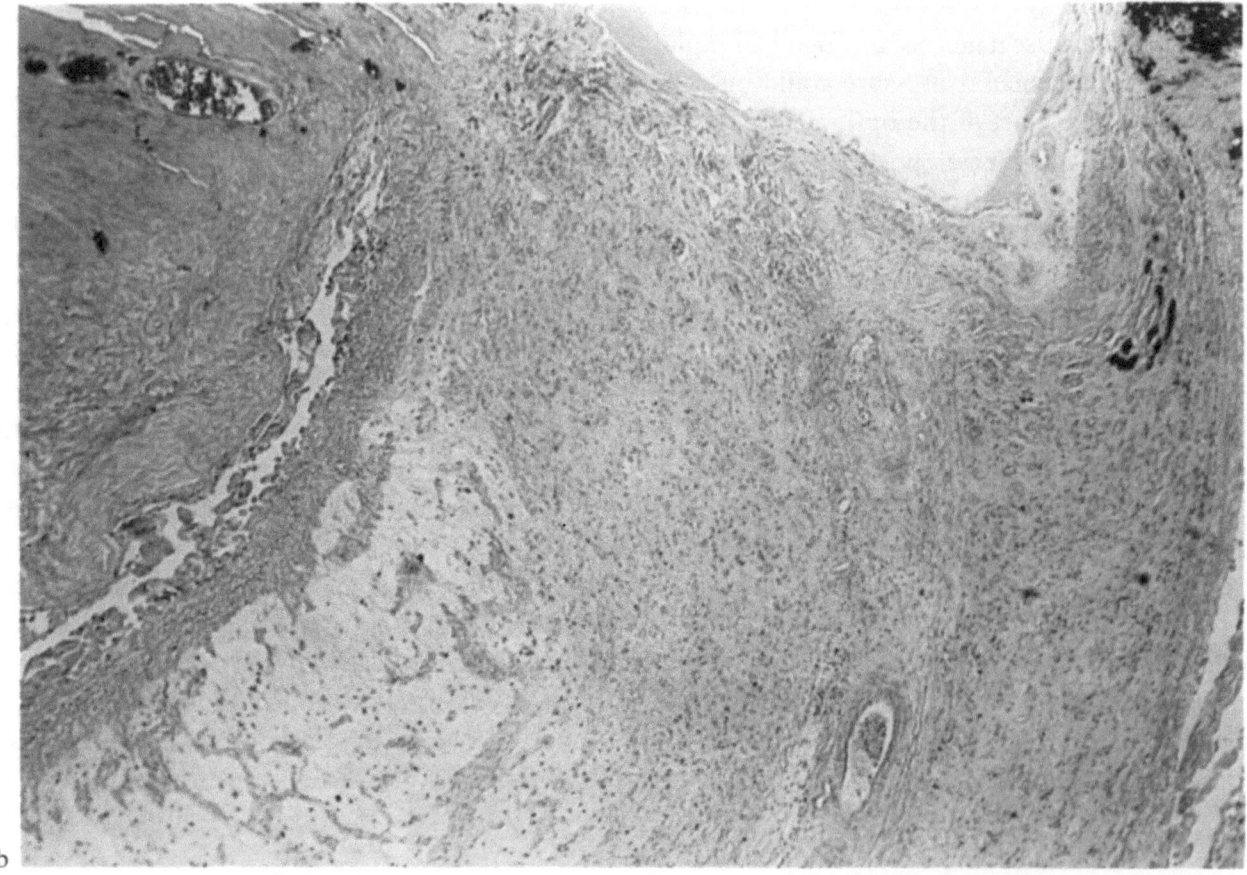

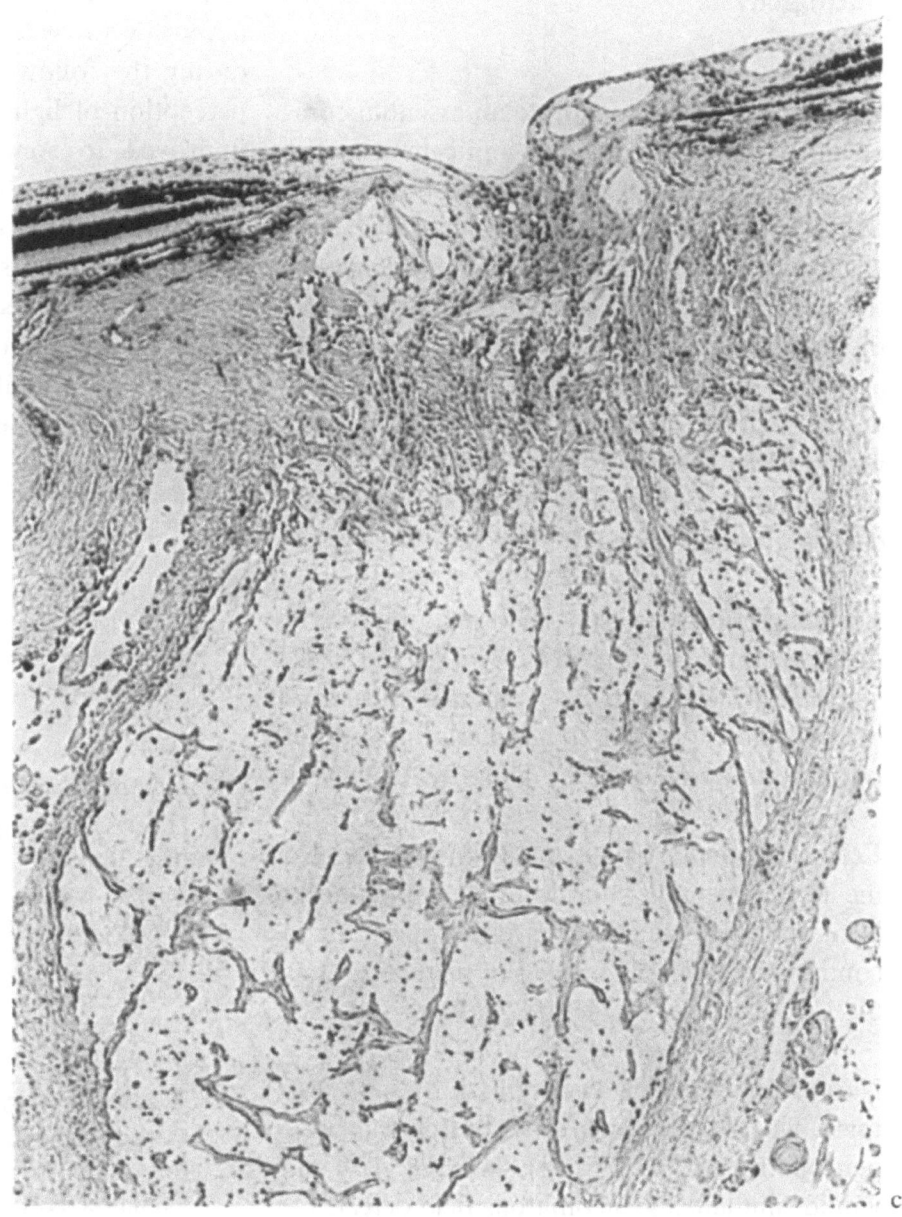

Fig. 36a–c. Microphotographs showing cavernous degeneration involving different parts of the optic nerve in glaucoma.

a) Cavernous degeneration involving the optic nerve head and retrolaminar optic nerve, being more extensive in a localized retrolaminar part with the corresponding part of the optic disc showing more cupping.

b) A 68-year-old patient with absolute glaucoma and very high intraocular pressure: Shows deep cupping of the optic disc, and cavernous degeneration localized to a part of the retrolaminar optic nerve at some distance posterior to the optic nerve head.

c) 81-year-old patient with marked glaucomatous cupping of the optic disc: Shows extensive cavernous degeneration involving the optic nerve head, retrolaminar optic nerve and the nerve for some distance posterior to that

Visual Field Defects and Their Pathogenesis

Visual field defects constitute an essential component of anterior ischemic optic neuropathy due to both temporal arteritis and other causes; the defects may be relative or absolute. They usually are of the optic nerve fiber bundle type— the size and site of a field defect depends upon the number and site of nerve fibers involved by ischemia and/or infarction. The visual field defects can be extremely variable and mimic many ocular and neurologic conditions. These field defects, although they may be very variable, can be grouped under the following headings:

Altitudinal Field Defects. There may be loss of the lower half [60, 61, 81, 151, 170, 339, 342, 388, 474] of the visual field. Inferior altitudinal defect is more common than superior in anterior ischemic optic neuropathy [60, 170, 342, 388].

Central Scotoma. This is due to involvement of the maculopapillar bundle in the optic nerve head and is frequently seen either alone or in combination with other types of field defect [60, 61, 170, 185, 322, 342, 388, 474].

Nerve Fiber Bundle Defect with an Arcuate Scotoma. This may be seen in anterior ischemic optic neuropathy [32, 61, 185, 247, 342, 388, 474] and would simulate a glaucomatous field defect.

Superior Nasal Quadrant Defect. Such a defect resembling glaucoma may be present [32, 151, 342, 474].

Segmental Field Defect. This is seen in sectoral anterior ischemic optic neuropathy [61, 474].

Contraction of Peripheral Visual Field. This is not uncommon in these cases [60, 185, 388].

Vertical Field Defects. The defects have been noticed, in these cases [247, 322, 342], to frequently involve the nasal half and are usually associated with central scotoma.

In the present study visual field defects were seen at some stage in all except seven eyes that never saw any better than no perception of light during the follow-up (of the ten eyes with no perception of light at first consultation, vision improved to some degree in three). In the remaining 23 eyes, the visual field defects varied from a nerve fiber bundle defect to only a small residual temporal island; not uncommonly these were relative defects, i.e., less extensive with larger targets than with smaller targets. Table 10 gives the details, and some of these field defects are shown in Fig. 37.

Table 10. Visual fields defects

Type of field defect	No. of eyes
(A) Inferior field defects (13 eyes)	
Defects involving the lower half field (Fig. 13a, b)	6
Inferior temporal defect	2
Inferior nasal defect (Fig. 31c)	1
Inferior nerve fiber bundle defect (Fig. 31d)	2
Could see HM/CF only in superior temporal field	2
(B) Superior field defects (3 eyes)	
Defects involving upper $1/2$[a] (Fig. 31e) to $1/3$ (Fig. 31f) field	2
Could see HM in lower temporal field	1
(C) Vertical defect (3 eyes)	
Defect involving temporal half or less of field	2
Defect involving nasal half of field (Fig. 30b)	1
(D) Central scotoma (5 eyes)	
Central scotoma only	2
Central scotoma associated with lower field loss	2
Central scotoma associated with nerve fiber bundle defect	1
(E) Lace-like defect	
Over whole field of one eye	1
(F) Small residual temporal field only	1

[a] This eye had NPL after one day

Fig. 37a–f. Visual field defects of some of patients of this series.

a) In the eye shown in Fig. 19 six months after onset and visual acuity 6/9.

b) In the eye shown in Fig. 22, 7 weeks after onset and visual acuity 6/9-pt.

c) In the eye shown in Fig. 21, 3¹/₂ months after onset and visual acuity 6/60.

d) In the eye shown in Fig. 25, 14 months after onset and visual acuity 6/36.

e) In the eye shown in Fig. 16 Two days after onset of visual disturbance and visual acuity of 6/9 which was reduced to no perception of light the next day.

f) In the eye of a 67-year-old man with no temporal arteritis and about 4 months after onset of partial anterior ischemic optic neuropathy and visual acuity of counting fingers

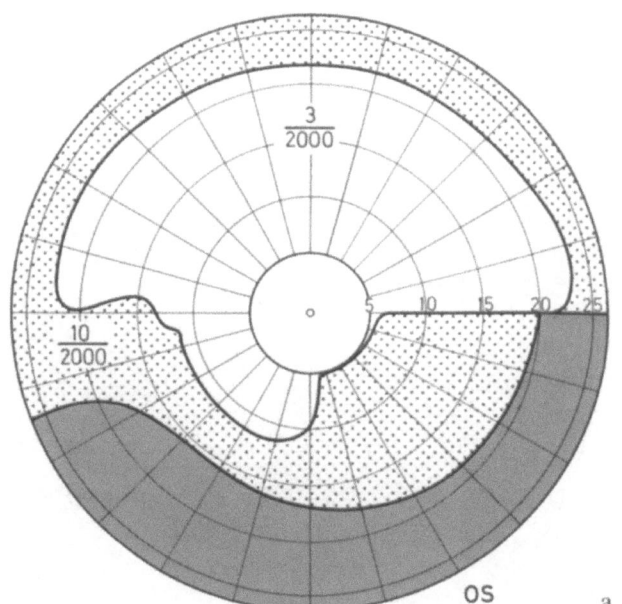

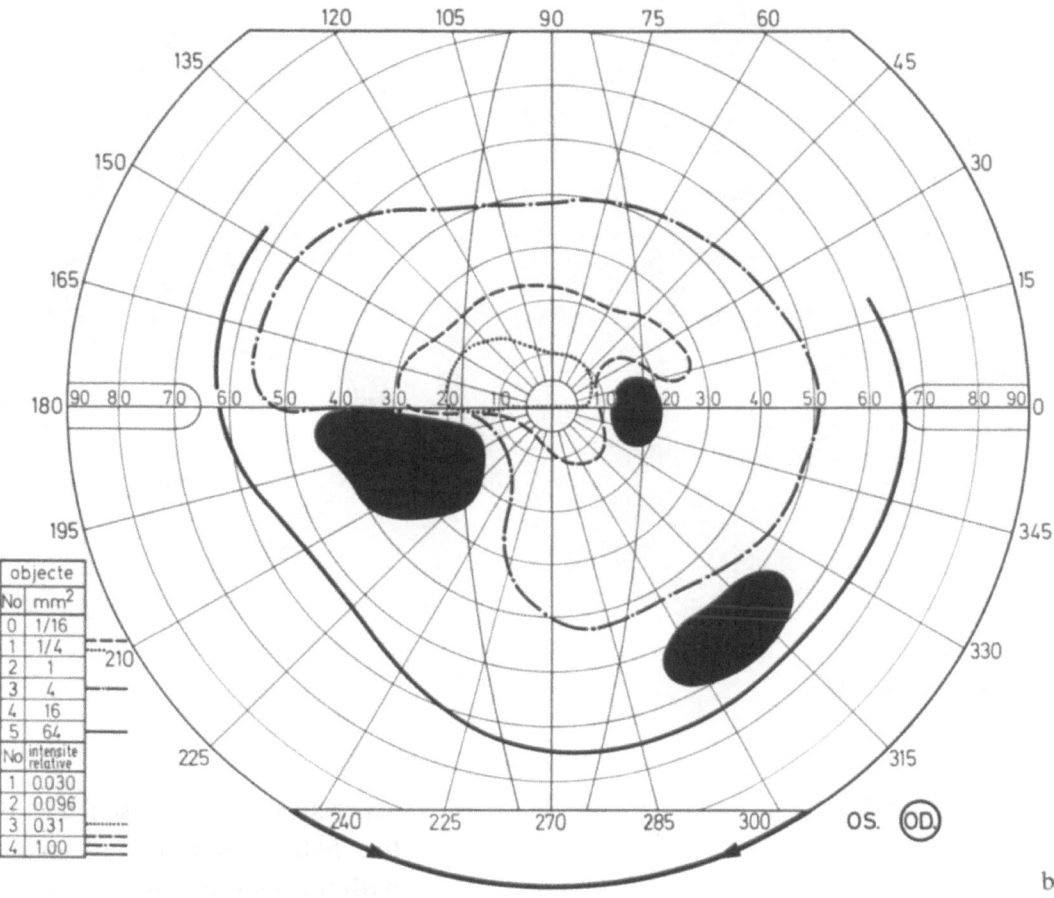

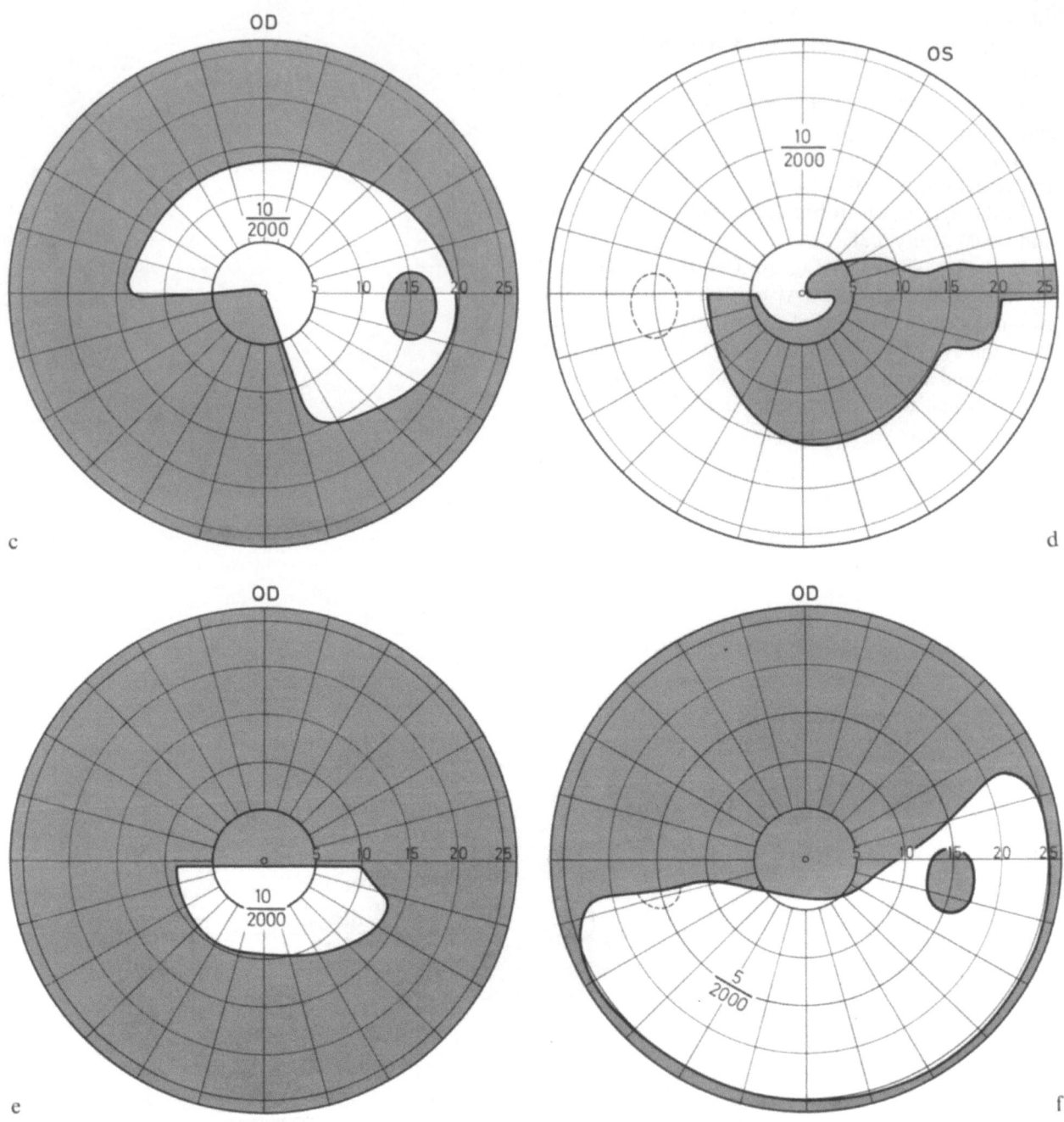

Fig. 37 (continued)

Pathogenesis

A good deal of controversy exists in the literature on the pathogenesis of the following visual field defects, which are seen not only in anterior ischemic optic neuropathy but also in other ophthalmic disorders. New information on the blood supply of the optic nerve head and on the patho-genesis of anterior ischemic optic neuropathy has helped in a better understanding of the pathogenesis of these visual field defects in general.

1. Prechiasmal Altitudinal Hemianopias

These are one of the well-known stigmata of vascular disease of the optic nerve, although some altitudinal hemianopias can result from occlusion of the superior or inferior branch of the central retinal artery. Prechiasmal altitudinal hemianopia without any retinal abnormality has been reported in anterior ischemic optic neuropathy due to temporal arteritis [36, 107, 441, 479, 548, 552] and arteriosclerosis [60, 81, 107, 151, 170, 171, 339, 342, 388, 441, 474]. These altitudinal defects have also been seen in other lesions of the optic nerve, most of which, in fact, represent manifestations of anterior ischemic optic neuropathy, e.g., arteriosclerotic optic atrophy [236, 291] following massive hemorrhages (p. 117); edema of the optic disc due to raised intracranial pressure [88, 554], angioma of the optic nerve head [292], arteriosclerosis of the internal carotid artery [321], primary optic atrophy due to Tabes [236, 555], and glaucoma and low-tension glaucoma. Hemianopia usually occurs in the lower visual field and less commonly in the upper half. The demarcation line lies horizontally and may not be absolutely straight. A generalized depression of the preserved field also may be seen.

The pathogenesis of these defects has evoked many ingenious hypotheses. The views of WOLFF [570] and HUGHES [292] are mentioned in the discussion on posthemorrhagic amaurosis (p. 118). PIPER and UNGER [441] thought that they were due to acute circulatory disorders of the optic nerve. They were of the opinion that occlusion of the distal part of the anterior branch of the central artery of the optic nerve caused an anemic infarct in the lamina cribrosa region, where fibers from the upper half of the retina run. However, it has now been fairly conclusively established, that the central artery of the optic nerve is rarely, if ever, present in man [241, 243]. HARRINGTON [236] suggested that injury to the blood supply of the optic nerve produced altitudinal hemianopia, usually inferior. He proposed a sharp division of the optic nerve into three areas based on its blood supply—superior peripheral, inferior peripheral, and central. He further stated that the vascular supply to the optic nerve came through a network of vessels in the arachnoid membrane, which passed through the subarachnoid space and entered the

optic nerve at right angles. In its upper part the space is narrow and the vessels that traverse it from the membrane to the nerve are short and easily damaged by torsion, edema, and other injury. This, according to HARRINGTON [236], gives rise to a unilateral altitudinal field defect, with horizontal border, steep edges, and great density. My detailed anatomic studies on the subject of the blood supply of the optic nerve, mentioned above [238, 240, 241, 243] and also those of the other workers on the subject, in no way support any of HARRINGTON's speculations. HUGHES [292] rightly pointed out that there was no evidence of a horizontal or vertical division of the blood supply of the optic nerve, apart from the central peripheral separation. He stated, however, that these field defects strongly suggested some segmental arterial supply in the optic nerve whereby the blood supply of one horizontal half of the nerve may be cut off by a single lesion. In many such cases the central area of the field is spared, but in some this is also affected. He stressed that none of the anatomic work reported could provide an explanation for the clinical experience.

WALKER and CUSHING [554] suggested that altitudinal hemianopia in optic disc edema was due to an intracranial lesion pressing against the upper rim of the optic foramen.

My studies have clearly demonstrated the sectoral distribution of the blood supply in the optic nerve head and choroid [245, 246, 247, 249, 259]. Sometimes, the posterior ciliary arteries supply the upper and lower parts of the choroid and the optic disc with a horizontal boundary line (Fig. 6). Occlusion of one of the two main posterior ciliary arteries, which supply half of the optic disc and the corresponding choroid, produces an altitudinal field defect with no retinal changes. More commonly, where the main posterior ciliary arteries supply the nasal and temporal halves of the choroid, nonfilling of the watershed zone between the posterior ciliary arteries, above or below the optic disc, would produce a filling defect in the corresponding half of the optic disc. Such filling defects were seen in the present study (Figs. 23c, 27). Watershed zones of the posterior ciliary arteries are highly susceptible to obliteration in the event of an imbalance between perfusion pressure in the posterior ciliary arteries and intraocular pressure [245, 246, 250, 263, 264]. However, I have no explanation as yet for the higher frequency with which the superior compared to the inferior watershed zone is involved. Gravity may play some role (as suggested by WOLFF [570]), but this is not definitely known. In acute occlusive disorders the corresponding half of the disc is edematous at first, with evidence of ischemic neuropathy in that part of the disc. Later, all cases show optic atrophy of the corresponding half of the disc (Figs. 19, 22, 27). Such a well-defined horizontal localization of blood supply exists only in the optic disc and that, too, in its posterior ciliary supply, not anywhere else in the optic nerve. Thus, altitudinal hemianopias of prechiasmal origin and without any retinal lesion are caused by interference with the posterior ciliary artery supply of the disc.

2. Prechiasmal Vertical Hemianopia

Vertical hemanopias are always considered to be due to chiasmal or suprachiasmal lesions and most often are expected to be bilateral. A unilateral hemianopia, when seen, is usually considered a precursor of ultimate bilateral hemianopias.

Unilateral vertical hemianopia has been reported in posthemorrhagic amaurosis [236, 486], in addition to anterior ischemic optic neuropathy; the line of hemianopia may be irregular [486].

The medial and lateral posterior ciliary arteries usually supply the medial and lateral halves, respectively, of the choroid and optic disc, with a sharp line of demarcation between the two (Figs. 4, 5, 24). The various lesions mentioned in altitudinal hemianopias, which produce occlusion of the main posterior ciliary arteries, may produce a vertical instead of an altidudinal hemianopia that may be nasal or temporal. If bilateral, it may result in homonymous or heteronymous hemianopias and may be confused with chiasmal or suprachiasmal

lesions. The border of the hemianopic field, instead of passing through the fixation point as in chiasmal and suprachiasmal hemianopias, will pass through the blind spot in optic disc hemianopias (Fig. 30b). The nasal hemianopia therefore, in these cases, is most likely to be accompanied by a central scotoma due to involvement of the papillomacular bundle (Fig. 30b). In acute onset, the temporal or nasal half of the disc may be edematous at first, with normal retinal vessels and fundus. Later, optic atrophy of the corresponding half of the disc will be seen in all these cases. Histopathologic examination in such a case would show infarction of the retrolaminar optic nerve involving the corresponding half of the nerve (Fig. 13a).

3. Segmental Visual Field Defects

It has already been seen that the main posterior ciliary artery frequently supplies half of the choroid and optic disc, the superior or inferior half (Fig. 6), or the temporal or nasal half [247, 249, 259] (Figs. 4, 5, 24n). Each posterior ciliary artery divides at some distance from the eyeball into further subdivisions. If it first divides into two, each of the subdivisions may supply a quadrant of the choroid and the disc. The same can happen when there are two medial posterior ciliary arteries (29 percent) [239] or two lateral posterior ciliary arteries (20 percent) [239] instead of one each. In that case, one posterior ciliary artery will supply about a quadrant instead of half of the choroid and optic disc. Such a quadrantic filling of the choroid by the dye has been seen (Figs. 3, 23c). Occlusion or stenosis of such an artery, due to any cause, would lead to a quadrantic or segmental field defect. During acute vascular occlusion of such an artery with resultant infarction, that segment of the disc may be edematous, but later it will be atrophic. The possibility of bilateral segmental defects due to this cause has to be borne in mind.

4. Nerve Fiber Bundle Defect

The term *"nerve fiber bundle"* refers to any small group of nerve fibers that lie together as they enter the optic disc [537]. The most classic visual field defect produced by nerve fiber bundle defects is the arcuate scotoma (Bjerrum scotoma, Comet scotoma, Scimitar scotoma). Though it is classically described in glaucoma, it can occur in a large variety of conditions [136, 235], including sectoral anterior ischemic optic neuropathy. The pathogenesis of the nerve fiber bundle defect has been discussed fully elsewhere [247].

Since the centripetal vessels in the optic disc and optic nerve are radial and have a segmental supply, these would involve nerve fibers in a sectoral fashion. In the optic nerve head there is no centrifugal vascular system, and the blood supply by the posterior ciliary arteries to the optic nerve head is of a better defined sectoral type than that in the retrobulbar optic nerve. Moreover, the arrangement of nerve fibers in the optic disc topographically is presumably more representative of the retinal arrangement than that in the intraorbital part of the optic nerve. A typical nerve fiber bundle defect is, therefore, far more likely to arise from an optic disc lesion than from a posterior optic nerve lesion. Occlusion of supply of one of the small subdivisions of the posterior ciliary arteries could involve a sector of the prelaminar, lamina cribrosa, and retrolaminar regions of the optic nerve. It is therefore not surprising to see the occurrence of nerve fiber bundle defects in sectoral anterior ischemic optic neuropathy.

5. Peripheral Contraction of Visual Fields

Peripheral contraction of the visual fields is not uncommon in anterior ischemic optic neuropathy [60, 185, 388]. It has also been mentioned as the most common type of field loss in arteriosclerotic optic atrophy, with multiple indentations in the peripheral field. These most commonly affect the lower field [292]. Depression of the peripheral fields in glaucoma is a well-known phenomenon. Involvement of the posterior ciliary arteries directly, or of the peripapillary choroid (via the recurrent pial branches arising from the peripapillary choroid), will interfere with the pial supply to the retrolaminar optic nerve. Since the pial branches in the retrolaminar part of the optic nerve contribute to the peripheral centripetal vascular system (p. 9), their involvement would cause the peripheral visual fields to contract.

Anterior Segment of the Eye

Usually the only abnormality detected in this part of the eye is an afferent pupil, with dilatation and absent or sluggish reaction to direct light. In one case with temporal arteritis and no perception of light (not included in this series), marked ocular hypotony, with folds in Descemet's membrane of the cornea, and anterior uveitis were seen. The findings very much resembled anterior segment necrosis and presumably resulted from occlusion of the ophthalmic artery by temporal arteritis. LANDBLAD [335] had reported iritis in temporal arteritis.

Intraocular Pressure

Although eyes with anterior ischemic optic neuropathy in uniocular cases of the present series had an intraocular pressure 2 to 3 mm Hg (8 mm Hg in one eye, 4 mm Hg in two eyes) lower than the opposite uninvolved eye, it was not considered to be significantly abnormal.

BEGG *et al.* [30, 31, 32], DRANCE *et al.* [132], FOULDS *et al.* [172], and FOULDS [171] described the association of chronic simple glaucoma and raised intraocular pressure with anterior ischemic optic neuropathy. In none of the patients of the present series was any abnormality of the intraocular pressure detected. Nevertheless, intraocular pressure is one of the two factors responsible for the development of anterior ischemic optic neuropathy, the other factor being perfusion pressure in the posterior ciliary arteries. Thus, intraocular pressure plays an extremely important role in the pathogenesis of anterior ischemic optic neuropathy (p. 23).

Electroretinal Responses in Anterior Ischemic Optic Neuropathy

Electro-oculographic and electoretinographic findings in both eyes of 16 patients of this series

are given in Table 11 and their relation to the following are summarized: (a) type of anterior ischemic optic neuropathy, (b) any associated retinal arterial occlusion, (c) the time interval between the onset of anterior ischemic optic neuropathy and the recording of these responses, (d) their visual acuity, and (e) visual fields.

1. Electro-Oculographic Studies

Using the same equipment, normal variations of the electro-oculographic ratio in normal subjects showed that in males and females above

Table 11. Electroretinal responses in anterior ischemic optic neuropathy

Pt. No.	Sex	Age	Diagnosis	Time interval from onset	EOG— Arden ratio[11] (%)		ERG— Maximum b-wave in μ		Visual Acuity	Visual fields	FFF—ERG (in Hz)	
					Rt. eye	Lt. eye	Rt. eye	Lt. eye			Rt. eye	Lt. eye
(A). Temporal arteritic anterior ischemic optic neuropathy												
1	M	72$\frac{1}{2}$	Right AION of upper one-half of OD and CRAO	5 days 7 days 11 days 17 days 4 months 12 months	flat — 220 189 182 243	200 — 246 156 207 207	40 90 — absent — 20	160 190 — — — 140	PL	A small island above present	20 20 — 20 — 10	40 40 — — — 80
2	F	72	Bilateral complete AION with right CRAO	6$\frac{1}{2}$ months 14 months	115 Visual acuity too poor	183	absent 80	240 240	Rt. NPL Lt. CF	Left—a small island present	— 20	— 60
3	F	72	Right complete AION with cilioret. art. occ. supplying upper $\frac{1}{2}$ retina	2 days 5 days 8 days 11 days 12 days 9 months	114 150 130 160 114 150	167 260 320 164 167 147	— — — — — 230	— — — — — 310	NPL		— — — — — 40	— — — — — 40
4	F	72	Right complete AION	2 days 4 days 11 days 29 days 5 months 14 months	— 210 167 191 154 213	— 218 167 200 159 200	300 — 340 280 — 320	300 — 260 200 — 120	NPL		60 — 60 60 — —	60 — 60 40 — —

Table 11 (continued)

No.	Sex	Age	Type	Time					Vision	Field		
5	F	80	Left complete AION	1 day	190	180	240	240	NPL		—	—
				6 months	218	194	160	130			60	60
6	F	75	Left complete AION	18 months	158	135	420	510	NPL		60	60
7	F	65	AION—bilateral complete	21 months	Visual acuity too poor		320	300	NPL in both eyes		60	60
8	F	78$^1/_2$	Right partial AION	7 months	275	200	230	240	CF	Central scotoma and generalized constriction	60	40

(B). *Non arteritic anterior ischemic optic neuropathy*

No.	Sex	Age	Type	Time					Vision	Field		
9	M	78	Bilateral partial AION	5 months	270	345	140	200	Rt. 6/6	Rt. constricted, more below	20	20
				16 months	225	257	230	260	Lt. CF	Lt. constricted, and central scotoma	—	—
				28 months	225	250	290	280			40	60
10	M	60	Bilateral complete AION	21 months	Visual acuity too poor		510	200	HM	Rt. lower temporal loss Lt. central scotoma	60	40
11	F	82	Left complete AION	12 months	207	146	—	—	CF	A small field near center	—	—
12	M	65	Right partial AION	19 days	225	250	200	180	HM/CF	Superior altitudinal defect	60	60
				7 months	320	320	160	180			—	—
13	M	61	Right partial AION	7 months	200	200	140	340	6/60	Lower nasal defect central scotoma	40	40
				20 months	214	250	160	180			40	20
14	M	59	Right partial AION	16 months	161	153	400	350	6/9	No defect detectable	60	60
15	F	79	Left partial AION	10 months	142	142	380	440	6/9	Lower temporal field loss	60	60
16	M	67	Left partial AION	30 months	269	256	590	430	6/9	Inferior altitudinal hemianopia	60	60

the age of 50 years, this ratio varied between 150 and 290 (mean = 212), with a normal difference between the two eyes of 80 [2]. In two cases (Patients 1 and 3) of this study, the electro-oculographic ratio was significantly lower in the eye with anterior ischemic optic neuropathy than in the opposite normal eye at the onset of anterior ischemic optic neuropathy, but the ratio normalized by the eleventh day in the affected eyes of both patients. In another case (Patient 4) the electro-oculogram was recorded on the fourth day after the onset of anterior ischemic optic neuropathy and its ratio was the same as in the opposite normal eye. In the former two eyes (Patients 1 and 3), there was additional retinal ischemia—occlusion of the central retinal artery in one and of the cilioretinal artery (supplying the upper half of the retina) in the second. In another case (Patient 2) with bilateral anterior ischemic optic neuropathy, the right eye (with additional evidence of old central retinal artery occlusion on electroretinogram) showed a lower electro-oculographic ratio than the left, which had only anterior ischemic optic neuropathy. These findings suggest that most probably the electro-oculographic ratio is low in an eye initially or permanently only when anterior ischemic optic neuropathy is accompanied by retinal ischemia. In the rest of the patients with anterior ischemic optic neuropathy due to temporal arteritis or arteriosclerosis, there was no abnormality on the electro-oculogram. FRANÇOIS et al. [185] also found normal electro-oculogram in patients with anterior ischemic optic neuropathy. This indicates that electro-oculogram in patients with anterior ischemic optic neuropathy is not of much help as a diagnostic aid. A normal electro-oculogram in these patients with anterior ischemic optic neuropathy is not unexpected, because they have an intact choroidal circulation, although there is no circulation in the optic nerve head (p. 72).

2. Electro-Retinographic Studies

In seven patients in the present series there was a difference of more than 30 percent between amplitudes of b-wave in the two eyes. Three of these cases (Patients 1, 2 and 3) had anterior ischemic optic neuropathy associated with retinal artery occlusion (central retinal artery occlusion in two and occlusion of the cilioretinal artery supplying the upper half of the retina in the third) and showed a smaller b-wave amplitude in the eye with retinal artery occlusion—a reduction of about 66 percent or more with central retinal artery occlusion and 35 percent with cilioretinal artery occlusion. In these three patients, the low amplitude of the b-wave was persistent. It was interesting to observe that one of these patients had bilateral anterior ischemic optic neuropathy, but only the eye with associated central retinal artery occlusion had a low b-wave amplitude. Patients 4, 9, 10, and 13 showed an isolated low reading of the b-wave in one or the other eye, and the reading was not persistently low. Such an isolated low b-wave reading seems to be an artefact and of no significance. Moreover, in the latter group there was no definite pattern. Flicker fusion frequency of the electroretinogram usually showed a photopic response (60 Hertz), and in a few eyes a mixed response (40 Hertz). The presence or absence of temporal arteritis or arteriosclerosis, complete or partial involvement of the optic nerve head, or the amount of visual loss (both of the visual acuity and visual fields) did not make any difference to this response. In two eyes with associated central retinal artery occlusion the response was scotopic (20 Hertz or less). These findings indicate that the electroretinogram is abnormal in anterior ischemic optic neuropathy only when there is associated retinal arterial occlusion; otherwise, it shows no significant abnormality. A normal electroretinogram in anterior ischemic optic neuropathy has also been reported by other workers [74, 149, 185, 381, 579]. BURIAN [74] described, in temporal arteritis, a very large a-wave, the bioelectric abnormality both in the affected and nonaffected eye, and normalization of the electroretinogram in both eyes with the steroid therapy, even though function in the affected eye may not be restored.

In our experimental studies [381], after cutting the posterior ciliary arteries in rhesus monkeys, we found a consistently subnormal electroretinogram. The difference between the clinical and experimental result is easy to explain. As mentioned above, in clinical fluorescein angiographic studies (p. 72) of anterior ischemic optic neuropathy, the choroidal circulation is almost always intact, although reduced. In contrast to this, in experimental studies in rhesus monkeys, angiography revealed a complete absence of choroidal filling during transit of the dye and later on ophthalmoscopic and histopathologic evidence of chorioretinal destruction in patches. Experimental studies showed that there was no abnormality in the configuration of the electroretinographic wave form, i.e., the amplitude of the a-wave was reduced proportionately to the b-wave with an overall subnormal response. The amplitude of the scotopic b-wave was lower in more marked choroidal ischemia. The generalized reduction of the electroretinogram was thought to be due primarily to a diminution in the P III component (due to receptor damage), with concurrent secondary diminution in the P II component (the bipolar layer being deprived of stimulation; recent studies indicate that the b-wave probably originates from the Müller cells [127]). However, P III is thought to be most resistant to ischemia [218]; the a-wave usually increases in amplitude when a reduction of the b-wave occurs, but this may be transitory.

Visually evoked responses were recorded in anterior ischemic optic neuropathy by FRANÇOIS et al. [185], and they found complete loss in total blindness but presence in segmental lesions.

Other Ocular Abnormalities

The only other ocular abnormality of significance, reported in some of the cases with temporal arteritis, was diplopia, which may be transient or constant (p. 114). Ptosis has also been reported [500]. Ophthalmoplegia has a better prognosis than blindness and is an indication for steroid therapy [384].

Palsies of the extraocular muscles, similar to those due to temporal arteritis, are also seen in patients with arteriosclerosis, hypertension, or diabetes, and have a similar mechanism.

In the present study I had no patient with diplopia.

Erythrocyte Sedimentation Rate

Erythrocyte sedimentation rate is a very important and essential investigation in all patients suspected of anterior ischemic optic neuropathy and must be carried out as a first priority. The primary object of this investigation is to detect patients with temporal arteritis as early as possible and to treat them energetically, at the earliest possible moment, with high doses of systemic corticosteroids since, if not treated, the possibility that the second eye will become involved is high.

Since patients with anterior ischemic optic neuropathy are elderly, many ophthalmologists are misled by the uncertainty as to what can be considered a normal erythrocyte sedimentation rate in this age group. It is well established that the erythrocyte sedimentation rate in normal elderly persons is higher than the usually accepted "normal" limit. BOYD and HOFFBRAND [66] consider an upper limit of 40 mm in one hour Westergren in persons over 65 years as normal, while BOTTIGER and SVEDBERG [64] described it as 30 mm in women and 20 mm in men over the age of 50. TOWNES and BLODI [536] found it over 60 mm in 12 of 45 cases with atherosclerotic anterior ischemic optic neuropathy and PAYNE [427] discovered that in 100 old patients with erythrocyte sedimentation rates of over 100 mm, only two had temporal arteritis. SCOTT [486] found an erythrocyte sedimentation rate in all of his arteriosclerotic anterior ischemic optic neuropathies of less than 30 mm.

In temporal arteritis, a high erythrocyte sedimentation rate usually is seen, and this has been well established by an enormous literature on the subject. An elevated erythrocyte sedimentation rate has been described as an invariable finding in active temporal arteritis [305, 389, 417, 467, 552]. However, cases of anterior ischemic optic neuropathy with temporal arteritis have been reported in whom the erythrocyte sedimentation rate was within normal limits [105, 220]. CULLEN [105] reported a patient with an erythrocyte sedimentation rate of 12 mm who, on postmortem, showed typical lesions of temporal arteritis in the eye and optic nerve.

In the present study, patients with a positive temporal artery biopsy for temporal arteritis had erythrocyte sedimentation rates of 50 to 135 mm in the first hour Westergren, although three patients with a negative temporal artery biopsy for arteritis had an erythrocyte sedimentation rate of 50 to 69 mm. In this study, every patient with an erythrocyte sedimentation rate of more than 40 mm was considered to suffer from temporal arteritis, unless proved otherwise; this may be considered a fairly safe practical rule, although exceptions are known.

No other relevant hematologic abnormality was detected in this series.

Temporal Artery Biopsy

To determine the presence or absence of temporal arteritis in a patient, it is considered that temporal artery biopsy examination for histopathologic evidence of temporal arteritis can confirm a diagnosis. However, there is some controversy about the diagnostic value of a negative temporal artery biopsy. Temporal artery involvement by arteritis is frequently spotty so that one part may be free and another positive for temporal arteritis [44]; a patient with negative biopsy could still have temporal arteritis [107, 417]. The latter statement was made by CULLEN [107] because he found it "difficult to see how arteriosclerosis, thrombosis, or embolism could produce this clinical picture" of anterior ischemic optic neuropathy, which, in light of present

knowledge of the pathogenesis of this disorder (p. 14) is not a valid statement. In a recent study of serial sections of temporal artery biopsy, it has been concluded that the chances of having a negative biopsy in temporal arteritis are practically nil [90]. CULLEN [107] emphasized that temporal artery biopsy should be taken from the side of anterior ischemic optic neuropathy, but I have seen biopsies from the side of the normal eye that showed evidence of temporal arteritis. CULLEN [109] pointed out that temporal artery biopsy is always positive for arteritis up to six months after the onset of the disorder and has seen it to be positive for up to 26 months. Classically, in temporal arteritis the temporal arteries are painful, tender, nodular, pulseless, and thickened. The relationship of temporal artery biopsy histopathologic changes to atherosclerotic anterior ischemic optic neuropathy is discussed on p. 115.

In the present study superficial temporal artery biopsy was carried out in all patients with an erythrocyte sedimentation rate higher than 20 mm. The biopsy findings and their relation to visual acuity and erythrocyte sedimentation rate are given in Table 12.

In group (a) seven patients reported within three days of onset of anterior ischemic neuropathy, three within two weeks and one after two months. In group (b) they were seen within 2 to 6 weeks after the onset of anterior ischemic optic neuropathy. In group (c) the first consultation was within one week by four patients, after two weeks by two, within 6 to 12 weeks by two, and $1^1/_2$ years by one patient. This suggests that patients with anterior ischemic optic neuropathy due to temporal arteritis were seen comparatively earlier than those with non-arteritic anterior ischemic optic neuropathy, mainly because their visual loss was more marked.

Table 12 indicates that visual loss was much less marked in patients without temporal arteritis, and they had a better prognosis than those with temporal arteritis. This is further illustrated by the following summary (Table 13).

Two of the patients in the present series had ulcerative necrosis of an area of scalp in the distribution of the superficial temporal artery.

Table 12. Relationship of temporal arteritis, erythrocyte sedimentation rate and visual acuity in anterior ischemic optic neuropathy

Temporal artery biopsy	Total number of		ESR in mm		Initial visual acuity (in eyes)							
	cases	eyes	Range	Mean	NPL	PL	HM	CF	6/60	6/36	6/18	6/12—6/6
(A) Positive	11	14	50—135	83±24	8	1	2	1	—	—	1	1
(B) Negative	5	6	20—69	46±18	—	—	1	—	1	1	—	3
(C) Biopsy not considered necessary	9	10	Less than 20	10±6	2	—	1	1	2	—	—	4

Table 13. Relationship of temporal arteritis and visual acuity

Temporal arteritis	Total number of		Initial/ final V.A.	Visual Acuity (% in eyes)								
	cases	eyes		NPL	PL	HM	C·F	6/60	6/36	6/18	6/12	6/9—6/5
Present	11	14	Initial	57	7	14	7	—	—	7	—	7
			Final	64	14	14	7	—	—	—	—	—
Absent	14	16	Initial	12[a]	—	12	6	19	6	—	25	19
			Final	—	—	12	25	6	12	—	6	39

[a] In this patient with bilateral NPL at first, the visual acuity improved to HM in both eyes within two weeks.

Systemic Examination

Most patients with anterior ischemic optic neuropathy have other systemic disorders that play an important role in its pathogenesis. The various systemic diseases, which can be associated with anterior ischemic optic neuropathy, are discussed later (Part III) and these include the following:

1. Generalized atherosclerosis and arteriosclerosis is the most common disorder.

2. Cardiovascular disorders, e.g., carotid artery disease, systemic arterial hypertension or hypotension, myocardial infarction or ischemia, heart failure, shock, etc., are also common.

3. Temporal arteritis is also an important (but less than 1 and 2) cause of anterior ischemic optic neuropathy.

4. Diabetes.

5. Collagen diseases, e.g., polyarteritis nodosa and lupus erythematous.

6. Massive or repeated blood loss.

7. Thromboangiitis obliterans.

8. Vasomotor disturbances, e.g., migraine, Raynaud's disease, cervical discopathies.

9. Syphilis.

10. Allergic disorders, e.g., serum sickness.

11. Hematologic disorders, e.g., polycythemia, thrombocytopenic purpura, sickle cell trait, leukemias and anemias, etc.

12. Pulseless disease.

There are, however, patients in whom it is not possible to pinpoint a systemic disorder to explain the development of anterior ischemic optic neuropathy.

In the present study the only abnormalities detected were in the cardiovascular system. Half of these patients suffered from arterial hypertension. A quarter, on the other hand, had a diastolic blood pressure of 60 to 70 mm Hg, with a systolic blood pressure of 100 to 110 mm Hg in three and 130 to 150 mm Hg in the other three. In only a quarter of them was blood pressure within normal limits. A third of the patients in this series had other cardiovascular disorders, e.g., carotid artery disease (in 2), intermittent claudication (in 1), migraine (in 1), previous history of venous stasis retinopathy in the contralateral eye (in 1), and congestive heart failure (in 2).

All of the above-mentioned cardiovascular diseases, in addition to low diastolic blood pressure (in 4) and hypertension (in 2), were seen in patients without temporal arteritis.

On investigating the correlation between abnormal systemic arterial blood pressure and visual loss, no perception of light was present in half of the patients with a diastolic blood pressure below 70 mm Hg and in only a quarter of those with hypertension.

Similarly BURDE [73] in his 45 patients with non-arteritic type of anterior ischemic optic neuropathy found a high incidence of associated cardiovascular disorders, e.g., diabetes mellitus in 13, hypertension in 7, both of them in 5, cardiac disease in 4, and cerebrovascular disease in 4.

These findings strongly emphasize that anterior ischemic optic neuropathy is generally an ocular manifestation of a systemic disease and every patient with this disorder requires a complete physical checkup by a physician, particularly for cardiovascular diseases. The onset of anterior ischemic optic neuropathy may be a clue to more serious cardiovascular disorders.

Differential Diagnosis

Anterior ischemic optic neuropathy, which is usually seen in persons past middle age, has the following essential features:

1. Visual disorders consisting of disturbance of visual acuity and/or a variety of visual field defects.

2. Edema of the optic disc which may be uniform or more marked in one sector during early stages and is followed by sectoral or complete optic atrophy a month or two later.

These features emphasize that this disorder must be differentiated from a large number of ocular, optic disc, optic nerve, intracranial, vascular and systemic diseases, which can produce one or more of the following:

1. Sudden or rapid loss of the entire or a part of the vision in one or both eyes, preceded by the presence or absence of amaurosis fugax.

2. Unilateral or bilateral edema of the optic disc associated with visual disorders and a variety of visual field defects.

3. Partial or complete unilateral or bilateral optic atrophy associated with visual disorders and a variety of visual field defects.

It is beyond the scope of this work to discusss all of the conditions that can have one or more of these three features, because there is such a large number of conditions that can present with these characteristics. However, I would like to stress that in patients who present for the first time with sectoral or complete optic atrophy of unknown etiology, anterior ischemic optic neuropathy should be considered as one of the diseases in differential diagnosis, particularly in elderly individuals. This is because every patient with anterior ischemic optic neuropathy about a couple of months after its onset has no edema of the disc but has optic atrophy (p. 31). LESSELL [352a] recently stated that "I am always dubious of the diagnosis (of anterior ischemic optic neuropathy) if there has been no phase of disc swelling. A surprising number of those patients who do not have swelling have turned out to have metastatic tumors of the optic nerve". This is a highly misleading and dangerous statement. As mentioned above, unless and until the patient with anterior ischemic optic neuropathy is seen during the early edematous phase, the short-lived edema of the optic disc may be completely missed. Thus, many patients with anterior ischemic optic neuropathy may be seen for the first time during the stage of optic atrophy. To imply that metastatic tumors of the optic nerve are a more common cause of optic atrophy than anterior ischemic optic neuropathy does not make sense to me because the occurrence of such tumors is exceptional whereas anterior ischemic optic neuropathy is seen not uncommonly. Unfortunately, many of the cases of anterior ischemic optic neuropathy are being missed because of lack of awareness of this disorder.

Treatment of Anterior Ischemic Optic Neuropathy

Anterior ischemic optic neuropathy is a serious blinding disease, with poor prognosis for the recovery of vision and a high probability that the second eye will be involved. Since we have only recently begun to understand its pathogenesis [255] (p. 14) and since most of the therapies tried so far have made no significant difference to any visual loss, such patients are generally given up as hopeless. The main therapeutic controversy lies in the management of non-arteritic type of anterior ischemic optic neuropathy, since patients with the temporal arteritis variety of this disorder are invariably treated with systemic corticosteroids, primarily to prevent the second eye from being involved. Most ophthalmologists do not treat patients with non-arteritic type of anterior ischemic optic neuropathy nor do they try to find a treatable associated systemic or ocular disorder, e.g., hypertension, diabetes, anemias, glaucoma, etc. (p. 22), but discard the patient with philosophic advice to accept the visual loss as a natural calamity.

In the present study, attempts were made to evaluate, systematically, systemic corticosteroid therapy in anterior ischemic optic neuropathy. When patients were treated early (i.e., while they still had edema of the optic disc) with large doses, there was visual improvement in a significant number of cases; almost all of these patients

had anterior ischemic optic neuropathy due to causes other than temporal arteritis. Since non-arteritic type of anterior ischemic optic neuropathy forms a much larger group than that with the temporal arteritis form of the disorder, there is a ray of hope in the gloomy picture of anterior ischemic optic neuropathy. Medical therapy to lower intraocular pressure, particularly acetazolamide (Diamox), also has been found helpful.

1. Review of Literature

There is a consensus of opinion that any patient suspected of having temporal arteritis must be treated immediately with high doses of systemic corticosteroids not to benefit the eye with anterior ischemic optic neuropathy, but to prevent the second eye from becoming involved [37, 44, 105, 384, 400, 417, 421, 467, 565]. The disorder has been reported to spread to the previously normal eye after the systemic corticosteroids were withdrawn; one such report is by CULLEN [105]. MILLER [389] reported the onset of central retinal artery occlusion in a patient whose temporal arteritis had apparently been controlled effectively with prednisone for three years. This report is very dubious and probably irrelevant because occlusion of the central retinal artery could have been totally unrelated to temporal arteritis and merely a coincidental finding; MILLER [389] made no mention of the state of the optic disc in this patient. Involvement of the second eye has been noticed within two weeks after steroid therapy had been started [384, 568]; presumably steroid therapy was started too late. In a dubious report, SCHIMEK et al. [477] claimed to have restored vision in temporal arteritis anterior ischemic optic neuropathy by retrobulbar injection of steroids. It has been claimed that vision in an eye with anterior ischemic optic neuropathy due to temporal arteritis improved when steroids were started less than a day after the disorder began [185, 431]. SCHNEIDER et al. [483a] reported recovery of vision in about 15 percent of eyes with steroid therapy for temporal arteritis, even from no perception of light. Steroids must be continued for at least six months and probably for 2 to 3 years [384].

As stated above, the main therapeutic controversy lies in the management of non-arteritic type of anterior ischemic optic neuropathy. Anticoagulants have been tried with claimed success in these cases [342, 474]. BONAMOUR [60] advised giving subtenon vasodilators and steroids during the early stages and claimed some success, while CALMETTES et al. [77] found vasodilators of no use, although others [185, 474] have claimed success by treating the patient on the day of occlusion. Another treatment that has been tried and that has been claimed to be successful, is the retrobulbar subtenon injection of atropine sulfate, 0.5–1 ml of a 1 percent solution twice weekly for 10–15 injections [95].

Interest has recently been shown in the possible use of diphenylhydantoin (DPH) in the treatment of anterior ischemic optic neuropathy. The basis for its use has been previous studies showing that it lowers intracellular concentrations of sodium in hypoxic nerves, possibly by activating the sodium extrusion process via sodium-potassium ATPase activity [438]. Electroretinographic studies on the hypoxic retina have shown that the antiepileptic drug, DPH, protected the activity of the retina from the inhibiting effect of oxygen deprivation by lowering intracellular sodium [287]. Diphenylhydantoin has been reported to improve the conduction of the action potential of Purkinje fibers during hypoxia [23]. The optic nerve contains an oxygen-dependent system for the accumulation of rubidium, and diphenylhydantoin partially protects this transport system in the optic nerve subjected to anoxia [28]. Diphenylhydantoin has been used with some preliminary success, in glaucoma, to counteract the effects of anoxia on nerve fibers and achieve functional recovery. A double blind study of this drug in anterior ischemic optic neuropathy has so far shown that it is not effective [73]; the cases included in the trial were late, with well-developed optic atrophy.

FOULDS [170] treated 11 of 21 patients with non-arteritic type of anterior ischemic optic neuropathy with systemic corticosteroids on the assumption that anoxia in the neuropathy leads to increased capillary permeability in the optic nerve head. This increased permeability is an important factor in the production of visual loss since it impedes further capillary circulation in the optic nerve head. He gave 60–80 mg of prednisolone for three to four days, after which dosage was reduced rapidly. In comparing his treated and untreated cases, he found that the former group had improved subjectively within 24 hours and objectively in 3 to 4 days. Of the treated group, eight patients showed significant improvement, while in the untreated group only two showed a similar degree of improvement. In a subsequent report FOULDS [171] found that visual acuity improved in 85 percent of the treated cases compared to 45 percent of the patients in the untreated group. He advocated [170], but did not try acetazolamide (Diamox) to lower intraocular pressure and thereby improve vascular perfusion in the optic disc. SANDERS [471] mentioned giving only retrobulbar steroids, but only in a single case.

2. Present Study

In the present series the following treatments were given:

a) Systemic Corticosteroid Therapy

To assess the efficacy of this treatment all patients with anterior ischemic optic neuropathy of the present series were divided into three groups. The results are given in Table 6.

Group 1. The group was composed of 11 patients with temporal arteritis, as confirmed by temporal artery biopsy, and who were treated with steroids.

These patients were usually given 40–60 mg of prednisolone orally, frequently combined with an initial dose of 40 units of adrenocorticotropic hormone. Dosage and duration of therapy were guided by the erythrocyte sedimentation rate; there was a rapid reduction of the dose initially (because of a rapid fall in the erythrocyte sedimentation rate at this stage) and a very slow tapering off later. Patients with temporal arteritis required prolonged steroid therapy because suddenly reducing or stopping the drug prematurely sometimes produced visual symptoms in the normal eye and a rise in erythrocyte sedimentation rate. Usually a maintenance dose of 5–10 mg daily for many months, if not years, was required to safeguard the normal eye. The steroids were still being given up to their last follow-up in six patients with temporal arteritis, five of whom had the disorder for 6 to 14 months and one for 29 months. In patients with no perception of light in both eyes and temporal arteritis, steroids were stopped as soon as the erythrocyte sedimentation rate settled down.

Group 2. Patients with no evidence of temporal arteritis and on steroid therapy; there were eight patients in this category.

This group was initially put on a regimen similar to that of Group 1, but steroids were given only for 2 to 3 months. In two patients with bilateral anterior ischemic optic neuropathy in whom some vision was retained this regimen was continued for 6 to 12 months by the ophthalmologist in charge.

Group 3. Patients with no evidence of temporal arteritis who were not treated with steroids; this group had six patients.

These patients were followed as those in Group 1 and 2 but without steroid therapy.

The results are summarized in Table 6. Comparing the outcome of visual acuity in the three groups, the best was in Group 2 patients where 75 percent showed improvement compared to only 17 percent in Group 3. Groups 2 and 3 are comparable, Group 3 serving as a control for Group 2. The outcome in eyes with anterior ischemic optic neuropathy due to temporal arteritis, i.e., Group 1, was the worst in the series. This study thus strongly suggests that systemic corticosteroids have a beneficial effect in patients with non-arteritic type of anterior ischemic optic neuropathy and confirms the results of FOULDS [170, 171]. Improvement with steroid therapy

has been further confirmed by 19 of 22 cases of Category II (p. 25) not included in Table 6.

The frequent accurate recording of visual fields with the Goldmann perimeter demonstrates more marked and constant improvement in visual fields during treatment. In some cases of partial anterior ischemic optic neuropathy, central vision may show no significant change, either because a central scotoma produced low visual acuity even when visual fields improved remarkably or because central visual acuity may have been normal all along despite marked visual field defects. This study indicates that visual fields are a much better guide in assessing improvement of anterior ischemic optic neuropathy than central visual acuity alone. If improvement in visual acuity and/or visual fields is used as a criterion of success, then the beneficial effect of steroid therapy in Group 2 is seen to be even greater than that shown in Table 6. It is most unfortunate that these are the cases that usually are abandoned without treatment by ophthalmologists. The following case report (belonging to Category II, p. 25) illustrates the efficacy of corticosteroids in Group 2-type patients.

A man, with unstable diabetes since 1938 and on insulin, was first seen on October 31, 1973. He reported that he woke up on September 15, 1973 to find that he "could not see from the inner half of the left eye"; he had a central scotoma. His visual symptoms had shown no significant change since onset, other than a questionable improvement 3 to 4 days before he sought treatment. Two weeks before attending this department, he had noticed that vision in his right eye had deteriorated to an inferior altitudinal field defect over the next 3 to 4 days and subsequently had not changed. The patient also reported that he had a right lateral rectus palsy for about one month, 4 to 5 years earlier. His right big toe had been amputated because of gangrene on July 10, 1973. He had also been taking thyroid for the last 3 to 4 years for hypothyroidism. He had smoked 1 to 1 1/2 packages of cigarettes daily since the age of 25.

On ocular examination, the patient's visual acuity in both eyes was limited to only counting fingers. His mid-dilated pupils reacted slug-gishly. Fundus examination revealed a mild degree of diabetic retinopathy in both eyes; the right optic disc showed generalized edema, maxi-mal in the superior temporal part and minimal in the inferior nasal part (Fig. 38a). There were flame-shaped hemorrhages in the optic disc and peripapillary region—maximal in the superior temporal area. The disc was slightly hyperemic, and there was no pallor. The left optic disc showed slight pallor in the temporal part, mild edema, and one flame-shaped hemorrhage nasally (Fig. 38b). In the left eye the visual fields showed nasal hemianopia with central scotoma (typical of lateral posterior ciliary artery occlu-sion) [247] (Fig. 38c_1) and in the right eye, an inferior nasal quadrantic field defect with central scotoma (Fig. 38d_1). The patient's disorder was diagnosed as bilateral anterior ischemic optic neuropathy and he was admitted to the hospital. In consultation with the diabetic department, he was put on prednisone, 15 mg four times daily, and long-acting acetazolamide (Diamox) 500 mg twice daily on November 1, 1973.

Follow-up. On November 6, 1973 visual acuity in both eyes was 6/120; this had improved to 6/30 in the left and 6/60 in the right by November 19, 1973. On November 26, 1973 both eyes, indi-vidually, could see better than 6/30; binocular vision was 6/21. When seen on January 14, 1974 his visual acuities were 6/18 and 6/24, with sco-toma in the right and left eyes respectively. They were not improving any more. Changes in the visual fields, shown in Figures 38c and d, demon-strate a very noticeable progressive improvement up to November 26, 1973 and have since been stationary. The improvement in visual acuity, although considerable, was not as evident because small central scotoma were present in both eyes.

Edema of the optic disc in the right eye started to subside on November 6th, while in the left eye no significant change in the disc was seen until November 19th. On November 26th, the left disc was not edematous; the right showed only a slight degree of edema. No marked pallor was visible in either disc. When seen on January 14, 1974, and subsequently both discs were

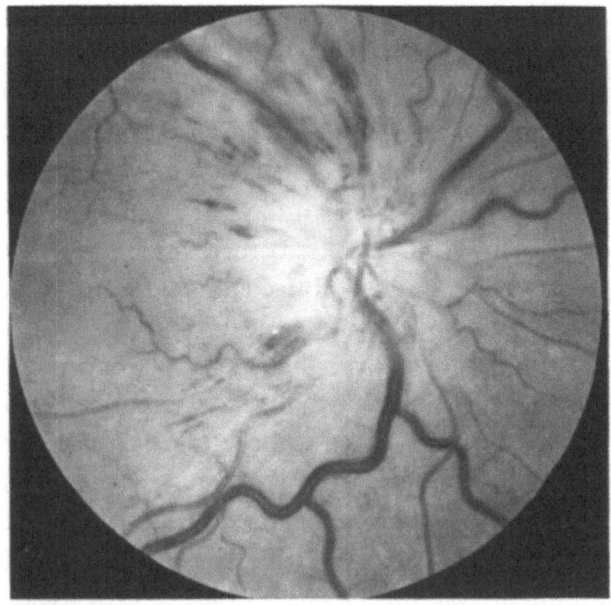 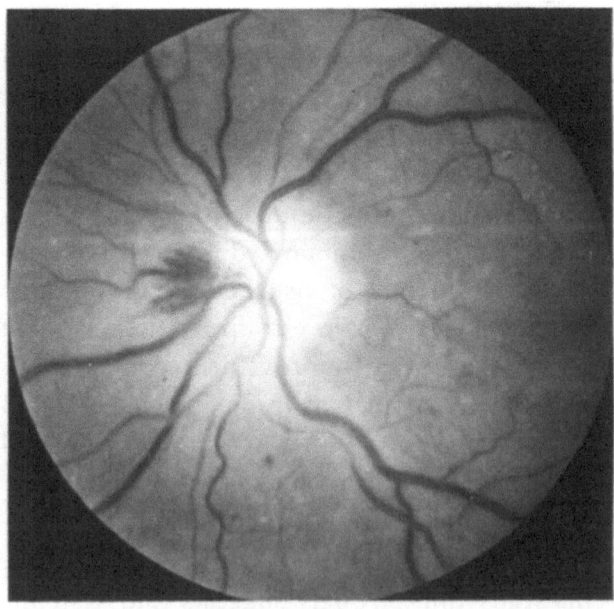

a   b

Fig. 38
a and b) Fundus photographs of right and left eyes respectively on October 31, 1973.
c and d) GOLDMANN perimetry records on November 1, 7 and 26, 1973 and June 6, 1974.
c) Left eye visual fields d) Right eye visual fields

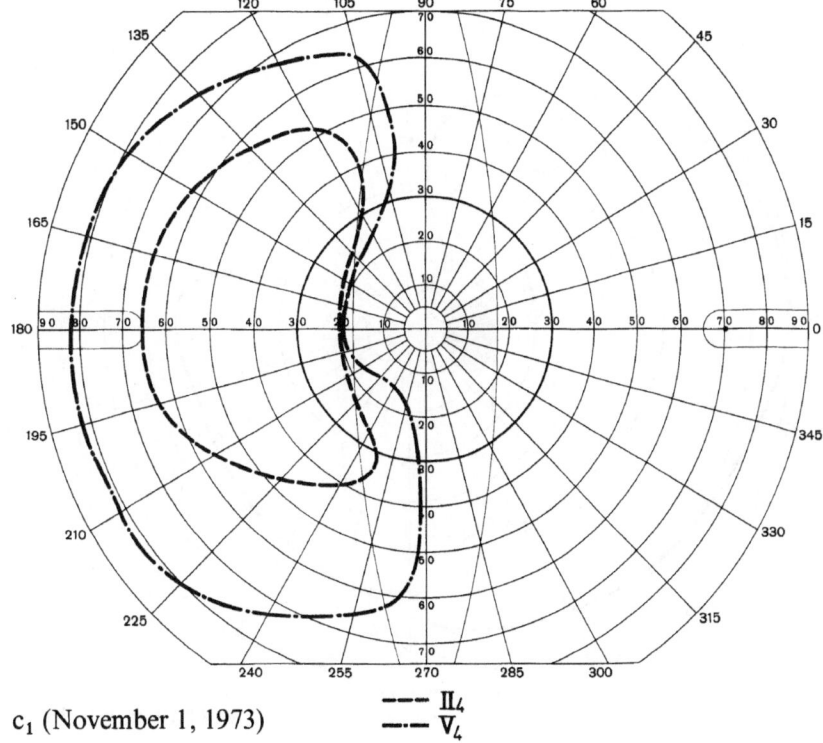

c_1 (November 1, 1973)

---- II_4
-·-·- V_4

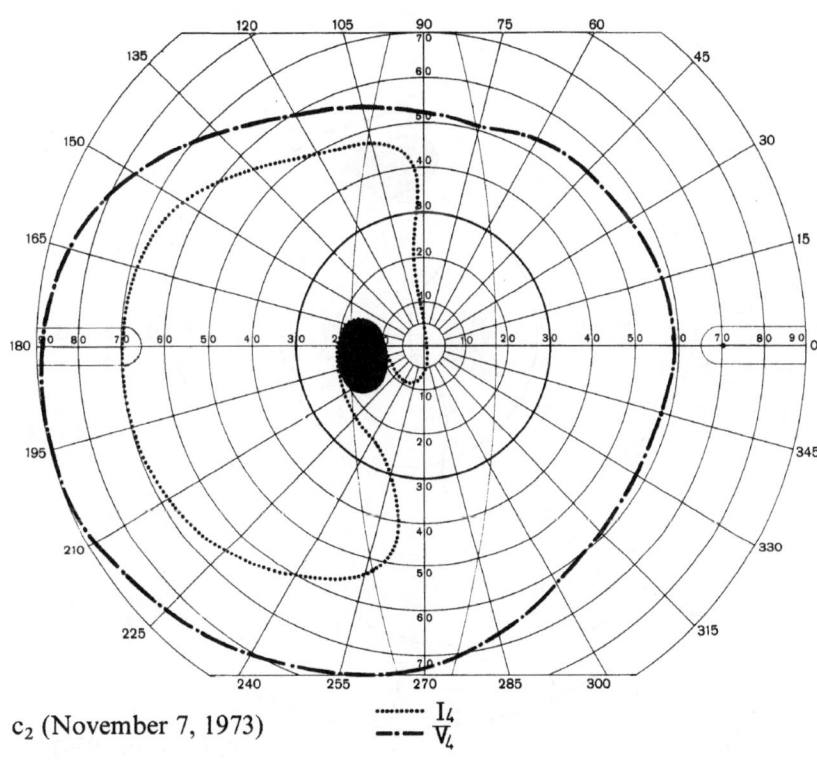

Fig. 38 (continued) c_2 (November 7, 1973)

··········· I_4
-·-·- V_4

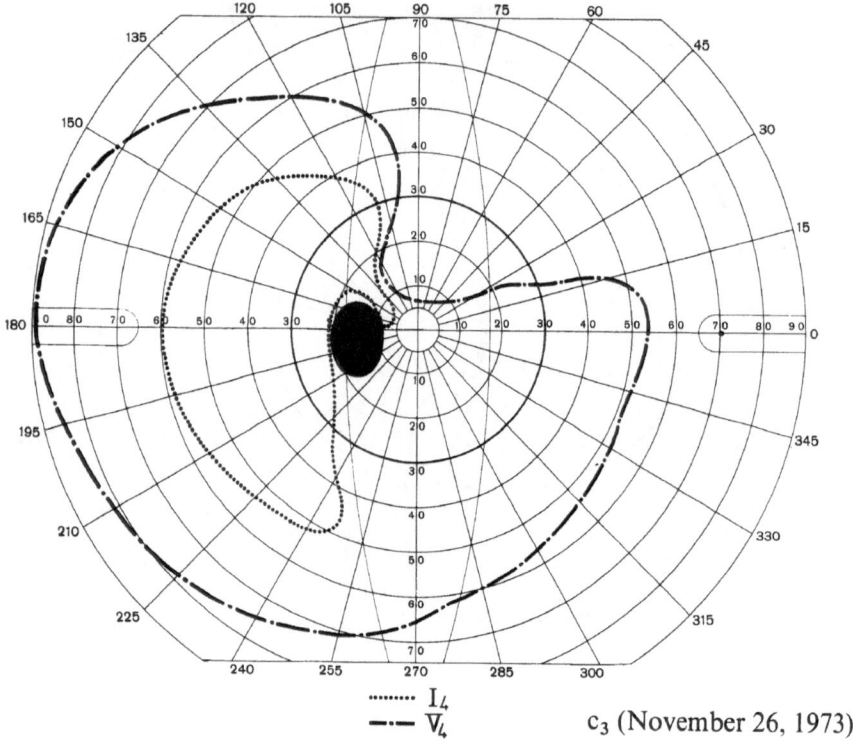

$\cdots\cdots$ I_4
$-\cdot-\cdot-$ V_4 c_3 (November 26, 1973)

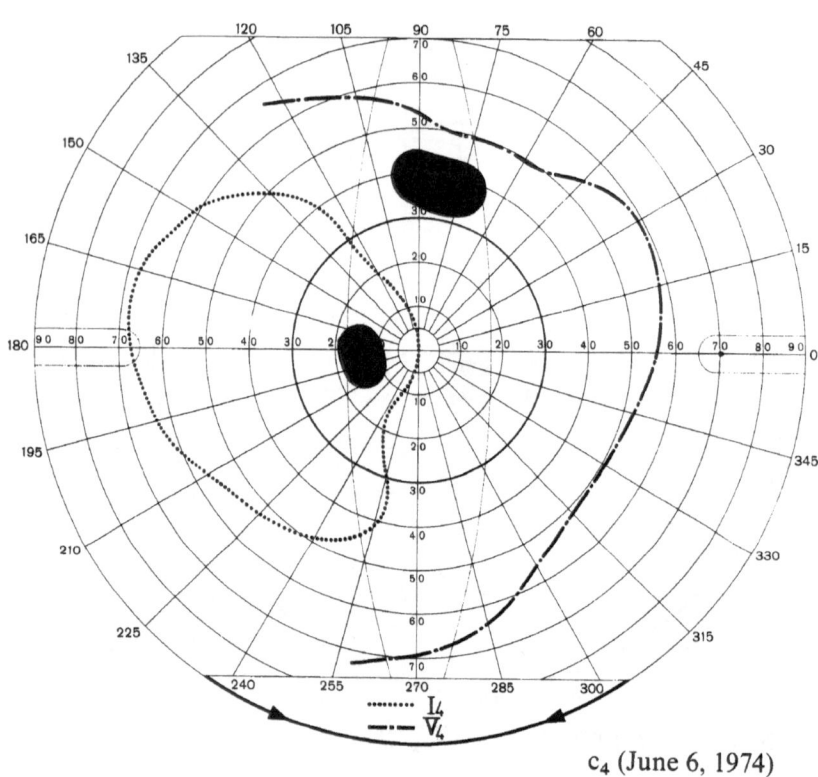

$\cdots\cdots$ I_4
$-\cdot-\cdot-$ V_4

c_4 (June 6, 1974)   **Fig. 38** (continued)

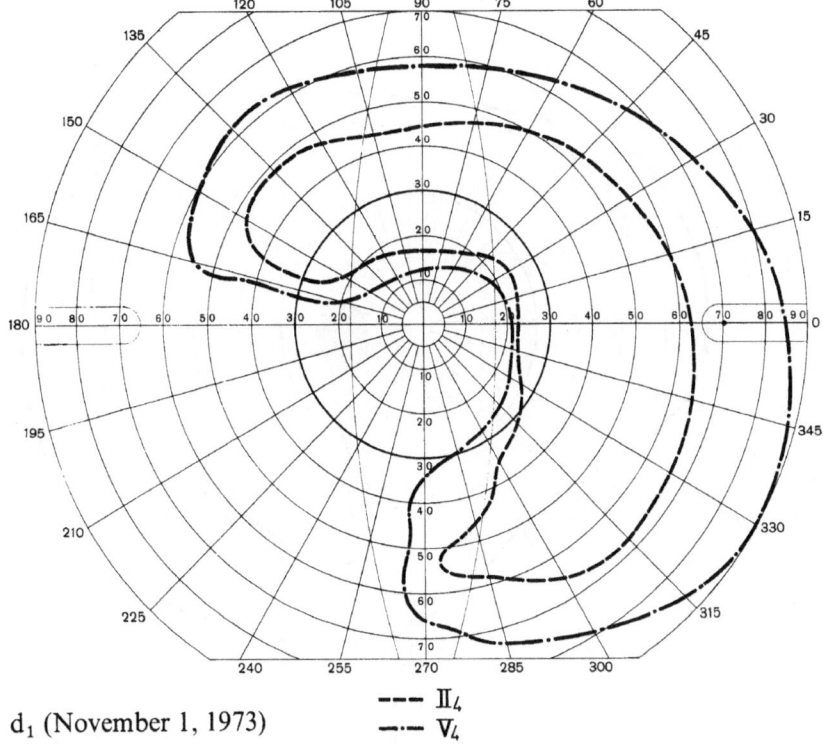

d₁ (November 1, 1973)

--- II_4
-.- V_4

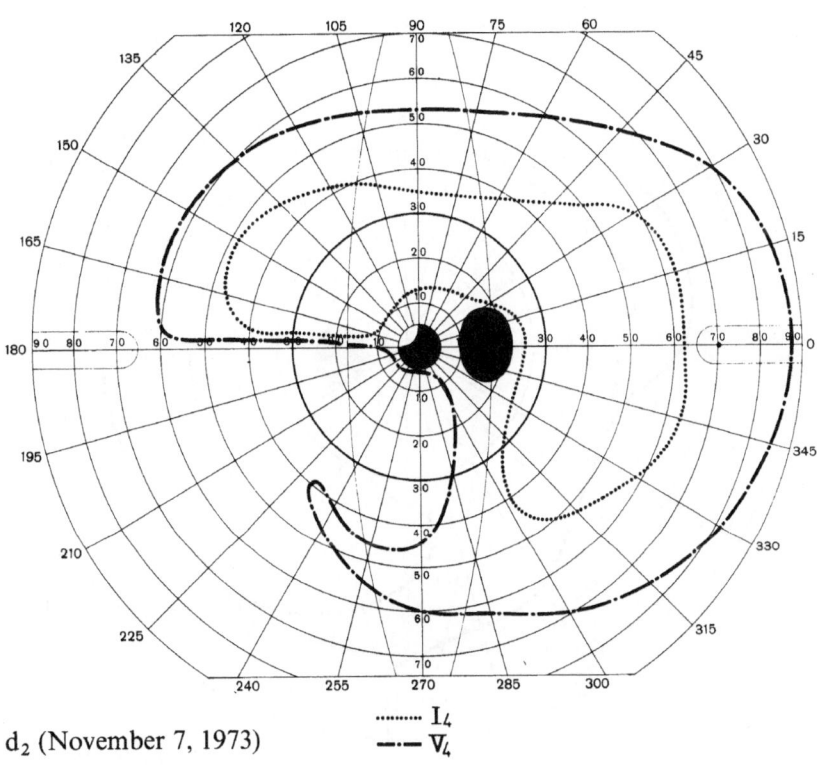

Fig. 38 (continued)   d₂ (November 7, 1973)

.... I_4
-.- V_4

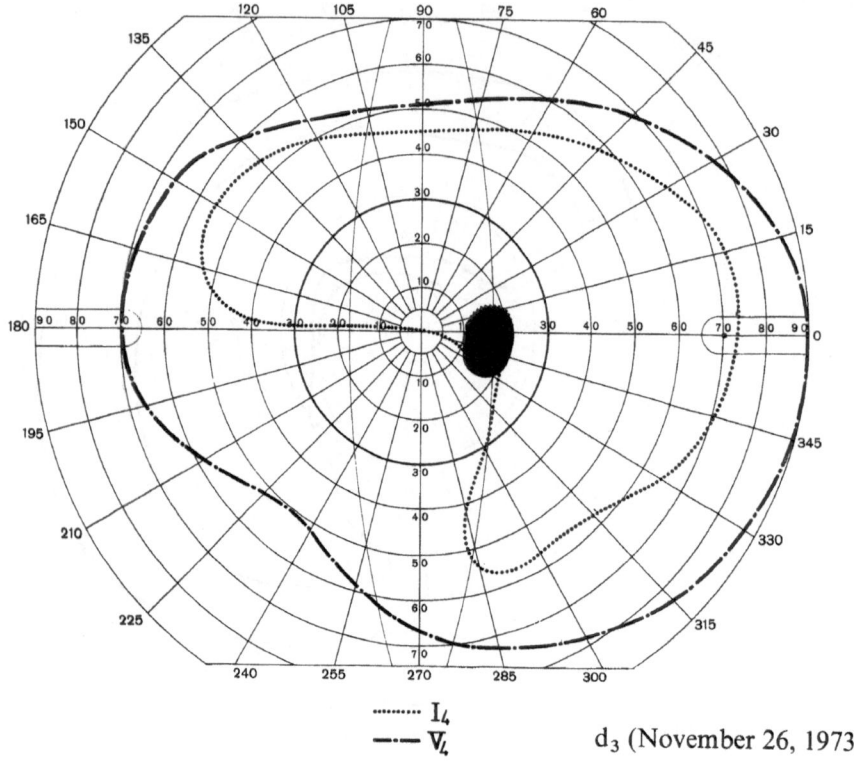

d$_3$ (November 26, 1973)

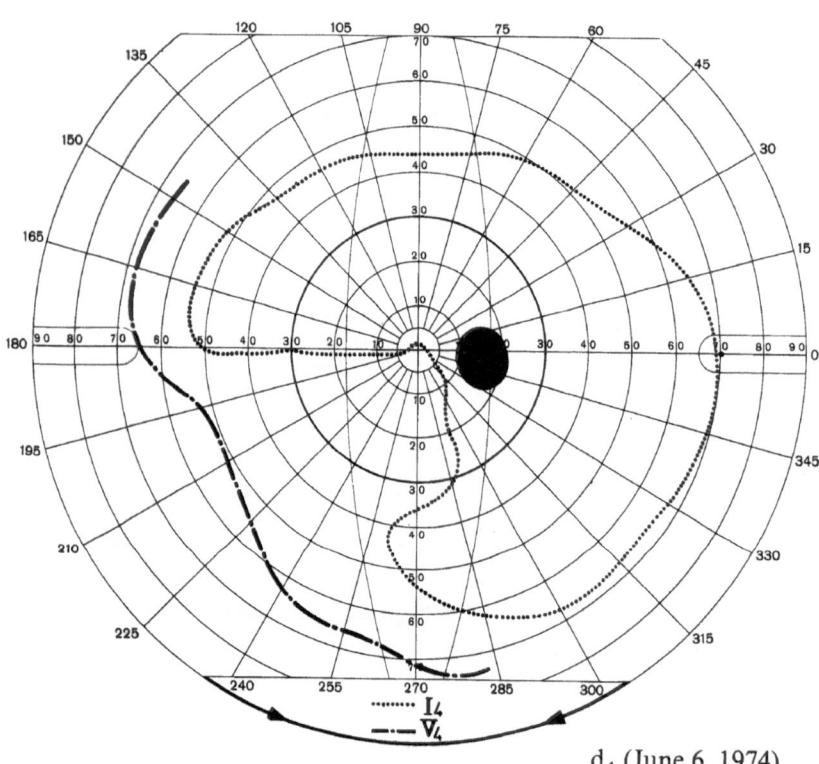

d$_4$ (June 6, 1974)

Fig. 38 (continued)

almost uniformly pale, with well-defined edges.

The patient was on 60 mg prednisone daily up to November 21st, when the dose was decreased by 5 mg daily to 30 mg daily; he was discharged on November 26th. He stopped his steroids on December 15, 1973, tapering gradually.

During the time the patient received corticosteroids, the diabetic department continuously supervised his diabetes but was unable to control it since the patient was not at all cooperative and, surprisingly, had frequent attacks of hypoglycemia.

Comments. This case clearly illustrates the great usefulness of corticosteroids in improving visual loss in anterior ischemic optic neuropathy. Moreover, it demonstrates the remarkable capacity of optic nerve fibers to recover their function when treatment was not started until six weeks after the ischemic process began in one eye (two weeks in the other). Visual loss in ischemia, therefore, should not be regarded as irreversible, and every possible effort must be made to resuscitate the nerve fibers. This case also points to the twin morals that all visual problems in the diabetic should not be ascribed to diabetic retinopathy, and that diabetes is not necessarily a contraindication to steroid therapy.

Critics will argue that my corticosteroid therapy trial in patients with anterior ischemic optic neuropathy not due to temporal arteritis has not been a double-blind randomized controlled study, and that the claims made for the efficacy of such a therapy may not be justified but may represent a natural recovery. Almost all the previous series of patients with anterior ischemic optic neuropathy not due to temporal arteritis reported in the literature have shown either no or insignificant recovery in large majority of their cases; those findings could be compared with those seen in group 3 of the present study. On the other hand, group 2 patients of the present series (i.e., treated with corticosteroids) showed improvement of visual acuity and/or visual fields in a significant number of cases. The decision to put some of the patients without temporal arteritis in Category I (p. 25) on corticosteroids and not others was more or less arbitrary. This was done by the ophthalmologists in charge of the patients, and main factors which influenced them were the initial suspicion of the possible presence of temporal arteritis in these cases, and a marked visual loss. I followed their fundus lesions, visual acuity and visual fields without knowing what therapy, if any, they were receiving from their ophthalmologists. The benificial effect of corticosteroids was not realised until the data of Category I were analysed three years after the start of the study. Thus no prejudice one way or the other was present while the study was in progress. In Category II (p. 25) there were two patients who had suffered a partial anterior ischemic optic neuropathy with no recovery and no treatment some years previously, and were referred to me because they had developed a similar lesion a few days previously in the follow eye. On treating these patients with corticosteroids, there was a significant improvement in the visual acuity and visual field defects in the eye with recent anterior ischemic optic neuropathy. Based on all these observations, I have been fairly convinced by the benificial effect of corticosteroids in these patients. However, to have still more definite evidence I am at present doing a double-blind randomized controlled trial of corticosteroids in patients with anterior ischemic optic neuropathy due to causes other than temporal arteritis and I hope to have a significant number of patients within the next few years.

b) Acetazolamide

Acetazolamide (Diamox) is administered to lower intraocular pressure so as to improve perfusion pressure in vessels of the optic nerve head, and to improve the imbalance between intraocular and perfusion pressure—the most important factor in the pathogenesis of anterior ischemic optic neuropathy. In the present series acetazolamide was given to six patients in the form of long-acting Diamox, 500 mg twice daily. It was given mainly in cases with a progressive loss of vision or visual fields after the initial insult and damage to the optic nerve head. The pretreatment intraocular pressure in all of these patients was less than 20 mm Hg on applanation tonometry. Further deterioration was prevented. Angiography in some of these patients showed poor perfusion pressure in the posterior ciliary artery system, even in the contralateral normal eye. Thus, intravenous fluorescein angiography can help to identify patients who could benefit from acetazolamide. This small trial has given some encouraging results, but to be effective acetazolamide must be used in conjunction with systemic steroids during the initial stages of anterior ischemic optic neuropathy.

Based on these observations from the present study, I would recommend the following regimen of therapy in patients with anterior ischemic optic neuropathy.

1. Patients with anterior ischemic optic neuropathy due to temporal arteritis should be given systemic corticosteroids to safeguard the second eye; they should be given high doses, e.g., up to 80 mg daily or higher, of prednisolone orally to begin with, and the dose should be regulated by the erythrocyte sedimentation rate. In addition, they should be given acetazolamide to lower intraocular pressure as much as possible so as to help the perfusion of blood vessels in the optic nerve head. The outcome in these cases is not good, but further treatment with acetazolamide is worth a trial for about four weeks from the onset of anterior ischemic optic neuropathy. The dose of steroids is guided by the erythrocyte sedimentation rate and the drug should be continued until the erythrocyte sedimentation rate remains normal even after the steroids are discontinued, and there are no symptoms.

2. In anterior ischemic optic neuropathy not due to temporal arteritis, systemic corticosteroids should be administered in an initial dose of 60 to 80 mg daily, and slowly tapered thereafter so that treatment is continued for about two months, i.e., during the time the disc is edematous. Reduction of edema by steroid therapy would relieve pressure on disc capillaries and restore some circulation in the vessels of the optic nerve head. At the same time acetazolamide therapy to lower intraocular pressure as far as pos-

sible would help further perfusion of the vessels. In ischemia of the optic nerve fibers, the function of the fibers may be impaired for some time before they undergo irreversible damage, just as a starving man who is unable to perform his job but is still alive can be restored to normal functional capacity by an adequate supply of food. *Thus, the fact that a person has marked visual loss with edema of the optic disc does not mean his loss of vision is irreversible unless all restorative methods have failed.* Once optic atrophy has been established, steroids are of no use. Acetazolamide has, in some cases, helped to prevent further deterioration due to a poor perfusion pressure in arteriosclerotic posterior ciliary arteries.

3. Prophylactic Measures against Anterior Ischemic Optic Neuropathy

Since anterior ischemic optic neuropathy, particularly in temporal arteritis, is a blinding disease with poor prognosis for recovery of vision, and the likelihood of the second eye being involved after the first, it is worthwhile to consider the possible preventive measures that could be taken to lower the incidence of blindness due to anterior ischemic optic neuropathy. These can be considered under the following two major causes of anterior ischemic optic neuropathy.

a) Temporal Arteritis Anterior Ischemic Optic Neuropathy

Preventive measures would include early and adequate systemic corticosteroid therapy in temporal arteritis. The following indicate that such therapy is needed.

a) Early diagnosis of temporal arteritis, i.e., before ocular symptoms develop; anterior ischemic optic neuropathy should be anticipated in all patients with temporal arteritis and polymyalgia rheumatica.

b) Amaurosis fugax should be considered a danger signal.

c) If a patient has anterior ischemic optic neuropathy in one eye, therapy should be started immediately even if the diagnosis of temporal arteritis is not conclusive. *This is an ophthalmic emergency.*

b) Arteriosclerotic Anterior Ischemic Optic Neuropathy

In patients with marked cardiovascular disease, the following features make them specially vulnerable to anterior ischemic optic neuropathy.

a) Hypertension, evidence of marked arteriosclerosis, and carotid artery disease, a tendency toward systemic arterial hypotension, congestive heart failure, myocardial ischemia, anesthesia, and surgical or nonsurgical shock.

b) Very low ophthalmodynamometric pressure in the ophthalmic artery, or easily induced pulsation with gentle pressure on the eyeball, may be indirect evidence of poor perfusion in the posterior ciliary arteries.

c) Amaurosis fugax. Usually this is considered to be due to migrating emboli in the retinal arteries. In the absence of ophthalmoscopic evidence of such emboli, posterior ciliary artery ischemia may be responsible. Moreover emboli can also become lodged in the posterior ciliary arteries. *Attacks of altitudinal hemianopia would suggest impending anterior ischemic optic neuropathy.*

d) Any tendency towards elevated intraocular pressure or glaucoma. In these patients anterior ischemic optic neuropathy should be anticipated because any sudden imbalance between perfusion pressure in the posterior ciliary arteries and intraocular pressure will precipitate anterior ischemic optic neuropathy.

Preventive measures should include:

1. Avoiding any sudden fall in systemic arterial blood pressure, e.g., hypotensive anesthesia, sudden lowering of blood pressure, congestive heart failure, etc.

2. Medical therapy to improve systemic circulatory hemodynamics.

3. Preventing any sudden rise in intraocular pressure, e.g., angle closure and after ocular surgery (e.g., cataract extraction and retinal detachment).

4. Keeping intraocular pressure as low as possible by medical means, e.g., miotics and acetazolamide.

5. In every patient with a visual disturbance that begins immediately after recovering from shock, anterior ischemic optic neuropathy should be considered a first possibility.

6. If anterior ischemic optic neuropathy does develop, its presence should be recognized and systemic corticosteroid therapy instituted immediately to reduce edema of the disc and assist residual circulation in the optic nerve head so that nerve fibers will survive. This can help toward recovery of vision. I am stressing this point because these cases are so often dismissed as hopeless and not worth treating.

Recurrence: SMITH [508a] claimed that "*ischemic optic neuropathy* virtually always occurs in the other eye, but it *never recurs in the same eye.*" I, however, have seen patients to have two successive attacks in the same eye. Occurrence of anterior ischemic optic neuropathy in the fellow eye is much more common than in the same eye but every patient does not always get involvement of the second eye.

Part III   Systemic and Ocular Diseases Associated with Anterior Ischemic Optic Neuropathy

From the discussion on the pathogenesis of anterior ischemic optic neuropathy (Part I) and its clinical picture (Part II), it is evident that anterior ischemic optic neuropathy is a manifestation of a systemic and/or ocular disease process. It would be desirable, therefore, to discuss briefly such diseases for a better understanding of anterior ischemic optic neuropathy.

A. Systemic Diseases

1. Temporal Arteritis or Giant Cell Arteritis

This is an important cause, though not the most common, of anterior ischemic optic neuropathy. This self-limited and rarely fatal disease, peculiar to the aged (55–80 years [94]; 60–83 years [552]) and of unknown etiology, was first noticed by HUTCHINSON [294] and SCHMIDT [471] but described as a definite clinical entity by HORTON et al. [289]. Ocular involvement frequently is seen in temporal arteritis (in 38 percent [62, 79], 40 percent [70, 382], 44 percent [552], 45 percent [40], 50 percent [506], 33 to 57 percent [564], more than half [36], and 70 percent [421]). The most common ocular complication is loss of vision in one or both eyes [3, 44, 62, 65, 94, 97, 117, 126, 288, 306, 307, 313, 325, 342, 345, 347, 368, 382, 400, 414, 417, 431, 461, 469, 487, 494, 511, 519, 552, 565]. The incidence of visual loss has been reported to be 20 percent [275], 25 percent [382], 26.3 percent [79], 33.3 percent [104], and 42 percent [36]; amaurosis fugax has been reported in 20 percent, visual impairment in 44 percent and bilateral blindness in 12 percent [552]; blindness was bilateral in 34 percent and

unilateral in 21 percent; bilateral moderate visual loss was reported in 6 percent [400]. When the vision in one eye is lost, chances that it will be lost in the other eye within the next few days or weeks are even [466]. However, if the second eye is not affected for two months, the prognosis is good [552]. The visual loss is usually sudden and permanent in temporal arteritis, though CROSBY et al. [104] reported that a patient who had been completely blind for one week recovered full vision. The loss of vision may be gradual and vary from mistiness and various field defects to complete blindness. It may be altitudinal [36, 549, 552] and the initial loss may occur in the lower half of the field [94, 113, 306, 307, 441].

The most frequent fundus finding is anterior ischemic optic neuropathy with a pale, edematous, and swollen disc [3, 36, 40, 44, 62, 65, 70, 81, 94, 96, 97, 106–108, 113, 117, 126, 151, 183, 189, 306, 307, 325, 342, 345, 347, 349, 368, 382–384, 396, 398, 400, 414, 417, 420, 421, 431, 432, 466, 468, 469, 494, 498, 500, 511, 519, 549, 552]. Frequently there are small hemorrhages on or near the swollen disc. In addition, other fundus changes may be seen, e.g., retinal vein congestion, central retinal artery occlusion [329, 421, 552], phlebitis of one of the retinal veins [94, 288], periarterial retinal exudates [318], and hemorrhages and exudates in the retina [494]. BIRKHEAD et al. [44] found signs of anterior ischemic optic neuropathy in 32.7 percent, retrobulbar neuritis in 1.8 percent, optic atrophy in 3.6 percent, transient amaurosis in 12.7 percent and, in the remainder, visual loss due to retinal involvement. PARSONS-SMITH [421], in his cases found anterior ischemic optic neuropathy in 14 percent, retrobulbar neuritis in 6 percent, optic atrophy in 4 percent, central retinal artery occlusion in 12 percent, retinal branch occlusion in

2 percent, central retinal vein thrombosis in 4 percent, and hemorrhages and exudates in 8 percent. WAGENER *et al.* [552] found anterior ischemic optic neuropathy in 64 percent, central retinal artery occlusion in 2 percent, central retinal artery occlusion plus central retinal vein occlusion in 2 percent, and optic atrophy in 24 percent. PALM [417] found anterior ischemic optic neuropathy in 74 percent, central retinal artery occlusion in 9 percent, a combination of anterior ischemic optic neuropathy and central retinal artery occlusion in 13 percent, and vascular constriction in 4 percent. MEADOWS [384] saw anterior ischemic optic neuropathy in 57.5 percent of cases of temporal arteritis.

In addition to anterior ischemic optic neuropathy, the eyes in temporal arteritis may show other lesions. Transient or constant diplopia due to extraocular muscle involvement, with or without visual disturbance, is seen in 10–15 percent [13, 38, 44, 285, 358, 384, 467, 500, 552]. The diplopia appears during the active phase of arteritis some weeks after the headache, although occasionally headache and diplopia appear together as the first signs [384]. Diplopia is thought to be due to ischemia of the III, IV, and VI cranial nerves or possibly to brain stem ischemia [384]. According to some authors, it involves the vertical eye muscles first and most often [285], while according to others, it involves VI nerve palsy [500]. The cranial nerve palsy is often incomplete, sparing the pupil, and may be unilateral or bilateral. Complete or partial recovery in some months is generally the rule [384]. Even proptosis has been recorded [500].

Iritis also has been reported [335]. I, too, have seen a patient with temporal arteritis with marked anterior uveitis and ocular hypotony, possibly due to marked ocular ischemia.

In addition to ocular symptoms, there are general symptoms in temporal arteritis to which a passing reference would not be out of place here. Headache is usually mentioned as a constant feature of temporal arteritis [169, 467] but it has been found to be inconstant [44], and even may be absent. When present, it is of recent onset and often located superficially in the scalp, in the temporal and periorbital regions. In addition to headache, there may be malaise, weakness, muscular and joint pains, anorexia, fever, night sweats, etc. Vertigo, tinnitus and hearing loss [169], hepatosplenomegaly and arthritis [347], weight loss [305], cerebral or brain stem infarction [384], and cardiac infarction [384, 511] may occur. Recently polymyalgia rheumatica has been emerging as an important disease because of its associations as a precursor of, or as part of, giant cell arteritis.

A frequent and striking feature in these patients is the degree of euphoria they have [382, 384], so that even bilateral complete blindness is accepted philosophically as if nothing significant had gone wrong with them; this may trick a beginner in estimating their visual loss, because even if the patient cannot perceive light, he may still say that he can see you and everything around. This euphoria may be due to coincidental cerebral ischemia, but visual symptoms of cerebral origin are rare [384]. A high erythrocyte sedimentation rate is typical of these cases, and is discussed on p. 97.

Systemic symptoms indicate a more generalized arteritis and this has been proven by necropsies [79, 84, 94, 103, 113, 203, 275, 325, 385, 511, 512]; the various arteries involved are the aorta, pulmonary, coronary, innominate, carotids, temporal, subclavian, radial, mesenteric, coeliac, renal, iliac, vertebral, femoral, popliteal, dorsalis pedis and, in the orbit, the ophthalmic, central retinal, and posterior ciliary arteries. Histologic changes are those of granulomatous panarteritis, infiltration with giant cells, lymphocytes, disruption of the internal elastic lamina due to focal necrosis in the media, and a lumen narrowed due to marked internal thickening and often occluded by an organized thrombus. Temporal artery biopsy showing these characteristic changes has been used as a test for the presence or absence of temporal arteritis. This is discussed on p. 98.

SIMMONS and COGAN [500] stressed the existence of a variety of anterior ischemic optic neuropathy in which the classic signs and symptoms of temporal arteritis are entirely missing and the first sign is a quiet ischemic blindness. This has been called "*Occult temporal arteritis*". Many cases belonging to this category have been recorded [105, 189, 325, 398, 417, 421, 468, 552], and some of the cases in the present series belonged to this group.

The disease is generally considered to be self-limiting and its duration has been reported as about three months [421], or 2 to 30 months [82], or several months to a year or more, with half of all patients suffering no long-term ill-effects even without therapy [384]. MILLER [389] and CULLEN [109] each reported a case in which ocular complications developed 3 and 7 years, respectively, after temporal arteritis was diagnosed and while the patient was being treated with corticosteroids.

2. Generalized Atherosclerosis and Arteriosclerosis

These and associated cardiovascular diseases are the most common cause of anterior ischemic optic neuropathy, and there are many reports of anterior ischemic optic neuropathy patients with these diseases [40, 50, 51, 60, 61, 77, 81, 124, 125, 170, 185, 190, 199, 309, 322, 325, 329, 342, 351, 352, 543]. In these cases, associated arteriosclerotic changes in the internal carotid artery (see below), ophthalmic artery, and posterior ciliary artery would cause either occlusion of or a marked fall in the perfusion pressure of the posterior ciliary arteries. There is also a significant incidence of ischemic heart disease in patients with anterior ischemic optic neuropathy.

It has been pointed out that temporal artery biopsy not only helps to differentiate the condition from temporal arteritis but also establishes the diagnosis of atherosclerotic and arteriosclerotic anterior ischemic optic neuropathy. In the latter cases the temporal artery shows severe atherosclerotic changes [50, 51, 185, 204, 388, 399, 474, 536], exceeding those expected according to the age of the patients [50, 51, 204]. TOWNES and BLODI [536] stated that the incidence of bilateral anterior ischemic optic neuropathy increases with the severity of temporal artery atherosclerosis. Also, severe loss of vision is associated with

marked temporal artery atherosclerosis. Prognosis with respect to life expectancy and vision is poor.

In the optic nerve, changes may involve the small nutrient vessels [39, 119, 183, 193, 274, 296, 297, 352, 359, 457, 515, 543]. IGERSHEIMER [297] observed severe endarteritis of the small vessels supplying the central bundle and of other branches in the optic nerve. RINTELEN [457] found arteriosclerotic optic atrophy mainly in the anterior third of the optic nerve. FRANÇOIS et al. [183] believed total or partial occlusion of the central artery of the optic nerve was responsible for anterior ischemic optic neuropathy. LEOPOLD [352] considered anterior ischemic optic neuropathy and optic atrophy, about three weeks later, were due to involvement of arterioles of the retrobulbar part of the optic nerve. PETERS [433] stated that anterior ischemic optic neuropathy may be a part of disseminated arteriosclerotic disease. It is worth stressing that arteriosclerotic changes in the retinal vasculature are no guide to the disease in the posterior ciliary arteries, as was noted by others [296, 542]. Thus, a patient with normal-looking retinal arteries may develop anterior ischemic optic neuropathy due to arteriosclerotic changes in the posterior ciliary arteries.

Anterior ischemic optic neuropathy, therefore, is an important manifestation of systemic atherosclerosis and arteriosclerosis, and such a patient requires a complete cardiovascular investigation for systemic arteriosclerosis, carotid artery disease, hypertension and ischemic heart disease.

3. Internal Carotid Artery Disease

Visual symptoms are known to occur in pathologic (arteriosclerosis being the most common cause) and sometimes surgical occlusion of the internal carotid artery [211, 330, 429, 499]. Although these symptoms do not occur frequently, [242], a great deal of literature is available on the subject. Unilateral optic atrophy with crossed hemiplegia and hemianopia is characteristic of carotid occlusion and is called the *optico-*

pyramidal [352] or Radovici syndrome [447]. This syndrome was described by ESPILDORA-LUQUE [161, 208, 555]. Anterior ischemic optic neuropathy, with swelling of the optic disc, (see below) may start with attacks of amaurosis fugax, which have been well-documented since PENZOLDT [429] described them first in 1881. The attacks are usually considered to be due to embolism [362, 377, 391, 407, 444, 561] or spasm of the central retinal artery [167, 293, 550, 578]. The incidence of amaurosis fugax in carotid insufficiency has been reported as 12.5 percent [150, 386]. Amaurosis fugax may be associated with signs of cerebral ischemia, particularly contralateral hemiplegia [12, 123, 167, 208, 510, 556]. Optic atrophy, in these cases, has been considered secondary to retinal ischemia. To explain retinal involvement, usually two theories were put forward:

1. extension of a thrombus of the internal carotid artery to the ophthalmic artery and central retinal artery [115, 330, 429, 518], and

2. embolism from internal carotid artery to central retinal artery, as mentioned above.

In addition to these two widely prevailing views, the following causes were also considered:

1. SMITH [510] postulated that pressure in the central retinal artery in these cases is less than intraocular pressure and leads to ischemia of the retina.

2. SARIN [475] hypothesized that in carotid artery occlusion, papilledema and blindness are due to anoxemia of the optic nerve and that optic atrophy follows within 7 to 10 days after papilledema. With partial optic atrophy and a patent central retinal artery of normal caliber, the nutrient artery of the optic nerve was thought to be blocked [518].

3. Some European workers believe the optic disc changes are a reflex vasomotor disturbance from the carotid artery disease [68, 342].

No doubt in some cases amaurosis fugax, and ultimately optic atrophy, may result from occlusion of the central retinal artery. But, in the light of new evidence, a much more frequent and important factor, which would start to operate much earlier than involvement of retinal circulation, is interference with the perfusion of vessels in the optic nerve head and peripapillary choroid due to the imbalance produced between perfusion pressure in the posterior ciliary arteries (due to carotid insufficiency) and intraocular pressure. With poor perfusion pressure, perfusion in the optic nerve head at normal intraocular pressure may be just sufficient to maintain the normal function of optic nerve fibers. Even a slight rise in intraocular pressure, induced by forceful blinking, sudden extreme ocular movement (extraocular muscles compressing the eyeball), rubbing the eye, or any other factor that increases venous pressure in the head and neck region, may produce amaurosis fugax. This would also apply to any sudden transitory fall in perfusion pressure, as on assuming an erect posture from a prone position. If the fall in perfusion pressure is profound and sudden, due to a drop in systemic blood pressure or other causes, anterior ischemic optic neuropathy may be complete or sectoral, producing complete or sectoral loss of vision that ultimately results in optic atrophy. Many such cases have been reported [42, 61, 63, 68, 87, 170, 233, 322, 324, 374, 392, 415, 416, 474, 475]. If ischemia of the optic nerve head is chronic, the presenting symptoms are those of "low-tension glaucoma".

The drop in perfusion pressure may be so great, even circulation in the central retinal artery may be compromised, producing ophthalmoscopic evidence of its occlusion. Ophthalmoscopy cannot assess interference with perfusion of the posterior ciliary artery circulation. In earlier studies ophthalmoscopy and ophthalmodynamometry focused the attention of almost all observers entirely on the retinal circulation. The role of the posterior ciliary artery circulation in producing these visual symptoms and optic disc changes was ignored completely.

4. Systemic Arterial Hypertension

Anterior ischemic optic neuropathy not due to temporal arteritis, correlated significantly with the incidence of systemic arterial hypertension.

The role of hypertension in anterior ischemic optic neuropathy has been mentioned by many workers [60, 81, 106, 107, 151, 170, 171, 342, 388]. Half of the patients in my series were hypertensive.

In malignant hypertension with hypertensive retinopathy IGERSHEIMER [297] found that degeneration may be quite independent of retinal changes because optic nerve changes occurred only in one eye of a patient with equally marked hypertensive retinopathy in both eyes. He found lesions of small vessels in the involved optic nerve. In another patient he found optic nerve degeneration without retinal involvement. Similar observations were made by RAUBITSCHEK [449]. IGERSHEIMER [297] found optic disc cupping with cavernous degeneration in the laminar and retrolaminar part of the optic nerve in a patient with hypertension and uremia. RINTELEN [457] believed that these changes were due to malacious areas in the anterior part of the nerve. KOYANAGI et al. [323] described hypertrophy or degeneration in small branches of the circle of Zinn and Haller in hypertensive retinopathy; these changes lead to degeneration of the nerve fibers in the affected part, with loss of vision in that part. PETERS [433] stated that ischemic optic neuropathy may be a part of systemic hypertension.

Hypertensive retinopathy and anterior ischemic optic neuropathy in malignant hypertension are unrelated, although both processes are related to hypertension. The remarkable dissociation of vascular disease of the optic nerve head and retrolaminar part of the optic nerve from that of the retinal vascular tree was noted by workers a long time ago [296, 542].

5. Systemic Arterial Hypotension

Anterior ischemic optic neuropathy may be produced by a sudden and profound drop in blood pressure, as in shock [133] or surgical hypotension [170, 171]. The fall may result from massive hemorrhages, myocardial infarction, cardiac arrest, heart failure, septicemia, syncope, surgical shock, hypotension during cardiac and thoracic surgery, or prolonged markedly hypoten-

sive anesthesias. The role of hypotension in anterior ischemic optic neuropathy has already been discussed (p. 22).

6. Posthemorrhagic Amaurosis

In a large number of cases reported in the literature, visual disturbances, even complete blindness, followed a marked loss of blood. It is interesting to note that Hippocrates was also aware of this when he wrote, "After the vomiting of blackish, sometimes bloody matter, the patient complains of headaches and his eyes do not see." The mechanism of the visual disturbances and field defects, particularly the altitudinal hemianopias, has remained obscure.

Amaurosis is mostly known to follow hemorrhages from the gastrointestinal tract and uterus and less often from the nose, lungs, kidneys, wounds, etc. [4, 47, 75, 86, 165, 171, 209, 212, 223, 232, 267, 279, 280, 336, 343, 353, 357, 361, 428, 437, 439, 441, 445, 446, 501, 526–530, 553, 566, 570]. Small recurrent hemorrhages rather than a single larger one, are mostly responsible for this process.

The visual disturbance varies from blurring to complete loss of vision. It is generally bilateral (in 85 percent [146], about 90 percent [98]). It may be permanent (in 45.9 percent [501], 50 percent [530], in 54 percent [430], in 83 percent [534]) or temporary. It usually starts between the third and seventh days after the hemorrhage [530, 570] but may develop within a few hours (within 24 hours in 30 percent [430], within 14 hours in 45 percent [224], within 12 hours in 34.1 percent [530]). The literature has been reviewed by SINGER [501], TERSON [530], HARBRIDGE [232], and LOCKET [357].

Clincially, the fundus is pale and anemic with narrow retinal arteries. The optic disc may show blurred margins [357, 555, 566] or edema [20, 22, 210, 357, 566, 570], which may be marked and may involve only the upper half of the disc [20]. There may be small superficial hemorrhages near the optic disc. The retinal veins may be congested. Later, all these cases show optic atrophy [209, 279, 280, 448, 580], which may involve only the upper half of the disc [20, 541]. There may, however, be pronounced loss of vision without any significant fundus changes during the early stages [292, 357, 404, 555], though later optic atrophy is almost always seen.

Altitudinal hemianopia, with loss of the lower visual fields, has been described [91, 92, 164, 195, 216, 225, 236, 291, 292, 357, 437, 441, 485, 526, 541, 570]. Less commonly it may involve loss of the upper visual fields [292]. In these cases, the hemianopia is irregular and the line of demarcation is along the horizontal meridian. The preserved field shows a generalized depression [292]. There may be vertical hemianopia [236, 485], bitemporal hemianopia [236], concentric contraction of fields [210, 225, 236], or central scotoma [22, 225]. SCOTT [485] described wide sectoral field defects in these cases, which may produce irregular hemianopias, either vertical or horizontal.

The pathologic lesions described in these cases are not definite. SEESE [488], GORLITZ [209] and ZEIGLER [580] reported them in 5, 11, and 22 days, respectively, after the onset of blindness. They found degeneration of ganglion cells, cytoid bodies in the nerve fiber layer, edema of the retina, and fatty degeneration in the optic nerve. GORLITZ [209] found the last change in the optic nerve situated behind the lamina cribrosa.

The pathogenesis of posthemorrhagic amaurosis, particularly that of the altitudinal and other field defects, has been the subject of much controversy. It has been considered to be due probably to primary ischemia of the retina [91, 96, 336, 580], focal anoxia of the retina [428], vasospasm of the retinal arteries [237, 570], lack of oxygen similar to quinine amblyopia [570], central retinal vein thrombosis [99], or ischemic fatty degeneration of the optic nerve [563]. Its prevalence after repeated hemorrhages and the lapse of time between hemorrhage and visual disorders suggest the possible role of some hemoclastic shock, anaphylactic crises, or toxemia due to profound hemolysis or other unknown causes [138, 224, 284, 327, 437, 463, 526, 530]. DUGGAN [138] thought the toxin was adrenaline. RISER

et al. [459] suggested that autointoxication was added to ischemia to cause visual loss. TERRIEN [526] thought the optic atrophy was due to the combined effect of hemorrhage and toxemia. Other workers have suggested hemorrhage into the optic nerve sheath [216], edema and multiple hemorrhages in the nerve [350], thrombotic foci causing degeneration and diffuse retinal edema [209], endothelial damage due to blood loss and thrombosis on damaged endothelium [541], endarteritis fibrosa [448], thrombosis of the central retinal artery [531], retrobulbar neuritis [281], a lesion in the optic nerve just behind the lamina cribrosa [428], exudation into the sheath of the optic nerve with associated cerebral edema sufficient to produce compression of the vascular supply of the optic nerve and retina [166], changed consistency of the blood [567], and hypoproteinemia leading to edema of the optic nerve and vascular compression [357]. WALSH and HOYT [555] postulated intravascular obstruction of microcirculation in the optic nerve and retina due to increased platelet aggregation following major hemorrhage.

Inferior altitudinal hemianopia, according to WOLFF [570], is due to the effect of gravity, the lower part of the retina receiving more blood than the upper part after severe hemorrhage. There is accompanying atrophy of the upper half of the disc and diminution in the caliber of the upper retinal arteries. WOLFF postulated that the edema of the optic disc in these cases was due to Starling's phenomenon, wherein the cutting-off of the blood supply injures the endothelium of the capillaries, so that when blood pressure is restored in them, an excessive amount of fluid is allowed to pass through the walls to produce edema. HUGHES [292] commented that in altitudinal hemianopia the horizontal line of demarcation would suggest a retinal origin. In one example he observed the fundus during the episode and found the retinal vessels were normal. In this case the horizontal line of demarcation did not exactly follow the horizontal meridian, and it seemed probable that the lesion lay in the optic nerve. He also reported another similar case. HARRINGTON [236] thought it to be due to ischemia of the anterior part of the optic nerve secondary to extreme hypotension or to stenosis or embolism of the optic nerve branches from the ophthalmic artery.

The possibility that in some cases the visual disturbances, especially total blindness, are due to occlusion of the central retinal artery cannot be ruled out. In these, however, a normal fundus and normal retinal vessels have frequently been reported, and one can hardly find a case report showing a fundus picture of classic central retinal artery occlusion. The presence of an extreme arterial hypotension has been reported in these cases. I feel the vast majority of these cases developed anterior ischemic optic neuropathy due to hypotension. The presence of an isolated edema of the optic disc without retinal edema is a further confirmation of this, because it can be produced only by occlusion of the posterior ciliary supply to the disc [247]. The altitudinal hemianopia, seen frequently in these cases, has the same pathogenesis as that discussed above (p. 91), i.e., it is due to involvement of the posterior ciliary circulation to one-half of the disc. In some cases, this could be the result of thrombosis affecting the posterior ciliary arteries because of extreme arterial hypotension. The presence of vertical hemianopia sometimes in these cases can be explained on the same basis as altitudinal hemianopia, where the main posterior ciliary artery supplies the temporal and nasal halves (Fig. 4, 5) instead of the superior and inferior halves (Fig. 6). Since smaller subdivisions of the posterior ciliary arteries would supply small sectors of the disc, their individual involvement would lead to a sectoral defect, as discussed above.

Thus, these cases represent a variety of anterior ischemic optic neuropathy, which is either due to systemic hypotension from massive hemorrhages or to marked anemia that causes anoxic damage by the mechanism discussed on p. 121 or most probably to increased platelet aggregation following hemorrhage, producing vascular occlusion in the optic nerve head.

7. Diabetes

Anterior ischemic optic neuropathy in diabetes has been mentioned in the literature [73, 106, 107, 151, 171, 185, 342, 388, 505, 535]. SKILLERN and LOCKHART [505] reported 14 cases of anterior ischemic optic neuropathy (20 eyes) with uncontrolled diabetes in the age group 40 to 69 years. Only two patients had diabetic retinopathy. They described the optic nerve changes as due to the toxic effect of prolonged hyperglycemia and failure of glucose utilization, together with relative anoxia and damage to the optic nerve of susceptible individuals. Decreased arterial circulation was not considered to be a significant factor.

In the series of 11 patients with anterior ischemic optic neuropathy, in the 45 to 69 age group reported by MILLER et al. [388], seven were very mildly diabetic, without diabetic retinopathy, and all but one had significant cardiovascular disease, e.g., hypertension, arteriosclerosis, and myocardial infarction.

The findings in these diabetic patients indicate that in all probability the primary factor responsible for their anterior ischemic optic neuropathy is associated cardiovascular disease, and the neuropathy is not significantly related to diabetes.

8. Collagen Diseases

Anterior ischemic optic neuropathy in polyarteritis nodosa [151, 171, 206, 319, 320, 555] and lupus erythematosus [314, 342, 464, 548] has been described. Temporal arteritis has also been considered to be a collagen disease. RUCKER [466] considered that polyarteritis nodosa is an extremely rare cause of anterior ischemic optic neuropathy, and that there is no clear difference, histopathologically, between it and temporal arteritis. The latter view was also expressed by other authors [79, 306, 318] but denied by some [288, 290, 494]. GOLDSTEIN et al. [206] described a case of polyarteritis nodosa with bilateral optic atrophy and histopathologic lesions of the posterior ciliary artery. The optic nerve head and retrolaminar optic nerve were infiltrated by many inflammatory round cells and glial tissue, which was attributed to disease of the posterior ciliary arteries. They described the ciliary arteries as most vulnerable to this disease—the choroidal arteries always and, sometimes, the short posterior ciliary arteries as well. They found typical lesions in choroidal arteries in another case [206]. BOCK [56] found lesions in the posterior ciliary vessels, at the entrance of the optic nerve, and in their course through the sclera to the suprachoroidal space. In another case he [57] found the lesions in the scleral and choroidal vessels and in the greater arterial circle of the iris. VON HERRENSCHWAN [277] stated that polyarteritis nodosa occurred particularly where the artery altered its direction, e.g., at its entrance into the sclera, and in its course from the sclera towards the ciliary body. KING [320] described anterior ischemic optic neuropathy in one eye, resulting in optic atrophy, and recurrent iritis and glaucoma in the fellow eye. However, he considered edema of the optic disc due to raised intracranial pressure secondary to cerebral arterial involvement. KERNOHAN et al. [317] described a case of choroidal lesions in one eye and severe hypertensive retinopathy with retinal detachment in the opposite eye. These retinal changes in polyarteritis nodosa have also been described by other workers [52, 56, 198, 344, 495, 555].

SVANE-KNUDSEN [520] found bilateral central scotoma and acutely increased intraocular pressure. In addition, reports are available in the literature of episcleritis, scleritis, extraocular muscle paresis, corneal ulceration, keratitis and uveitis, etc., in polyarteritis nodosa.

9. Thromboangiitis Obliterans or Bürger's Disease

A disease of obscure etiology, described by VON WINIWARTER [569] in 1879, was brought into prominence by BÜRGER [72] in 1908. It affects generally males of 30 to 50 years. Classically, there is intermittent claudication in the lower limbs; but it can affect arteries in other parts

of the body. ANTONI [14] reported thrombosis of the internal carotid artery and vertebral artery. SEGAL et al. [489] described unilateral thrombosis of the internal carotid artery with hypertensive disease, generalized atherosclerosis, fundus changes, and thromboangiitis obliterans of the lower limbs. Relative to the eye, there are many reports of retinal arterial involvement and closure [46, 222, 228, 356, 370, 376, 436, 478, 544], but no definite case of anterior ischemic optic neuropathy. HOGAN and ZIMMERMAN [283] described transient blindness and partial or total obliteration of the vascular supply to the optic nerve. In this disease, since thrombosis of the internal carotid artery and central retinal artery are recorded, the possibility that the posterior ciliary arteries may be involved cannot be ruled out. It is conceivable that some cases of optic atrophy attributed to central retinal artery occlusion may, in fact, be due to anterior ischemic optic neuropathy. WALSH and HOYT [555] believe that this disease is a thromboembolic disease and not an independent entity, so that the ocular manifestations of this disease are examples of carotid vascular insufficiency or carotid thromboembolism.

10. Vasomotor Disturbances

The possibility that vasomotor disturbances may involve the posterior ciliary arteries, resulting in anterior ischemic optic neuropathy, cannot be excluded.

a) Migraine

Sectoral anterior ischemic optic neuropathy with inferonasal arcuate field defect has been reported in a 53-year-old lady suffering from migraine [378, 471]. The cases of PASTEUR et al. [422] and those of CONNOR [93] represent posterior ciliary ischemia in migraine.

b) Raynaud's Disease

Retinal arterial caliber changes, including spasm and occlusion, have been recorded in this disease since RAYNAUD [450], in 1874, described such changes [11, 15, 18, 24, 49, 80, 327, 395, 497, 551, 560]. The only definite case of anterior ischemic optic neuropathy in Raynaud's disease has been reported by LASCO [342]. A 40-year-old patient with Raynaud's disease developed an inferior temporal field defect with pale and blurred optic disc, with two hemorrhages on the nasal border and normal-looking retinal vessels. This patient later developed optic atrophy.

In Raynaud's disease the possibility of posterior ciliary artery involvement similar to retinal arterial involvement has to be borne in mind. BLAAUW [48] saw a normal fundus in a patient with temporary dimness of vision in the eye. He believed the dim vision was due more to the involvement of the uveal than of the retinal vessels.

c) Cervical Discopathies

Anterior ischemic optic neuropathy has been mentioned in cervical discopathies [342, 424, 425, 426, 524]. In this condition there is degeneration of the fourth through seventh cervical intervertebral discs, which is associated with sympathetic nervous system disorders, e.g., heterochromic irides, Horner's syndrome, Adies' syndrome, acrocyanosis, parasthesia of upper extremity, etc., due to irritation of the cervical sympathetic nerves. This produces changes in the reflex capillary permeability of the optic nerve, which are irreversible and which produce anterior ischemic optic neuropathy [342]. The ocular symptoms disappear after surgery. Strangely enough, there does not seem to be any report on this entity in the English literature.

11. Syphilis

Syphilitic optic neuritis is well-documented [147, 219, 229, 295]. Some of the cases reported were possibly anterior ischemic optic neuropathy and not true optic neuritis. COGAN [88] described syphilis as a major cause of anterior ischemic optic neuropathy in the past. SANDERS [471]

reported syphilitic ischemic optic neuropathy in a 44-year-old man. SMITH et al. [507] reported finding Treponema pallidum in 5 of 10 temporal artery biopsies from patients with temporal arteritis who had a positive serology for syphilis. They suggested that patients with temporal arteritis should be screened carefully for evidence of syphilis. However, none of the eight patients, from the same institute, with anterior ischemic optic neuropathy due to causes other than temporal arteritis showed a positive serology for syphilis [388].

12. Allergic Disorders

The development of anterior ischemic optic neuropathy has been reported after serum sickness [29, 68, 226, 315, 342, 373, 375], B.C.G. vaccination [197], T.A.B. [83], urticaria [69], and with Quincke's edema [342, 345]. Altered capillary permeability has been postulated as the cause. It is more likely that in some cases of serum sickness, the element of shock and consequent hypotension may be a much more important factor than capillary changes in the production of anterior ischemic optic neuropathy. The other possibility in these cases is the development of vasculitis.

13. Hematologic Disorders

Optic disc edema is known to occur in various types of blood dyscrasias, e.g., sickle-cell trait, polycythemia, thrombocytopenic purpura, leukemias, and various types of anemia. Reports of frank anterior ischemic optic neuropathy are very rare, but it has been reported in pernicious anemia [153, 231, 406]. FRIEDENWALD [188] and LASCO [342] reported anterior ischemic optic neuropathy in idiopathic polycythemia. GOWERS [212] described low-grade optic disc edema and decreased central vision in severe anemias and chlorosis, resembling anterior ischemic optic neuropathy. FOULDS [171] postulated that oxygenation of the optic nerve depends not only upon the amount of blood flowing through the capillaries in the optic nerve head, but also on the oxygen-carrying capacity of the blood, so that in severe anemia unexplained visual disturbances may be due to some degree of anterior ischemic optic neuropathy. In chronic bronchitis with polycythemia, poor oxygen pressure in the blood and slow circulation from increased viscosity may produce anterior ischemic optic neuropathy.

14. Pulseless Disease

This is a disease discovered by H. John DAVY [118] in 1839, described by TURK [540] in 1901, and first described in Japanese by TAKAYASU [523], under whose name it is commonly known. The condition is seen most often in women under 40 and is due to gradual closure of the large arteries that arise from the aortic arch—hence is also called the *aortic arch syndrome*. Most often idiopathic in origin, with considerable evidence that it is an autoimmune disease [308], pulseless disease may be due to syphilitic aortitis or to trauma from crushing injuries of the chest. Bürger's disease, polyarteritis nodosa, temporal arteritis, upper mediastinal tumors, and suspected congenital anomaly may be all considered possible etiologies.

The most prominent and common symptoms are due to carotid artery insufficiency, which includes amaurosis fugax or blindness [112], episodes of visual loss, frequently related to minor changes in posture [496], and cerebral symptoms. PINKHAM [440] has reviewed the ocular signs and symptoms in this disease. The main stress in ocular signs has been the inadequate retinal arterial supply producing characteristic retinopathy [495a]. However, there must be generalized hypoxia of the ocular tissue, with the optic nerve head as vulnerable as, if not more than, the retinal circulation (p. 116). Although no definite patient with anterior ischemic optic neuropathy has been reported so far, the optic disc edema with central scotoma reported by BEGUE and GRAZZIANI [33] may represent a case of anterior ischemic optic neuropathy in pulseless disease.

15. Herpes Zoster Ophthalmicus

WALSH and HOYT [555] considered that reports of optic neuritis in herpes zoster ophthalmicus really represent anterior ischemic optic neuropathy. They cited three reports [419, 423, 546], but a review of these does not lend much support to their speculations [555] since the classic picture of anterior ischemic optic neuropathy in the fundus was not observed. Two of the reports had optic atrophy [423, 546], and the third report strongly suggested retrobulbar neuritis [419]. The optic atrophy and narrow retinal vessels reported could be due to occlusion of the retinal artery. I have seen a young girl of 14 who, while under my care for herpes zoster ophthalmicus, developed central retinal artery occlusion and later optic atrophy as well as marked loss of vision with attenuated vessels (a small island of vision corresponding to a patent cilioretinal artery was intact). I feel that so far there is no definite report of anterior ischemic optic neuropathy in herpes zoster ophthalmicus.

16. Optic Neuropathy of Graves' Disease

Following thyroidectomy or other antithyroid treatment, with or without thyroid dysfunction, an optic neuropathy may develop. The neuropathy consists of edema of the optic disc with decreased visual acuity and visual field defects (e.g., central scotoma, nerve fiber bundle defects, peripheral field defects), with or without exophthalmos [67, 116, 120–122, 157, 163, 196, 200, 207, 266, 269, 270, 276, 298, 405, 484, 533, 562, 568]. This has been thought to be caused by interference with the blood supply of the optic nerve [120, 121, 266, 269, 270, 298, 405, 443], presumably due to a rise in pressure of the muscle cone or of swollen extraocular muscles. COGAN [88] speculated that the cause was edema and lymphocytic infiltration of the optic nerve. These cases may develop optic atrophy with permanent visual loss. The clinical picture suggests a variety of anterior ischemic optic neuropathy, and I feel that in eyes with exophthalmos it may be due to either direct pressure on the posterior ciliary arteries in the retrobulbar part or to elevated intraocular pressure due to pressure on the eye by tight inferior rectus and pressure by retrobulbar tissue. I have seen two or three patients in whom occlusion of the central artery of the retina was caused by very high intraocular pressure. As discussed above, circulation of the posterior ciliary arteries within the eyeball is obliterated long before the central retinal artery is occluded. In eyes with no exophthalmos, involvement of the posterior ciliary arteries is difficult to explain; presumably lymphocytic infiltration of the arteries may be responsible.

17. No Systemic Abnormality

There are always some cases in which no systemic abnormality can be detected to account for anterior ischemic optic neuropathy. In the older age groups arteriosclerosis usually is considered to be the cause.

This long list of diseases with which anterior ischemic optic neuropathy can be associated stresses the necessity for a thorough search for causative factors and, hence, the scientific management of such patients.

B. Ocular Diseases

1. Glaucoma and Low-Tension Glaucoma

The association of anterior ischemic optic neuropathy with glaucoma [31, 32, 132, 170, 171, 471] and low-tension glaucoma [286] is not surprising, in view of the pathogenesis of anterior ischemic optic neuropathy discussed on p. 21. Any imbalance between perfusion pressure in the posterior ciliary artery and intraocular pressure would produce anterior ischemic optic neuropathy. In patients with glaucoma (elevated intraocular pressure) and in low-tension glaucoma a fall in perfusion pressure is already present. Only

minor changes in one or the other are required to tip the balance to produce anterior ischemic optic neuropathy. Anterior ischemic optic neuropathy following cataract extraction and intraocular surgery is rare, though often not recognized. It has been reported by REESE and CARROLL [454] and LAVY and NEUMAN [348], and I have encountered three similar cases. I feel this is due to a rise in intraocular pressure during the postoperative period, which is not uncommon, although it is frequently unrecognized unless the patient's intraocular pressure is checked by applanation tonometry. In arteriosclerotic individuals in whom perfusion pressure in the posterior ciliary arteries is already poor, a slight rise in intraocular pressure is enough to compromise vessels in the optic disc. The other possible factor, although of minor importance, is compression by a retrobulbar injection on the extraocular part of the posterior ciliary arteries. Since, during the immediate postoperative period, it is frequently difficult to assess any fall in visual acuity or optic disc change, these cases are likely to be missed or misdiagnosed.

2. Compression Anterior Ischemic Optic Neuropathy

Any lesion that compresses the blood vessels in the optic nerve head and retrobulbar part can result in anterior ischemic optic neuropathy. It has been mentioned with peripapillary malignant melanoma, glioma infiltrating the optic nerve head, and other tumors compressing the disc [68]. In this category could be included the anterior ischemic optic neuropathy due to massive optic disc edema of long duration, where the edema compresses vessels in the optic nerve head. Segmental anterior ischemic optic neuropathy with drusen of the optic nerve [312] may be due to compression of vessels in the optic nerve head by the drusen.

Pseudotumor, endocrinal exophthalmos, and retrobulbar tumor pressing on the retrobulbar optic nerve and posterior ciliary arteries, could produce anterior ischemic optic neuropathy.

3. Traumatic Anterior Ischemic Optic Neuropathy

No definite case of anterior ischemic optic neuropathy due to trauma has so far been reported. A dubious report of a case claimed to be "traumatic ischemic optic neuropathy" following injury to the orbit from a kick has been reported [577]. The authors postulated injury to the posterior ciliary arteries in this case, but without any proof of posterior ciliary artery occlusion, in angiographic studies, to support their hypothesis.

Conclusions

1. Causes

Anterior ischemic optic neuropathy, in most cases, is due to either arteriosclerosis or temporal arteritis, more often the former than the latter. There is also a large variety of systemic, local vascular, and ocular disorders that can produce anterior ischemic optic neuropathy (see Part III).

2. Age

In patients with temporal arteritis anterior ischemic optic neuropathy is seen most often in those over the age of 60 years (75 ± 9 years). In arteriosclerosis it is found most often in a comparatively younger age group (69 ± 8 years). Anterior ischemic optic neuropathy due to other causes can be seen even in much younger persons.

3. Laterality

Bilateral anterior ischemic optic neuropathy can occur in about one-quarter to one-third of those cases due to temporal arteritis, with a time interval of usually less than two months. In other types of anterior ischemic optic neuropathy, the incidence of bilateral disease varies.

4. Visual Symptoms

Transient blurring or loss of vision as a prodromal symptom was seen in about three-quarters of the temporal arteritis and in about one-fourth of the non-arteritic type of cases a few hours to several days before the onset of more permanent, partial, or complete loss of vision.

5. Visual Acuity

Visual acuity in these cases may vary from no perception of light to perfectly normal central vision, being much worse in temporal arteritis than in those without arteritis.

6. Optic Disc Changes

The main ocular abnormality on examination is in the optic disc. In temporal arteritic anterior ischemic optic neuropathy, half of the patients show chalky-white swelling of the optic disc with a rare hemorrhage. The other half show pink or pale-pink edema of the optic disc with frequent flame-shaped hemorrhages. In non-arteritic type of anterior ischemic optic neuropathy, it is rare to see chalky-white swelling of the disc; the pale-pink edema with hemorrhages is more common. Swelling of the optic disc usually starts to subside in about 7 to 10 days and optic atrophy develops after a month or two. The edema and atrophy may involve the entire disc or only a sector of it. The vast majority of optic discs with anterior ischemic optic neuropathy due to temporal arteritis develop cupping of the disc; this is not common in non-arteritic cases.

7. Retinal Changes

On occasion there may be associated infarction of a sector or the entire retina due to additional involvement of the cilioretinal or central retinal arteries respectively.

8. Chorioretinal Lesions

About one-third of the cases with anterior ischemic optic neuropathy may show peripheral chorioretinal degenerative patches.

9. Intravenous Fluorescein Angiography

In complete anterior ischemic optic neuropathy, the optic disc shows no filling of vessels of posterior ciliary artery origin during the first and second weeks after onset or during the atrophic stage; some filling is seen during the intermediate period. In sectoral anterior ischemic optic neuropathy, staining is seen in only the normal part during the first week but in the whole disc towards the end of the second week, until the ischemic part becomes atrophic and shows no fluorescence. Markedly delayed and poor filling of the choroid is seen during the first week, the filling defect being very pronounced in the peripapillary choroid. In sectoral anterior ischemic optic neuropathy this choroidal and peripapillary choroid filling defect is localized to the corresponding sector. After a few weeks, the choroidal circulation is restored to normal. In the event of retinal arterial occlusion, angiography shows evidence of occlusion during the early stages.

10. Visual Field Defects

A variety of visual field defects are seen, mainly of nerve fiber bundle patterns that include altitudinal field defects (commonly inferior), central scotoma, segmental defects, arcuate scotoma, vertical defects, and peripheral contraction.

11. Electro-Oculogram and Electro-Retinogram

These are usually normal unless there is associated retinal infarction.

12. Erythrocyte Sedimentation Rate (ESR)

ESR estimation is important to determine the presence or absence of temporal arteritis. A Westergren higher than 40 mm the first hour suggests temporal arteritis and a temporal artery biopsy is indicated.

13. Associated Systemic Diseases

Systemic examination reveals a very high incidence of cardiovascular disorders in non-arteritic anterior ischemic optic neuropathy.

14. Treatment of Anterior Ischemic Optic Neuropathy

Patients with anterior ischemic optic neuropathy due to temporal arteritis should be given high doses of systemic corticosteroids as soon as possible to safeguard the second eye. In non-arteritic type of anterior ischemic optic neuropathy systemic corticosteroids should be administered in an initial dose of 60 to 80 mg daily, slowly tapered thereafter so that the treatment is continued for about two months. This regimen produced improvement in 75 percent as compared to only 17 percent in untreated cases. Acetazolamide, to lower intraocular pressure, has been found beneficial in these cases.

15. Visual Prognosis

Prognosis is worst in patients with anterior ischemic optic neuropathy due to temporal arteritis. In non-arteritis patients treated with systemic corticosteroids, the prognosis is comparatively better. It is not as good for untreated as for treated cases. Perhaps it is better than for temporal arteritis because anterior ischemic optic neuropathy is more often partial in the former group and more often total in the latter. In general, a very cautious visual prognosis should be given in all these cases. Since arteriosclerotic anterior ischemic optic neuropathy is usually associated with marked cardiovascular disorders, the neuropathy may be a warning signal of a poor systemic prognosis. Patients with temporal arteritis, on the other hand, suffer no long-term systemic ill-effects.

16. Course of Anterior Ischemic Optic Neuropathy

Initially, patients have edema of the optic disc, which may involve the entire disc or a sector of it. The edema usually starts to subside in about 7 to 10 days and results in atrophy of the involved part of the optic disc after about a month or two.

17. Pathogenesis of Anterior Ischemic Optic Neuropathy

Occlusion of the posterior ciliary arteries (due to any cause) is responsible for the development of anterior ischemic optic neuropathy because the lamina cribrosa, prelaminar, and retrolaminar regions are supplied by the posterior ciliary arteries. Usually there is a partial occlusion of the posterior ciliary arteries, which reduces the perfusion pressure. The perfusion pressure may also fall due to marked systemic arterial hypotension, e.g., in shock, hemorrhage, etc. As the perfusion pressure falls to a significant low level,

the optic disc circulation is the first to compromise, then the peripapillary choroid, and finally the rest of the choroid. This explains the frequent presence of anterior ischemic optic neuropathy without a chorioretinal lesion. Since a cilioretinal artery arises from a posterior ciliary artery and, sometimes, a central retinal artery may arise with a posterior ciliary artery from the ophthalmic artery by a common trunk, retinal arterial occlusion may be associated with anterior ischemic optic neuropathy.

18. Pathogenesis of Cupping of the Optic Disc

Disc cupping in anterior ischemic optic neuropathy is most probably due to destruction of neural tissue in the prelaminar region, backward bowing of the lamina cribrosa, due to retrolaminar fibrosis, and to the absence of normal support of the lamina cribrosa posteriorly by the disappearance of retrolaminar neural tissue, as well as to weakness of the lamina cribrosa.

19. Pathogenesis of Visual Field Defects

In anterior ischemic optic neuropathy altitudinal and vertical hemianopias, central scotoma, nerve fiber bundle defect, segmental field defects, and peripheral contraction are due to interference with the posterior ciliary supply to the optic nerve head, which is sectoral in distribution.

References

1. ABELSDORFF, G.: Sehnervenatrophie durch athero-sklerotischen Verschluß der Zentralarterie. Zt. Augenheilk. **52**, 273–276 (1924)

2. ADAMS, A.: Normal variation in the human elec-tro-oculogram. Internat. Res. Commun. System (73–5) 24–19–1 (1973)

3. ALLAN, E., BARKER, N., HINES, E.: Peripheral vas-cular diseases, 2nd, ed. p. 346–351. Philadelphia: W.D. Saunders 1955

4. ALT, A.: A case of optic nerve atrophy after severe hemorrhage from the stomach. Amer. J. Ophthal. **29**, 74–75 (1912)

5. ANDERSON, D.R.: Ultrastructure of meningeal sheaths. Arch. Ophthal. (Chic.) **82**, 659–674 (1969)

6. ANDERSON, D.R.: Ultrastructure of human and monkey lamina cribrosa and optic nerve head. Arch. Ophthal. (Chic.) **82**, 800–814 (1969)

7. ANDERSON, D.R.: Ultrastructure of the optic nerve head. Arch. Ophthal. (Chic.) **83**, 63–73 (1970)

8. ANDERSON, D.R.: Vascular supply to the optic nerve of primates. Amer. J. Ophthal. **70**, 341–351 (1970)

9. ANDERSON, D.R.: Pathology of the glaucomas. Brit. J. Ophthal. **56**, 146–156 (1972)

9a. ANDERSON, D.R., DAVIS, E.B.: Retina and optic nerve after posterior ciliary artery occlusion. Arch. Ophthal. (Chic.) **92**, 422–426 (1974)

10. ANDERSON, D.R., HOYT, W.F.: Ultrastructure of intraorbital portion of human and monkey optic nerve. Arch. Ophthal. (Chic.) **82**, 506–530 (1969)

11. ANDERSON, R.G., GRAY, E.B.: Spasm of the cen-tral retinal artery in Raynaud's disease. Arch. Oph-thal. (Chic.) **17**, 662–665 (1937)

12. ANDRELL, P.O.: Thrombosis of the internal carotid artery. Acta med. scand. **114**, 336–372 (1943)

13. ANDREWS, J.M.: Giant cell (temporal) arteritis. Neurology (Minneap.) **16**, 963–971 (1966)

14. ANTONI, N.: Buerger's disease, thromboangiitis in the brain. Acta med. scand. **108**, 502–528 (1941)

15. APPELBAUM, S.J., LERNER, M.C.: Raynaud's dis-ease with ocular complication. Amer. J. Ophthal. **9**, 569–573 (1926)

16. ARDEN, G.B., BARRADA, A., KELSEY, J.H.: New clinical test of retinal functions based upon the standing potential of the eye. Brit. J. Ophthal. **46**, 449–467 (1962)

17. AXENFELD, T.: Kavernöse (lakunäre) Sehnerven-atrophie und multiple Dehiscenzen der Sklera bei hochgradiger Myopie. Ber. dtsch. ophthal. Ges. Heidelberg **32**, 303–305 (1905)

18. BAILLIART, M.: Cécités par spasme vasculaire. Ann. Oculist. (Paris) **161**, 382 (1924)

19. BAILLIART, P.: La pression artérielle rétinienne. Ann. Oculist. (Paris) **165**, 321–348 (1928)

20. BALLANTYNE, A.J.: Case presenting multiple struc-tural anomalies in eye, probably of embryonic ori-gin. Trans. ophthal. Soc. U.K. **55**, 349 (1935)

21. BARBER, V.C., GRAZIADEI, P.: The fine structure of cephalopod blood vessels. II. Z. Zellforsch. Mikrosk. Anat. **77**, 147–161 (1967)

22. BARR, A.S.: Amblyopia after hemorrhage. Amer. J. Ophthal. **17**, 396–399 (1934)

23. BASSETT, A.L., BIGGER, J.T., HOFFMAN, B.F.: "Protective" action of diphenylhydantoin on canine Purkinje fibers during hypoxia. J. Pharm. exp. Ther. **173**, 336–343 (1970)

24. BATTEN, B.: A case of Raynaud's disease, with retinal haemorrhage and changes in the retinal ves-sels. Trans. ophthal. Soc. U.K. **30**, 238 (1910)

25. BEAUVIEUX, J.: L'excavation de la papille dans le glaucome. Etude histo-pathologique et pathogéni-que. Bull. Soc. Ophtal. (Paris) 476–501 (1948)

26. BEAUVIEUX, J., RISTITCH, K.: Les vaisseaux cen-traux du nerf optique. Arch. Ophtal. (Paris) **41**, 352–369 (1924)

27. BECKER, B., SHAFFER, R.N.: Diagnosis and therapy of the glaucoma, 2nd ed., p. 125. St. Louis: Mosby 1965

28. Becker, B., Stamper, R.L., Asseff, C., Podos, S.: Effect of diphenylhydantoin on glaucomatous field loss: A preliminary report. Trans. Amer. Acad. Ophthal. Otolaryng. **76**, 412–422 (1972)

29. BEDELL, A.J.: Traumatic retinal angiopathy. Arch. Ophthal. (Chic.) **22**, 351–359 (1939)

30. BEGG, I.S., DRANCE, S.M., GOLDMANN, H.: Fluo-rescein angiography in the evaluation of focal cir-culatory ischaemia of the optic nerve head in rela-tion to the arcuate scotoma in glaucoma. Canad. J. Ophthal. **7**, 68–74 (1972)

31. BEGG, I.S., DRANCE, S.M., SWEENEY, V.P.: Haem-orrhage on the disc.—A sign of acute ischaemic optic neuropathy in chronic simple glaucoma. Canad. J. Ophthal. **5**, 321–330 (1970)

32. BEGG, I.S., DRANCE, S.M., SWEENEY, V.P.: Ischaemic optic neuropathy in chronic simple glaucoma. Brit. J. Ophthal. **55**, 73–90 (1971)

33. BEGUE, H., GRAZZIANI, A.: La maladie sans pouls. Arch. Ophtal. (Paris) **18**, 571–572 (1958)

34. BEHR, C.: Beitrag zur Anatomie und Klinik des septalen Gewebes und des Arterieneinbaus im Sehnervenstamm. Albrecht v. Graefes Arch. Ophthal. **134**, 227–267 (1935)

35. BEHRMAN, S.: Optic neuritis, papillitis, and neuronal retinopathy. Brit. J. Ophthal. **48**, 209–217 (1964)

36. BENEDICT, W.L., WAGENER, H.P., HORTON, B.T.: Temporal arteritis. Ophthal. ibero-amer. **19**, 160–164 (1957)

37. BENNETT, G.: Cortisone therapy of visual loss in temporal arteritis. Brit. J. Ophthal. **40**, 430 (1956)

38. BERGOUIGNAN, M., JULIEN, R.G.: Constatations ophtalmoscopiques dans 2 cas d'artérite temporale. Rev. Oto-neuro-ophtal. **22**, 540–545 (1950)

39. BESELIN, O.: Subakute Funktionsstörung des Sehnerven beziehungsweise der Netzhaut durch Arteriosklerose. Klin. Mbl. Augenheilk. **75**, 363–368 (1925)

40. BESSIERE, E., JULIEN, R.G.: Les manifestations papillaires dans le syndrome dit "artérite temporale": fréquence de l'oedème papillaire ischémique. Arch. Ophtal. (Paris) **10**, 701–714 (1950)

41. BEST, M., BLUMENTHAL, M., GALIN, M.A., TOYOFUKU, H.: Flurescein angiography during induced ocular hypertension in glaucoma. Brit. J. Ophthal. **56**, 6–12 (1972)

42. BETTELHEIM, H. VON: Zur Ätiologie der ischämischen Papillenschwellung. Ophthalmologica (Basel) **150**, 241–251 (1965)

43. BETTETO, G.: Modificazioni strutturali dell' arteria centrale della retina e delle arteriole del nervo ottico in rapporto all'arterio ed arteriosclerosi renale. Ann. Ottal. **84**, 61–79 (1958)

44. BIRKHEAD, N.C., WAGENER, H.P., SHICK, R.M.: Treatment of temporal arteritis with adrenal corticosteroids. J. Amer med. Ass. **163**, 821–827 (1957)

45. BIRNBACHER, A., CZERMAK, W.: Beiträge zur pathologischen Anatomie und Pathogenese des Glaucoms. Albrecht v. Graefes Arch. Ophthal. **32** (4), 1–94 (1886)

46. BIRNBAUM, W., PRINZMETAL, M., CONNOR, C.L.: Generalised thromboangiitis obliterans. Arch. intern. Med. **53**, 410–422 (1934)

47. BISTIS, J.: Sur l'amblyopie et l'amaurose consécutives à des hémorragies. Arch. Ophtal. (Paris) **28**, 34–40 (1908)

48. BLAAUW, E.E.: Etwas über Augensymptome bei der Raynaudschen Krankheit. Ber. über d. 39. Versamml. d. Ophthal. Ges., S. 278, 1913.

49. BLAND, W.C.: Case of Raynaud's disease following acute mania. Brit. med. J., **1889 I**, 1227

50. BLODI, F.C.: The temporal artery biopsy as a diagnostic procedure in ophthalmology. Trans. Aust. College Ophth. **1**, 26–33 (1969)

51. BLODI, F.C.: The temporal artery biopsy as a diagnostic procedure in ophthalmology. Trans. ophthal. Soc. N.Z. **22**, 26–33 (1970)

52. BLODI, F.C., SULLIVAN, P.B.: Involvement of the eyes in periarteritis nodosa. Trans. Amer. Acad. Ophthal. Otolaryng. **63**, 161–165 (1959)

53. BLUMENTHAL, M., BEST, M., GALIN, M.A., GITTER, K.A.: Ocular circulation: Analysis of the effect of induced ocular hypertension on retinal and choroidal blood flow in man. Amer. J. Ophthal. **71**, 819–825 (1971)

54. BLUMENTHAL, M., BEST, M., GALIN, M.A., TOYOFUKU, H.: Peripapillary choroidal circulation in glaucoma. Arch. Ophthal. (Chic.) **86**, 31–38 (1971)

55. BLUMENTHAL, M., GITTER, K.A., BEST, M., GALIN, M.A.: Fluorescein angiography during induced ocular hypertension in man. Amer. J. Ophthal. **69**, 39–43 (1970)

56. BÖCK, J.: Über einen Fall von Periarteriitis Nodosa mit histologisch nachgewiesenen Veränderungen von Muskel und Ziliargefäßen des Auges. Z. Augenheilk. **69**, 225–230 (1929)

57. BÖCK, J.: Ein Beitrag zur Periarteriitis Nodosa am Auge. Z. Augenheilk. **78**, 28–40 (1932)

58. BONAMOUR, G.: Les atrophies optiques chez les hypertendus artériels. Conf. Lyon. Ophtal. **1**, 1–20, janvier (1954)

59. BONAMOUR, G.: Troubles vaso-moteurs oculaires dans les traumatismes craniens fermes. Entretien d'Opht., 1955

60. BONAMOUR, M.G.: A propos de »pseudo-papillites vasculaires«. Bull. Soc.. Ophtal. Fr. **66**, 846–850, Sept. (1966)

61. BONAMOUR, G., BREGEAT, P., BONNET, M., JUGE, P.: La Papille Optique, p. 8, 264–283, 362–363, 426. Paris: Masson & Cie. 1968

62. BONNET, P.: L'artérite temporale et ses manifestations oculaires. Arch. Ophtal. (Paris) **14**, 24–27 (1954)

63. BONNET, P., BONAMOUR, M.G.: La thrombose spontanée de la carotide interne. J. Méd. Lyon, 575–595, 5 juillet (1954)

64. BOTTIGER, L.E., SVEDBERG, C.A.: Normal erythrocyte sedimentation rate and age. Brit. med. J. **1967 II**, 85–87

65. BOUDET, CH.: Artéritie temporale avec oedéma papillaire bilateral. Bull. Soc. Ophtal. Fr. **11**, 748–750 (1959)

66. BOYD, R.V., HOFFBRAND, B.I.: Erythrocyte sedimentation rate in elderly hospital in-patients. Brit. med. J. **1966 I**, 901–902

67. BRALEY, A.E.: Malignant exophthalmos. Amer. J. Ophthal. **36**, 1286–1290 (1953)

68. BREGEAT, P.: L'oedéma papillaire. Bull. Soc. franç. Ophtal., p. 441–472. Paris: Masson & Cie. Suppl., 1956

69. BROWN, A.L.: Ocular manifestations in serum sickness. Amer. J. Ophthal. 8, 614–618 (1925)

70. BRUCE, G.M.: Temporal arteritis as a cause of blindness. Trans. Amer. ophthal. Soc. 47, 300–316 (1949)

71. BRUCE, G.M.: Temporal arteritis as a cause of blindness. Amer. J. Ophthal. 33, 1568–1573 (1950)

72. BUERGER, L.: The pathology of the vessels in cases of gangrene of the lower extremities due to so-called endarteritis obliterans. Proc. N.Y. path. Soc. 8, 48–68 (1908)

73. BURDE, R.M.: Ischemic optic neuropathy. Neuro-ophthalmology Symposium of the University of Miami and the Bascom Palmer Eye Institute (ed. J.L. Smith and J.S. Glaser), vol. VII, pp. 38–62. St. Louis: Mosby 1973

74. BURIAN, H.M.: Electro-retinography in temporal arteritis. Amer. J. Ophthal. 56, 796–800 (1963)

75. CALHOUN, F.P.: The report of a case of "optic atrophy caused by uterine hemorrhage". J. med. Ass. Ga. 3, 73–75 (1913)

76. CALMETTES, L., DEODATI, F., BECHAC, G.: Pseudo-papillite vasculaire. Rev. Oto-neuro-ophtal. 35, 64–65 (1963)

77. CALMETTES, L., DEODATI, F., BEC, P., BECHAC. G.: L'artériosclérose du nerf optique. Rev. Oto-neuro-ophtal. 35, 365–372 (1963)

78. CALMETTES, L., DEODATI, F., GAYRAL, L., BECHAC, G.: Pseudo-papillite vasculaire bilatérale. Rev. Oto-neuro-ophtal. 36, 371–373 (1964)

79. CARDELL, B.S., HANLEY, T.: A fatal case of giant cell or temporal arteritis. J. Path. Bact. 63, 587–597 (1951)

80. CARPENTER, W.M., CARPENTER, E.W.: Raynaud's disease with intermittent spasm of the retinal artery and veins. Arch. Ophthal. (Chic.) 19, 111–113 (1938)

81. CARROLL, F.D.: Optic neuritis: A 15 year study. Amer. J. Ophthal. 35, 75–82 (1952)

82. CECIL, R.L., LOEB, R.F.: Cranial "temporal" arteritis. In: A textbook of medicine (ed. P.B. Beeson and W. McDermott), 11 ed., vol. 1, p. 485, 1963

83. CHABOT, MME: Sur un cas de papillite après vaccination par le »D.T.T.A.B.«. Ann. Oculist. (Paris) 190, 140 (1957)

84. CHASNOFF, J., VORZIMER, J.J.: Temporal arteritis: a local manifestation of a systemic disease. Ann. intern. Med. 20, 327–333 (1944)

85. CHAVALLEREAU: Sur l'hémianopsie consécutive à des hémorragies utérines. France méd. 1, 321–324 (1890)

86. CHEVALLEREAU: Sur l'hémianopsie consécutive à des hémorragies utérines. Arch. de tocol 17, 722–728 (1890)

87. CHRAST, B., GOTTWALD, O.: Ocni poruchy pri thrombose arteria carotis. Čs. Oftal. 12, 358–377 (1956)

88. COGAN, D.G.: Neurology of the visual system, p. 137, 173, 185–188. Springfield, Ill.: C.C. Thomas 1966

89. COHEN, H., HARRISON, C.V.: Temporal arteritis: A report of 3 cases. J. clin. Path. 1, 212 (1948)

90. COHEN, D.N., SMITH, T.R.: Skip areas in temporal artery biopsies. Trans. Amer. Acad. Ophthal. Oto-laryng. 77, op. 526 (1973)

91. COLLINS, E.T.: In discussion of paper by Whiting, M. Trans. ophthal. Soc. U.K. 49, 150 (1929)

92. COMBERG, W.: Bisher nicht beachtete Möglichkeiten mechanischer Einwirkung auf Sehnerven und Netzhaut. Klin. Mbl. Augenheilk. 129, 284 (1956)

93. CONNOR, R.C.R.: Complicated migraine. Lancet 1962 II, 1072–1075

94. COOKE, W.T., CLOAKE, P.C.P., GOVAN, A.D.T., COLBECK, J.C.: Temporal arteritis: A generalized vascular disease. Quart. J. Med. 15, 47–75 (1946)

95. CORDES, F.C.: Retrobulbar injections of atropine in arteriosclerotic atrophy. Amer. J. Ophthal. 20, 53–55 (1937)

96. CORDES, F.C.: Retinal ischemia with visual loss. Amer. J. Ophthal. 45 (2), 79–88 (1958)

97. CORDIER, J., ARNOULD, C., ROUBIER, J., TRIDEN, P., SCHMITT, J.: Maladie de Horton et cécité. Rev. Oto-neuro-ophtal. 32, 173–178 (1960)

98. COSTON, T.O.: Ocular manifestations of blood diseases. Int. Clin. 45th Ser. 3, 252–265 (1935)

99. COX, R.A.: Amblyopia resulting from hemorrhage. Arch. Ophthal. (Chic.) 32, 368–371 (1944)

100. CRISTINI, G.: Exploration de la fonction pré-capillaire et capillaire dans le glaucome. Ann. Oculist. (Paris) 180, 530–541 (1947)

101. CRISTINI, G.: The rationale of ocular hypertension in glaucoma. The common pathological basis for hypertension and nervous atrophy. XVI Conc. Ophthal. 1950 Britannia, Acta, vol. 2, p. 865–871

102. CRISTINI, G.: Common pathological basis of the nervous ocular symptoms in chronic glaucoma. Brit. J. Opthal. 35, 11–20 (1951)

103. CROMPTON, M.R.: The visual changes in temporal (giant-cell) arteritis: Report of a case with autopsy findings. Brain 82, 377–390 (1959)

104. CROSBY, R.C., WADSWORTH, R.C.: Temporal arteritis: Review of the literature and report of five additional cases. Arch. intern. Med. 81, 431–464 (1948)

105. CULLEN, J.F.: Occult temporal arteritis. Trans. ophthal. Soc. U.K. 83, 725–736 (1963)

106. CULLEN, J.F.: Ischaemic optic neuropathy. Trans. ophthal. Soc. U.K. 87, 759–774 (1967)

107. CULLEN, J.F.: Occult temporal arteritis; a common cause of blindness in old age. Brit. J. Ophthal. 51, 513–525 (1967)

108. CULLEN, J.F.: Ischaemic optic neuropathy—temporal arteritis. Proc. Wm. Mackenzie Cent. Symp. on the Ocular circulation in health and disease, ed. J.S. Cant, p. 142–146. London: Kimpton 1968

109. CULLEN, J.F.: Temporal arteritis. Brit. J. Ophthal. **56**, 584–588 (1972)

110. CUNHA-VAZ, J.G., SHAKIB, M., ASHTON, N.: Studies on the permeability of the blood-retinal barrier: I. Brit. J. Ophthal. **50**, 441–453 (1966)

111. CÜPPERS, C.: Über die Mitbeteiligung des Auges bei der Arteriitis temporalis. Klin. Mbl. Augenheilk. **118**, 645–647 (1951)

112. CURRIER, R.D., DEJONG, R.N., BOLE, G.G.: Pulseless disease: central nervous system manifestations. Neurology (Minneap.) **4**, 818–830 (1954)

113. CURTIS, H.C.: Cranial arteritis. Amer. J. Med. **1**, 437–446 (1946)

114. DALSGAARD-NIELSEN, E.: Glaucoma-like cupping of the optic disc and its etiology. Acta ophthal. (Kbh.) **15**, 151–178 (1937)

115. DANDY, W.E.: Intracranial aneurysm of the internal carotid artery cured by operation. Ann Surg. **107**, 654–659 (1938)

116. DANIS, P., BASTENIE, P.: Les atteintes du nerf optique au cours de exophtalmies oedémateuses endocriniennes. Ophthalmologica (Basel) **126**, 65–90 (1953)

117. DAVIDSON, P., SCHLEZINGER, N.S., MULLER, C.R.: Temporal arteritis. Report of a case treated with cortisone. Penn. med. J. **62**, 1835–1838 (1959)

118. DAVY, J.H.: Researches: Physiological and anatomical, vol. 1, p. 426–436. London 1839

119. DAWSON, B.H.: On the blood vessels of the human optic chiasma, hypophysis and hypothalmus. M.D. Thesis, Manchester, 1948

120. DAY, R.N., CARROLL, F.D.: Optic nerve involvement associated with thyroid dysfunction. Trans. Amer. ophthal. Soc. **59**, 220–238 (1961)

121. DAY, R.M., CARROLL, F.D.: Optic nerve involvement associated with thyroid dysfunction. Arch. Ophthal. (Chic.) **63**, 43–51 (1962)

122. DAY, R.M., CARROLL, F.D.: Corticosteroids in the treatment of optic nerve involvement associated with thyroid dysfunction. Arch. Ophthal. (Chic.) **79**, 279–282 (1968)

123. DENNEY-BROWN, D.: The treatment of recurrent cerebrovascular symptoms and the question of "vasospasm". Med. Clin. N. Amer. **35**, 1457–1474 (1951)

124. DESVIGNES, P., BRUN, M.: Névrite optique aiguë avec artériosclérose de l'artère ophthalmique. Ann. Oculist. (Paris) **185**, 990 (1952)

125. DESVIGNES, P., BRUN, M.: Névrite optique aiguë avec artériosclérose de l'artère ophthalmique. Bull. Soc. franç. Ophthal. **65**, 110–113 (1952)

126. DICK, G.F., FREEMAN, G.: Temporal arteritis. J. Amer. med. Ass. **114**, 645–647 (1940)

127. DOWLING, J.E.: Organization of vertebrate retinas. Invest. Ophthal. **9**, 655–680 (1970)

128. DRANCE, S.M.: Studies in the susceptibility of the eye to raised intraocular pressure. Trans. ophthal. Soc. U.K. **82**, 73–89 (1962)

129. DRANCE, S.M.: Studies in the susceptibility of the eye to raised intraocular pressure. Arch. Ophthal. (Chic.) **68**, 478–485 (1962)

130. DRANCE, S.M.: Some factors involved in the production of low tension glaucoma. Proc. 2nd Wm. Mackenzie Mem.. Symp. on the Optic Nerve, ed. J.S. Cant, p. 339–366. London: Kimpton 1972

132. DRANCE, S.M., BEGG, I.S.: Sector Haemorrhage—A probable acute ischaemic disc change in chronic simple glaucoma. Canad. J. Opthal. **5**, 137–141 (1970)

133. DRANCE, S., MORGAN, R.M., SWEENEY, V.P.: Shock-induced optic neuropathy. New Engl. J. Med. **288**, 392–395 (1973)

134. DRANCE, S.M., WHEELER, C., PATTULLO, M.: Uniocular open-angle glaucoma. Amer. J. Ophthal. **65**, 891–902 (1968)

135. DUBOIS-POULSEN, A.: Reproduction expérimentale du ressant de Rönne et du scotome de Bjerrum. Ann. Oculist. (Paris) **189**, 37–52 (1956)

136. DUBOIS-POULSEN, A., MAGIS, C.: Le Scotome de Bjerrum est-il d'origine extra-oculaire? Acta XVII Conc. ophthal, vol. 2, 1954, p. 1136–1144

137. DUBOIS-POULSEN, A., MAGIS, C.: Pathogénie du scotome de Bjerrum. Ann. Oculist. (Paris) **189**, 174–184 (1956)

138. DUGGAN, W.F.: Clinical vascular physiology of the eye. Amer. J. Ophthal. **26**, 354–368 (1943)

139. DUKE-ELDER, S.: Fundamental concepts in glaucoma. Arch. Ophthal. (Chic.) **42**, 538–545 (1949)

140. DUKE-ELDER, S.: The dependence of surgery on physiology. Amer. J. Ophthal. **33**, 11–18 (1950)

141. DUKE-ELDER, S.: Primary glaucoma as a vascular disease. Ulster med. J. **22**, 1–16 (1953)

142. DUKE-ELDER, S.: The aetiology of simple glaucoma. Trans. ophthal. Soc. U.K. **77**, 205–228 (1957)

143. DUKE-ELDER, S.: The diagnosis and treatment of simple glaucoma. Canad. med. Ass. J. **82**, 293–297 (1960)

144. DUKE-ELDER, S.: System of ophthalmology, vol. 2, p. 286–293. London: Kimpton 1961

145. DUKE-ELDER, S.: The problems of simple glaucoma. Trans. ophthal. Soc. U.K. **82**, 307–313 (1962)

146. DUKE-ELDER, S., DOBREE, J.H.: System of ophthalmology, vol. X, p. 60–63. London: Kimpton 1967

147. EARL, C.J., ZILKHA, K.J.: Syphilitic visual failure. Brit. J. Ophthal. **48**, 630–632 (1964)

148. ECHTE, K., PAPST, W.: Vorteile der Linsen-Haftschale für die Registrierung des Elektroretinogramms. Acta ophthal. (Kbh.), Suppl. 70, 176–181 (1962)

149. EDMUND, J., JENSEN, S.F.: E.R.G. in temporal arteritis. Acta ophthal. (Kbh.) 45, 601–609 (1967)

150. EDWARDS, C.H., GORDON, N.S., ROB, C.: The surgical treatment of internal carotid artery occlusion. Quart. J. Med. 29, 67–84 (1960)

151. ELLENBERGER, C. JR., NETSKY, M.G.: Infarction in the optic nerve. J. Neurol. Neurosurg. Psychiat. 31, 606–611 (1968)

152. ELLIS, C.J., HAMER, D.B., HUNT, R.W., LEVER, A.F., LEVER, R.S., PEART, W.S., WALKER, S.M.: Medical investigation of retinal vascular occlusion. Brit. med. J. 1964 II, 1093–1098

153. ELLIS, P.P., HAMILTON, H.: Retrobulbar neuritis in pernicious anemia. Amer. J. Ophthal. 48, 95–97 (1959)

154. ELSCHNIG, A.: Bemerkungen über die glaucomatöse Excavation. Ber. dtsch. ophthal. Ges. Heidelberg 24, 149–154 (1895)

155. ELSCHNIG, A.: Glaukom ohne Hochdruck und Hochdruck ohne Glaukom. Z. Augenheilk. 52, 287–296 (1924)

156. ELSCHNIG, A.: In: Handbuch der speziellen pathologischen Anatomie und Histologie, ed. F. Henke und O. Lubarsch, vol. II (Auge), pt. I, p. 917. Berlin: Springer 1928

157. ENGEL, F.L.: An unusual case of malignant exophthalmos and postoperative hypothyroidism complicating Graves' disease. J. clin. Endocr. 13, 1132–1139 (1953)

158. ERNEST, J.T., ARCHER, D.: Fluorescein angiography of the optic disk. Amer. J. Ophthal. 75, 973–978 (1973)

159. ERNEST, J.T., POTTS, A.M.: Pathophysiology of the distal portion of the optic nerve, II. Amer. J. Ophthal. 66, 380–387 (1968)

160. ERNEST, J.T., POTTS, A.M.: Pathophysiology of the distal portion of the optic nerve. III. Amer. J. Ophthal. 68, 594–604 (1969)

161. ESPILDORA-LUQUE, C.: Sindrome Oftalmico-silviano. Arch. Oftal. hisp.-amer. 34, 616–621 (1934)

162. EVANS, P.J.: The underlying causes of glaucoma. Brit. J. Opthal. 23, 745–783 (1939)

163. FALCONER, M.A., ALEXANDER, W.S.: Experiences with malignant exophthalmos. Brit. J. Ophthal. 35, 253–283 (1951)

164. FERREIRA, C. DE, PARREIRA, F.: Hemianópsia bilateral inferior por hemorragia uterina. Gaz. med. Port. 10, 357–369 (1957)

165. FINK, K.: Akute transitorische Erblindung post partum. Zbl. Gynäk. 48, 1188–1191 (1924)

166. FISHER, J.H.: Optic atrophy following haemorrhage. Trans. ophthal. Soc. U.K. 49, 151 (1929)

167. FISHER, M.: Transient monocular blindness associated with hemiplegia. Arch. Opthal. (Chic.) 47, 167–203 (1952)

168. FLEISCHER, B.: Zur Pathologie und Therapie der Hypophysis Tumoren. Klin. Mbl. Augenheilk. 52, 625–653 (1914)

169. FONT, J.H.: Otorhinolaryngological considerations of the temporal arteritis syndrome. J. Amer. med. Ass. 174, 853–856 (1960)

170. FOULDS, W.S.: Ischaemic optic neuropathy. Proc. Wm. Mackenzie Cent. Symp. on the ocular circulation in health and disease, ed. J.S. Cant, p. 136–141. London: Kimpton 1968

171. FOULDS, W.S.: Visual disturbances in systemic disorders—optic neuropathy and systemic disease. Trans. ophthal. Soc. U.K. 89, 125–146 (1969)

172. FOULDS, W.S., CHISHOLM, I.A., REID, H.C.R.: The effects of raised intra-ocular pressure on visual function. Proc. 2nd Wm. Mackenzie Symp. on the optic nerve, Glasgow, ed. J.S. Cant, p. 323–330. London: Kimpton 1972

173. FRANÇOIS, J.: Les pseudo-papillites vasculaires. Rapport Soc. franç. Ophthal. (1956)

174. FRANÇOIS, J., NEETENS, A.: Vascularization of the optic pathway. I. Brit. J. Ophthal. 38, 472–488 (1954)

175. FRANÇOIS, J., NEETENS, A., COLLETTE, J.M.: Vascular supply of the optic pathway. II. Brit. J. Opthal. 39, 220–232 (1955)

176. FRANÇOIS, J., NEETENS, A.: Vascularization of the optic pathway. III. Brit. J. Ophthal. 40, 45–52 (1956)

177. FRANÇOIS, J., NEETENS, A.: Central retinal artery and central optic nerve artery. Brit. J. Ophthal. 47, 21–30 (1963)

178. FRANÇOIS, J., NEETENS, A.: Vascularity of the eye and the optic nerve in glaucoma. Arch. Ophthal. (Chic.) 71, 219–225 (1964)

179. FRANÇOIS, J., NEETENS, A.: Increased intraocular pressure and optic nerve atrophy, p. 38–93, 124–145. Brüssels: Editions Arscia 1966

180. FRANÇOIS, J., NEETENS, A.: Physio-anatomy of the axial vascularization of the optic nerve. Docum. ophthal. (Den Haag) 26, 38–49 (1969)

182. FRANÇOIS, J., VERRIEST, G., BARON, A.: Pseudo-papillites. Bull. Soc. franç. Ophtal. 69, 36–57 (1956)

183. FRANÇOIS, J., VERRIEST, G., BARON, A.: Pseudo-papillites vasculaires. Acta ophthal. (Kbh.) 35, 32–52 (1957)

184. FRANÇOIS, J., VERRIEST, G., DEROUCK, A.: L'électro-oculographie en tant qu'examen functionnel de la rétine. Progr. en Ophtal. 7, 1–67 (1957)

185. FRANÇOIS, J., VERRIEST, G., DEROUCK, A., HANSSENS, M.: Pseudonévrites optiques oedémateuses d'origine vasculaire. Ann. Oculist. (Paris) 195, 830–885 (1962)

186. FRANÇOIS, J., VERRIEST, G., NEETENS, A., DE-
ROUCK, A.: Pseudopapillites vasculaires. Bull.
Soc. belge Ophtal. **129**, 413–427 (1961)

187. FREITAS DE, F., MORIN, J.D.: The changes in the
blood supply of the posterior pole of rabbits with
ocular hypertension. Canad. J. Ophthal. **6**, 139–
142 (1971)

188. FRIEDENWALD, H.: Visual disturbances in poly-
cythaemia Vera. Contr. med. biol. Res. **1**, 495–501
(1919)

189. FRIEDMAN, J.J.: Occult temporal arteritis. Amer.
J. Ophthal. **60**, 333–335 (1965)

190. FRONIMOPOULOS, J., COFINAS, H.: A case of
pseudo-papilloedema (en grec). Bull. Soc. Hell.
Opht. **25**, 10–15 (1957)

191. FUCHS, E.: Glaucoma simplex. Z. Augenheilk. **25**,
108–110 (1911)

192. FUCHS, E.: Über die Lamina cribrosa. Albrecht
v. Graefes Arch. Ophthal. **91**, 435–485 (1916)

193. FUCHS E.: Über senile Veränderungen des Sehnerven. Albrecht v. Graefes Arch. Ophthal **103**,
304–330 (1920)

194. GAFNER, F., GOLDMANN, H.: Experimentelle Untersuchungen über den Zusammenhang von
Augendrucksteigerung und Gesichtsfeldschädi-
gung. Ophthalmologica (Basel) **130**, 357–377
(1955)

195. GÁLVEZ MONTES, J.: Sobre las affeciones vascu-
lares del nervio optico. Arch. Soc. Oftal. hisp.-
amer. **19**, 208–220 (1959)

196. GARBER, M.I.: Methylprednisolone in the treatment of exophthalmos. Lancet **1966 I**, 958–960

197. GATH, L., MANDI, L.: Das Auftreten von Papillo-
retinitis bei BCG-Geimpften. Ophthalmologica
(Basel) **122**, 143–153 (1951)

198. GAYNON, I.E., ASBURY, M.K.: Ocular findings in
a case of periarteritis nodosa. Amer. J. Ophthal.
26, 1072–1076 (1943)

199. GAYRAL., L., BECHAC, G.: Pseudo-névrite optique
oedémateuse aiguë d'origine vasculaire. Rev.
neurol. **112**, 128–131 (1965)

200. GEDDA, P.O., LINDGREN, M.: The hyperophthal-
mopathic type of Graves' disease. Acta med.
scand. **148**, 385–403 (1954)

201. GEORGIADES, G., KONSTAS, P., STANGOS, N.: Réfle-
xions issues de l'étude de nombreux cas de pseudo-
papillite vasculaire. Bull. Soc. franç. Ophtal. **79**,
506–539 (1966)

202. GILBERT, W.: Beiträge zur Lehre vom Glaukom.
II. Pathologische Anatomie. Albrecht v. Graefes
Arch. Ophthal. **90**, 76–97 (1915)

203. GILMOUR, J.R.: Giant-cell chronic arteritis. J.
Path. Bact **53**, 263–277 (1941)

204. GODER, G.: Durchblutungsstörungen des Auges
und Biopsie der Arteria temporalis. Leipzig:
V.E.B. Georg Thieme 1968

205. GOLDMANN, H.: Some basic problems of simple
glaucoma. Amer. J. Ophthal. **48** (2), 213–220 (1959)

206. GOLDSTEIN, I., WEXLER, D.: Bilateral atrophy of
the optic nerve in periarteritis nodosa. Arch. Ophthal. (Chic.) **18**, 767–773 (1937)

207. GOLDZIEHER, M.A., McGAVACK, T.H., PETERSON,
C.A., GOLDZIEHER, J.W., MILLER, H.R.: Retro-
bulbar neuritis associated with hyperthyroidism.
Arch. Neurol. Psychiat. (Chic.) **65**, 189–196 (1951)

208. GORDON, N.: Ocular manifestations of internal
carotid artery occlusion. Brit. J. Ophthal. **43**, 257–
267 (1959)

209. GOERLITZ, M.: Histologische Untersuchung eines
Falles von Erblindung nach schwerem Blutverlust.
Klin. Mbl. Augenheilk. **64**, 763–782 (1920)

210. GOULDEN, C.: Discussion of optic atrophy following haemorrhage. Trans. ophth. Soc. U.K. **49**, 151–
152 (1929)

211. GOWERS, W.R.: A manual of diseases of the nervous system, 2nd ed., p. 412. London: Churchill 1893

212. GOWERS, W.R.: A manual and atlas of medical
ophthalmoscopy, 4th ed., p. 224–232. Philadelphia: Blakiston's Son and Co. 1904

213. GRADLE, H.S.: Glaucoma simplex without per-
ceptible rise in tension. Arch. Ophthal. (Chic.) **46**,
117–125 (1917)

214. GRAEFE, A. VON: Vorläufige Notiz über das Wesen
des Glaucoma. Albrecht v. Graefes Arch. Ophthal,
1, abt. 1, 371–382 (1854)

215. GRAEFE, A. VON: Amaurose mit Sehnervenexcava-
tion. Albrecht v. Graefes Arch. Ophthal. **3** (2),
484–487 (1857)

216. GRAEFE, A. VON: Über Complication von Sehner-
venentzündung mit Gehirnkrankheiten. Albrecht
v. Graefes Arch. Ophthal. **7** (2) 58–71 (1860)

217. GRAEFE, A. VON: Beiträge zur Pathologie und
Therapie des Glaucoms. Albrecht v. Graefes Arch.
Ophthal. **15**, abt. 3, 108–252 (1869)

218. GRANIT, R.: The components of the retinal action
potential in mammals and their relation to the
discharge in the optic nerve. J. Phys. **77**, 207–239
(1933)

219. GRAVESON, G.S.: Syphilitic optic neuritis. J.
Neurol. Neurosurg. Psychiat. **13**, 216–224 (1950)

220. GREAVES, D.P.: Ophthalmic manifestations of
giant-cell arteritis. Trans. ophthal. Soc. U.K. **81**,
427–436 (1961)

221. GREENFIELD, J.G.: A case of giant-cell arteritis.
Proc. roy. soc. Med. **44**, 855–857 (1951)

222. GRESSER, E.B.: Partial occlusion of retinal vessels
in a case of thrombo-angiitis obliterans. Amer.
J. Ophthal **15**, 235–237 (1932)

223. GRIMMINGER, W.: Über Atrophia nervi optici par-
tialis nach schweren Blutungen. Z. Augenheilk.
57, 106–120 (1925)

224. GROENOUW, A.: Intrasklerale Nervenschleifen.
Klin. Mbl. Augenheilk. **43**, 637–639 (1905)

225. GROUT, G.H.: A case of permanent impairment
of vision following gastrointestinal hemorrhage.
Arch. Ophthal. (Chic.) **43**, 234–236 (1914)

226. GUTTMAN-FRIEDMAN, A.: Blindness after snakebite. Brit. J. Ophthal. **40**, 57–59 (1956)

227. HAAB, O.: System of the diseases of the eye, ed. W.F. Norris and C.A. Oliver, vol. IV, p. 481–537. London: Lippincott 1900

228. HAGER, H.: Weiterer Beitrag zur Augenbeteiligung bei Thromboangiitis obliterans. Klin. Mbl. Augenheilk. **118**, 147–155 (1951)

229. HAHN, R.D.: Some remarks on the management of neurosyphilis. J. chron. Dis. **13**, 1–5 (1961)

230. HAMASAKI, D.I., FUJINO, T.: Effect of intra-ocular pressure on ocular vessels. Arch. Ophthal. (Chic.) **78**, 369–379 (1967)

231. HAMILTON, H.E., ELLIS, P.P., SHEETS, R.F.: Visual impairment due to optic neuropathy in pernicious anemia. Blood **14**, 378–385 (1959)

232. HARBRIDGE, D.F.: Optic atrophy manifested by visual disturbance following distant hemorrhage. Amer. J. Ophthal. **7**, 192–196 (1924)

233. HARRINGTON, D.O.: In: Discussion of "Igersheimer (1958)"

234. HARRINGTON, D.O.: The pathogenesis of the glaucoma field: clinical evidence that circulatory insufficiency in the optic nerve is the primary cause of visual field loss in glaucoma. Amer. J. Ophthal. **47**(2), 177–185 (1959)

235. HARRINGTON, D.O.: The Bjerrum scotoma. Trans. Amer. ophthal. Soc. **62**, 324–348 (1964)

236. HARRINGTON, D.O.: The visual fields, 2nd ed., p. 109, 136–137, 155, 160, 167, 171, 186–187, 195, 205–209, 231–232, 242. St. Louis: Mosby 1964

237. HARTMANN, E., PARFONRY, J.: Cécité part perte de sang améliorée par l'acétylcholine mais conservant un netrecissement binasal du champ visuel. Bull. Soc. Ophtal. (Paris) 56–61 (1934)

238. HAYREH, S.S.: A study of the central artery of the retina in human beings. Thesis for Master of Surgery, Panjab University, India, 1958

239. HAYREH, S.S.: The ophthalmic artery. III. Brit. J. Ophthal. **46**, 212–247 (1962)

240. HAYREH, S.S.: Blood supply of the optic nerve and its clinical significance. Acta XIX Conc. Ophthal. New Delhi **2**, 1194–1199 (1962)

241. HAYREH, S.S.: Blood supply and vascular disorders of the optic nerve. An. Inst. Barraquer **4**, 7–109 (1963)

242. HAYREH, S.S.: Arteries of the orbit in the human being. Brit. J. Surg. **50**, 938–953 (1963)

243. HAYREH, S.S.: The central artery of the retina—its role in the blood supply of the optic nerve. Brit. J. Ophthal. **47**, 651–663 (1963)

244. HAYREH, S.S.: The central artery of the retina. Acta XX Conc. Ophthal. Germania **1**, 104–105 (1966)

245. HAYREH, S.S.: Blood supply of the optic nerve head and its role in optic atrophy, glaucoma and oedema of the optic disc. Brit. J. Ophthal. **53**, 721–748 (1969)

246. HAYREH, S.S.: Blood supply of the optic nerve head and its role in optic atrophy, glaucoma and oedema of the optic disc. Proc. Int. Symp. Fluorescein Angiography—Albi, ed. P. Amalric p. 510–530. Basel: Karger 1969

247. HAYREH, S.S.: Pathogenesis of visual field defects—role of the ciliary circulation. Brit. J. Ophthal. **54**, 289–311 (1970)

248. HAYREH, S.S.: Pathogenesis of occlusion of the central retinal vessels. Amer. J. Ophthal. **72**, 998–1011 (1971)

249. HAYREH, S.S.: Posterior ciliary arterial occlusive disorders. Trans. ophthal. Soc. U.K. **91**, 291–303 (1971)

250. HAYREH, S.S.: Optic disc changes in glaucoma. Brit. J. Ophthal. **56**, 175–185 (1972)

251. HAYREH, S.S.: Colour and fluorescence of the optic disc. Ophthalmologica (Basel) **165**, 100–108 (1972)

252. HAYREH, S.S.: Optic disc vasculitis. Brit. J. Ophthal. **56**, 652–670 (1972)

253. HAYREH, S.S.: Occlusion of the posterior ciliary arteries. Trans. Amer. Acad. Ophthal. Otolaryng. **77**, OP–300–309 (1973)

254. HAYREH, S.S.: Anatomy and physiology of the optic nerve head. Trans. Amer. Acad. Ophthal. Otolaryng. **78**, OP–240–254 (1974)

255. HAYREH, S.S.: Anterior ischaemic optic neuropathy I. Terminology and Pathogenesis. Brit. J. Ophthal. **58**, 955–963 (1974)

256. HAYREH, S.S.: Anterior ischaemic optic neuropathy, II. Fundus on Ophthalmoscopy and Fluorescein Angiography. Brit. J. Ophthal. **58**, 964–980 (1974)

257. HAYREH, S.S.: Anterior ischaemic optic neuropathy. III. Treatment, prophylaxis, and differential diagnosis. Brit. J. Ophthal. **58**, 981–989 (1974)

258. HAYREH, S.S.: Pathogenesis of cupping of the optic disc. Brit. J. Ophthal. **58**, 863–876 (1974)

258a. HAYREH, S.S.: The long posterior ciliary arteries. An experimental study. Albrecht v. Graefes Arch. klin. exp. ophthal. **192**, 197–213 (1974)

259. HAYREH, S.S., BAINES, J.A.B.: Occlusion of the posterior ciliary artery. I. Effects on choroidal circulation. Brit. J. Ophthal. **56**, 719–735 (1972)

260. HAYREH, S.S., BAINES, J.A.B.: Occlusion of the posterior ciliary artery. II. Chorio-retinal lesions. Brit. J. Ophthal. **56**, 736–753 (1972)

261. HAYREH, S.S., BAINES, J.A.B.: Occlusion of the posterior ciliary artery. III. Effects on the optic nerve head. Brit. J. Ophthal. **56**, 754–764 (1972)

262. HAYREH, S.S.,, PERKINS, E.S.: Clinical and experimental studies on the circulation at the optic nerve head. Proc. The William Mackenzie Centenary Symposium on the Ocular Circulation in Health and Disease. Glasgow, 1968, ed. J.S. Cant, p. 71–86. London: Kimpton

263. HAYREH, S.S., PERKINS, E.S.: The effects of raised intra-ocular pressure on the blood vessels of the

retina and optic disc. Proc. Int. Symp. Fluorescein Angiography. Albi, 1969, ed. P. Amalric, p. 323–328. Basel: Karger

264. HAYREH, S.S., REVIE, I.H.S., EDWARDS, J.: Vasogenic origin of visual field defects and optic nerve changes in glaucoma. Brit. J. Ophthal. **54**, 461–472 (1970)

265. HAYREH, S.S., VRABEC, F.: The structure of the head of the optic nerve in rhesus monkey. Amer. J. Ophthal. **61**, 136–150 (1966)

266. HEDGES, T.R., SCHEIE, H.G.: Visual field defects in exophthalmos associated with thyroid disease. Arch. Ophthal. (Chic.) **54**, 885–892 (1955)

267. HEGNER, C.A.: Über Sehstörungen bei schweren Blutverlusten. Klin. Mbl. Augenheilk. **50**(1), 119 (1912)

268. HEILMANN, K.: Augendruck, Blutdruck und Glaukomschaden. Stuttgart: Ferdinand Enke 1972

269. HENDERSON, J.W.: Optic neuropathy of Graves, disease. Trans. Amer. ophthal. Soc. **55**, 353–367 (1957)

270. HENDERSON, J.W.: Optic neuropathy of exophthalmic goiter (Graves' disease). Arch. Ophthal. (Chic.) **59**, 471–480 (1958)

271. HENKIND, P.: Radial peripapillary capillaries of the retina. I. Anatomy: Human and comparative. Brit. J. Ophthal. **51**, 115–123 (1967)

272. HENKIND, P., CHARLES, N.C., PEARSON, J.: Histopathology of ischemic optic neuropathy. Amer. J. Ophthal. **69**, 78–90 (1970)

273. HENKIND, P., LEVITZKY, M.: Angioarchitecture of the optic nerve. I. The papilla. Amer. J. Ophthal. **68**, 979–986 (1969)

274. HENSCHEN, S.E.: Über circumscripte arteriosklerotische Nekrosen (Erweichungen) in dem Sehnerven, im Chiasma und in dem Tractus. Albrecht v. Graefes Arch. Ophthal. **78**, 212–223 (1911)

275. HEPTINSTALL, R.H., PORTER, K.A., BARKLEY, H.: Giant-cell (temporal) arteritis. J. Path. Bact. **67**, 507–519 (1954)

276. HERMANN, K.: Pituitary exophthalmos. Brit. J. Ophthal. **36**, 1–19 (1952)

277. HERRENSCHWAND, F. VON: Über morphologische Befunde am Auge bei Periarteriitis nodosa im Vergleich zu denen bei Sepsis leuta. Klin. Mbl. Augenheilk. **83**, 419–432 (1929)

278. HIPPEL, E. VON: Über die Schnabelsche Lehre von der Entstehung der glaukomatösen Excavation. Albrecht v. Graefes Arch. Ophthal. **74**, 101–167 (1910)

279. HIRSCHBERG, J.: Amaurose nach Blutverlust. Ber. XIII Vers. Ophthal. Ges. Heidelberg **19**, 69–72 (1881)

280. HIRSCHBERG, J.: Über Amaurose nach Blutverlust. Z. klin. Med. IV, 216–222 (1882)

281. HOFFMAN (cit. by Theobald, 1889)

282. HOGAN, M.J., ALVARADO, J.A., WEDDELL, J.E.: Histology of the human eye, p. 527–606. Philadelphia: Saunders 1971

283. HOGAN, M.J., ZIMMERMAN, L.E.: "Circulatory disturbances" of optic nerve. In: Ophthalmic pathology, 2nd ed., p. 602–604. London and Philadelphia: Saunders 1962

284. HOLDEN, W.A.: The pathology of the amhlyopia following profuse hemorrhage and of that following the ingestion of methyl alcohol, with remarks on the pathogenesis of optic nerve atrophy in general. Arch. Ophthal. (N.Y.) **28**, 125–134 (1899)

285. HOLLENHORST, R.W., BROWN, J.R., WAGENER, H.P., SHICK, R.M.: Neurologic aspects of temporal arteritis. Neurology (Minneap.) **10**, 490–498 (1960)

286. HOLLOW, F.C., GRAHAM, P.A.: The Ferndale glaucoma survey. Proc. Symp. at the Roy. Coll. Surg. of England, ed. L.B. Hunt, p. 24–44. Edinburgh: Livingstone 1965

287. HONDA, Y., PODOS, S.M., BECKER, B.: The effect of diphenylhydantoin on the electroretinogram of rabbits. II. Invest. Ophthal. **12**, 573–578 (1973)

288. HORTON, B.T., MAGATH, T.B.: Arteritis of the temporal vessels. Proc. Mayo Clin. **12**, 548–553 (1937)

289. HORTON, B.T., MAGATH, T.B., BROWN, G.E.: An undescribed form of arteritis of the temporal vessels. Proc. Mayo Clin. **7**, 700–701 (1932)

290. HORTON, B.T., MAGATH, T.B., BROWN, G.E.: Arteritis of the temporal vessels; a previously undescribed form. Ach. intern. Med. **53**, 400–409 (1934)

291. HUGHES, B.: The visual fields, p. 67–71, 76–79. Oxford: Blackwell 1954

292. HUGHES, B.: Blood supply of the optic nerve and chiasma and its clinical significance. Brit. J. Ophthal. **42**, 106–125 (1958)

292a. HUMMELSHEIM, LEBER, T.: Ein Fall von atrophischer Degeneration der Netzhaut und des Sehnerven mit hochgradiger Endarteriitis der Arteria centralis retinae bei Diabetes mellitus. Albrecht v. Graefes Arch. Ophthal. **52**(2), 336–357 (1901)

293. HUTCHINSON, E.C., YATES, P.O.: Carotico-vertebral stenosis. Lancet **1957** I, 2–8

294. HUTCHINSON, J.: On the peculiar form of thrombotic arteritis of the aged which is sometimes productive of gangrene. Disease of Arteritis. Arch. Surg. (Lond.) **1**, 323–329 (1890)

295. IGERSHEIMER, J.: Syphilis und Auge. Berlin: Springer 1918

296. IGERSHEIMER, J.: Sehnervenerkrankung bei maligner Sklerose. Z. Augenheilk. **69**, 47–59 (1929)

297. IGERSHEIMER, J.: General hypertension and peripheral optic pathways. Amer. J. Ophthal. **23**, 1243–1254 (1940)

298. IGERSHEIMER, J.: Visual changes in progressive exophthalmos. Arch. Ophthal. (Chic.) **53**, 94–104 (1955)

299. IGERSHEIMER, J.: Serious visual troubles caused by unusual circulatory disturbances in the region of the optic nerve. Trans. Amer. Ophthal. soc. **56**, 275–287 (1958)

300. IGERSHEIMER, J.: Serious visual troubles caused by unusual circulatory disturbances in the region of the optic nerve. Amer. J. Ophthal. **47**, 767–772 (1959)

301. ISHIKAWA, T.: Fine structure of retinal vessels in man and the Macaque monkey. Invest. Ophthal. **2**, 1–15 (1963)

302. JACOBSON, T.: Dissertation, Königsberg, 1853

303. JACOBY, E.: Über die Neuroglia des Sehnerven. Klin. Mbl. Augenheilk. **43**, 129–137 (No. 1) (1905)

304. JAEGER, E.: Über Star und Staroperationen. Wien: Seidel 1854

305. JAGER, B.V.: In Harrison, T.B., Principles of internal medicine, p. 1708. New York: McGraw-Hill Book Co. 1958

306. JENNINGS, G.H.: Arteritis of the temporal vessels. Lancet **I**, 424–428, **1938**

307. JOHNSON, R.H., HARLEY, R.D., HORTON, B.T.: Arteritis of the temporal vessels associated with loss of vision. Amer. J. Ophthal. **26**, 147–151 (1943)

308. JUDGE, R.D., CURRIER, R.D., GRACIE, W.A., FIGLEY, M.M.: Takayasu's arteritis and the aortic arch syndrome. Amer. J. Med. **32**, 379–392 (1962)

309. KADLECOVÁ, V.: Oedema papillae ischaemicum. Čsl. Ofthal. **7**, 388–394 (1951)

310. KALVIN, N.H., HAMASAKI, D.I., GASS, J.D.M.: Experimental glaucoma in monkeys. Arch. Ophthal. (Chic.) **76**, 82–93, 94–103 (1966)

311. KAPUSCINSKI, W.: Contribution à l'etude du développement de l'excavation et de l'atrophie du nerf optique dans le glaucome simple. Arch. Ophtal. (Paris) **47**, 779–787 (1930)

312. KAREL, I., OTRADOVEC, J., PELESKA, M.: Fluorescence angiography in circulatory disturbances in drusen of the optic disk. Ophthalmologica (Basel) **164**, 449–462 (1972)

313. KAYE, S.L.: Temporal arteritis. Lancet **1949 I**, **1039–1042**

314. KEIL, H.: Dermatomyositis and systemic lupus erythematosus. Arch. intern. Med. **66**, 339–383 (1940)

315. KENNEDY, F.: Cerebral symptoms induced by angioneurotic oedema. Arch. Neurol. Psychiat. (Chic.) **15**, 28–33 (1926)

316. KENNEDY, F.: Certain nervous complications following the use of therapeutic and prophylactic sera. Amer. J. Med. Sci., **177**, 555–559 (1929)

317. KERNOHAN, J.W., WOLTMAN, H.W.: Periarteritis nodosa: A clinicopathological study with special reference to the nervous system. Arch. Neurol. Psychiat. (Chic.) **39**, 655–686, 1938

318. KILBOURNE, E.D., WOLFF, H.G.: Cranial arteritis: A critical evaluation of the syndrome of "temporal arteritis" with report of a case. Arch. intern. Med. **24**, 1–10 (1946)

319. KIMBRELL, O.C., WHELISS, J.A.: Polyarteritis nodosa complicated by bilateral optic neuropathy. J. Amer. med. Ass. **201**, 61–62 (1967)

320. KING, E.F.: Ocular involvement in a case of periarteritis nodosa. Trans. ophthal. Soc. U.K. **55**, 246–256 (1935)

321. KNAPP, A.: Course in certain cases of atrophy of the optic nerve with cupping and low tension. Arch. Ophthal. (Chic.) **23**, 41–47 (1940)

322. KNOX, D.L., DUKE, J.R.: Slowly progressive ischemic optic neuropathy: A clinico-pathologic case report. Trans. Amer. Acad. Ophthal. Otolaryng. **75**, 1065–1068 (1971)

323. KOYANAGI, Y., TAKAHASHI, T.: Kavernöse Sehnervenatrophie bei Orbitaltumoren. Albrecht v. Graefes Arch. Ophthal. **115**, 596–619 (1925)

324. KRAYENBUHL, H., RICHTER, H.R.: Cerebrale Angiographie, S. 217. Stuttgart: Georg Thieme 1952

325. KREIBIG, W.: Optikomalazie, die Folge eines Gefäßverschlusses im retrobulbären Abschnitt des Sehnerven. Klin. Mbl. Augenheilk. **122**, 719–731 (1953)

326. KUHNT, H.: Zur Kenntnis des Sehnerven und der Netzhaut. Albrecht v. Graefes Arch. Ophthal. **25**(3), 179–288 (1879)

327. KÜMMELL, R.L.: Die Sehstörungen nach Blutverlust. In: Kurzes Handbuch der Ophthalmologie, ed. F. Schieck and A. Brückner, vol. 7, p. 62–68. Berlin: Springer 1932

328. KURZ, O.: Zur Pathogenese des Glaucoms ohne Hochdruck. Arch. Augenheilk. **109**, 108–123 (1935)

329. KURZ, O.: Über Papillitis arteriosclerotica. Ophthalmologica (Basel) **116**, 281–285 (1948)

330. KUSSMAUL A.: Zwei Fälle von spontaner allmäliger Verschliessung großer Halsarterienstämme. Dtsch. Klin. **24**, 461–473 (1872)

331. LAATIKAINEN, L.: Fluorescein angiographic studies of the peripapillary and perilimbal regions in simple, capsular and low-tension glaucoma. Acta ophthal. (Kbh.), Suppl. III (1971)

332. LAGRANGE, F., BEAUVIEUX, J.: Anatomie pathologique et pathogénie de l'excavation glaucomateuse. Arch. Ophtal (Paris) **42**, 129–145 (1925)

333. LAKER, C.: Ein experimenteller Beitrag zur Lehre von der glaucomatösen Excavation. Klin. Mbl. Augenheilk. **24**, 187–201 (1886)

334. LAMPERT, P.W., VOGEL, M.H., ZIMMERMAN, L.E.: Pathology of the optic nerve in experimental acute glaucoma. Invest. Ophthal. **7**, 199–213 (1968)

335. LANDBLAD, Y.: Temporal arteritis complicated by iritis. Nord. med. **56**, 1794 (1956)

336. LANGDON, H.M.: Amaurosis after uterine hemorrhage. Arch. Ophthal. (Chic.) **10**, 99–102 (1933)

337. LANGE, O.: Zur Lehre vom Glaukom. Klin. Mbl. Augenheilk. **14**, 540–553 (1912)

338. LARMANDE, A.M.: Les pseudo-syndrome de Fos-

ter Kennedy d'origine vasculaire. Rev. Oto-neuro-ophtal. **20**, 483–485 (1948)

339. LARMANDE, A.M.: Oedèmes papillaires purs d'origine vasculaire en dehors de l'hypertension artérielle. Bull. Soc. Ophtal. (Paris) **8**, 541–546 (1948)

340. LASANSKY, A.: The pathway between hyaloid blood and retinal neurons in the toad. J. Cell. Biol. **34**, 617–626 (1967)

341. LASANSKY, A., WALD, F.: The extracellular space in the toad retina as defined by the distribution of Ferrocyanide. J. Cell. Biol. **15**, 463–479 (1962)

342. LASCO, F.: Les affections vasculaires du nerf optique et leurs manifestations cliniques. I. Ophthalmologica (Basel) **142**, 429–455 (1961)

343. LASCO, F., CONSTANTINESCO, G.: L'amaurose post-hémorragique. Comm. Soc. roum. Ophtal. (1948)

344. LASCO, F., NICOLESCO, M.: Les localisations ophtalmologiques des collagénoses. Arch. Ophtal. (Paris) **20**, 602–615 (1960)

345. LASCO, F., RICONTE, H.: Manifestations papillaires de l'oedème de Quincky. Oftalmologia (Buc.) **3**, 17–18 (1959)

346. LAUBER, H.: Treatment of atrophy of optic nerve. Arch. Ophthal. (Chic.) **16**, 555–568 (1936)

347. LAVY, S., LIBAN, E.: An unusual case of temporal arteritis. Harefuah **54**, 6–9 (1958). Cit. from Ophthal. Lit. (Lond.) **12**, 98 (1958)

348. LAVY, S., NEUMAN, E.: Changes of the optic nerve after cataract extraction simulating the Foster Kennedy syndrome. Confm. neurol. (Basel) **19**, 383–389 (1959)

349. LE BEAU, J., TAPTAS, J.N., BLATRIX, C.: Un nouveau cas d'artérite Temporale thrombosante. Bull. Soc. méd. Hôp. Paris **64**, 397–399 (1948)

350. LEBER, T.: Die Amaurose nach Blutverlusten. In: Handbuch der Gesamten Augenheilkunde (A. Graefe und T. Saemisch), Bd. V, S. 901–906. Leipzig: Engelmann 1877

351. LEGRAND, J., BARON, A., BIGA, S., BILLET: A propos de 3 cas d'oedéma papillaire. Bull. Soc. Ophtal. Fr. **4**, 235–240 (1957)

352. LEOPOLD, M.: Les signes ophthalmologiques de l'athérosclérose. J. Méd. Lyon **40**, 683–691 (1959)

352a. LESSELL, S.: Neuro-ophthalmology. Ann. Rev. Arch. Ophthal. (Chic.) **91**, 66–80 (1974)

353. LEVATIN, P.: Atrophy of the optic nerve following hemorrhage. Arch. Ophthal. (Chic.) **37**, 18–24 (1947)

354. LEVITZKY, M., HENKIND, P.: Angioarchitecture of the optic nerve—II. Lamina cribrosa. Amer. J. Ophthal. **68**, 986–996 (1969)

355. LEYDHECKER, W.: Glaucoma. Symposium by the Council for International Organization of Medical Sciences. Ed. Sir Stewart Duke-Elder, p. 41. Oxford: Blackwell 1955

356. LISCH, K.: Embolie der Zentralarterie bei der Buergerschen Krankheit. Klin. Mbl. Augenheilk. **99**, 812–813 (1937)

357. LOCKET, S.: Blindness associated with haemorrhage. Brit. J. Ophthal. **33**, 543–555 (1949)

358. LOCKSHIN, M.D.: Diplopia as early sign of temporal arteritis: Report of two cases. Arthr. and Rheum. **13**, 419–421 (1970)

359. LOEWENSTEIN, A.: Cavernous degeneration, necrosis and other regressive processes in the optic nerve with vascular disease of the eye. Arch. Ophthal. (Chic.) **34**, 220–226 (1945)

360. LOEWENSTEIN, A., GARROW, A.: Thrombosis of the retinal, choroidal and optic nerve vessels. Amer. J. Ophthal. **28**, 840–851 (1945)

361. LONG, A.E.: Amaurosis following nasal Hemorrhage. Amer. J. Ophthal. **26**, 1179–1182 (1943)

362. LORING, E.G.: Remarks on embolism. Amer. J. med. Sci. **67**, 313–328 (1874)

363. MACFAUL, P.A.: Ciliary artery involvement in giant cell arteritis. Brit. J. Ophthal. **51**, 505–512 (1967)

364. MACMICHAEL, I.M., CULLEN, J.F.: Pathology of ischaemic optic neuropathy. Proc. 2nd Wm. Mackenzie Symp. on the optic nerve. Glasgow, Ed. J.S. Cant, p. 108–116. London: Kimpton 1972

365. MAGITOT, A.: La symptomatologie du glaucome et le problème pathogénique. Ann. Oculist. (Paris) **166**, 356–376, 439–468, 565–580, 609–639 (1929)

366. MAGITOT, A.: Sur l'origine intra-cranienne de l'atrophie optique glaucomateuse. Ann. Oculist. (Paris) **180**, 321–341 (1947) (Ophthal. Lit. (Lond.) **1**, 291–292 (1947)

367. MAGITOT, A.: L'atrophie optique du glaucome primaire; considérations neuro-vasculaires. Ann. Oculist. (Paris) **186**, 385–414 (1953)

368. MANSCHOT, W.A.: The eye in relation to collagen diseases. Trans. ophthal. Soc. U.K. **80**, 137–151 (1960)

369. MANSCHOT, W.A.: A fatal case of temporal arteritis, with ocular symptoms. Ophthalmologica (Basel) **149**, 121–130 (1965)

370. MARCHESANI, O. VON: Thromboangiitis obliterans am Auge. Arch. Augenheilk. **109**, 124–138 (1935)

371. MARCHESANI, O. VON: In „Über den Wert der Röntgendiagnose bei unklaren Sehnervenleiden" Klin. Mbl. Augenheilk. **95**, 389–390 (1935)

372. MARQUEZ, M.: Old and new theories on ocular hypertension and glaucoma. Ophthal. ibero-amer. **9**, 148–169 (1947)

373. MASON, V.R.: Optic neuritis in serum sickness. J. Amer. med. Ass. **78**, 88–89 (1922)

374. MASPES, P.E., FASSANÒ: la thrombos della carotide interna al collo. Sist. nerv. **2**, 75–118 (1953)

375. MATHUR, S.P.: Allergy to antivenine serum. Brit. J. Ophthal. **43**, 50–51, (1959)

376. MAUL, G.H.: Über die Thromoangiitis obliterans (Bueger) unter dem Bild einer Embolie der arteria centralis retinae. Klinische und anatomische Beobachtungen. Dissertation, Univ. Münster, 1938

377. MAUTHNER, L.: Transient embolism of the central artery of the retina. Amer. J. med. Sci. **68**, 273 (1874)

378. McDONALD, W.I., SANDERS, M.D.: Migraine complicated by ischaemic papillopathy. Lancet **1971 II**, 521–523

379. McGUIRE, W.P.: The effect of dicumarol on the visual fields in glaucoma. Trans. Amer. ophthal. Soc. **46**, 96–121 (1948)

380. McLEAN, J.M.: Management of the primary glaucomas. Amer. J. Ophthal. **44**, 323–334 (1957)

381. McLEOD, D., HAYREH, S.S.: Occlusion of the posterior ciliary artery. IV. Electroretinographic studies. Brit. J. Ophthal. **56**, 765–769 (1972)

382. MEADOWS, S.P.: Temporal arteritis and loss of vision. Trans. ophthal. Soc. U.K. **74**, 13–24 (1954)

383. MEADOWS, S.P.: Temporal or giant cell arteritis. Proc. roy. Soc. Med. **59**, 329–333 (1966)

384. MEADOWS, S.P.: Temporal or giant cell arteritis—ophthalmic aspects. Proc. Neuro-Opthal. Symp. of the Univ. of Miami and Bascom Palmer Eye Institute, IV, ed. J.L. Smith, p. 148–157. St. Louis: Mosby

385. MENEELY, J.K., JR., BIGELOW, N.H.: temporal arteritis. Amer. J. Med. **14**, 46–51 (1953)

386. MERKULOV, I.I.: Vascular neuro-ophthalmological syndromes. In: Vop. Neirooftal. Moscow, Medgiz, **4**, 5–79 (1959). Cit. from Excerpta med. XII, **15**, 110 (1961)

387. MICHAELSON, I.C., CAMPBELL, A.C.P.: The anatomy of the finer retinal vessels, and some observations on their significance in certain retinal diseases. Trans. ophthal. Soc. U.K. **60**, 71–112 (1940)

388. MILLER, G.R., SMITH, J.L.: Ischaemic optic neuropathy. Amer. J. Ophthal. **62**, 103–115 (1966)

389. MILLER, H.: Headache. Trans. ophthal. Soc. U.K. **84**, 627–636 (1964)

390. MILLER, S.: The enigma of glaucoma simplex. Trans. ophthal. Soc. U.K. **92**, 563–584 (1972)

391. MINTON, J.: A clinical study of fifty-four cases of occlusion of the central artery of the retina and its branches. Proc. roy. Soc. Med. **30**, 285–300 (1936)

392. MONIZ AND EGAS: Thrombosis of the internal carotid artery and its branches. Meet. Soc. Brit. Neurol. Surgeons, Lisbonne **1**, 30 (1947)

393. MONIZ LIMA, A., DE LACERDA: Les himiplégies par thrombose de la carotide interne. Presse méd. **45**, 977–980 (1937)

394. MORAX, V.: Glaucome simple ou atrophie avec excavation. Ann. Oculist. (Paris) **153**, 25–36 (1916)

395. MORGAN, J.E.: Raynaud's symmetrical gangrene in a patient suffering from constitutional syphilis-Lancet **1889 II**, 9–11

396. MORO, F.: Sulle manifestazioni occulare delle forme occulte di arterite temporale. Ann. Ottal. **89**, 631–650 (1963)

397. MORO, F.: Affezioni vascolari del nervo ottico e della retina e biopsia dell'arteria temporale superficiale. Ann. Ottal. **89**, supp. a dic., 1167–1198 (1963)

398. MORO, F.: Pseudo-papillite vascolare in arterite temporale occulta. Atti Soc. oftal. lombarda **18**, 74–80 (1963)

399. MORO, F.: Considérations sur une sérese de biopsii de l'artère temporale superficielle dans quelques affections vasculaires del'œil. Bull. Soc. franç. Ophtal. **76**, 226–241 (1963)

400. MOSHER, H.A.: The prognosis in temporal arteritis. Arch. Ophthal. (Chic.) **62**, 641–644 (1959)

401. MUGNAINI, E., WALBERG, F.: The fine structure of the capillaries and their surroundings in the cerebral hemispheres of Myxine Glutinosa. Z. Zellforsch. Mikrosk. Anat. **66**, 333–351 (1965)

402. MÜLLER, H.: Sitzungsberichte der physikalisch-medizinischen Gesellschaft in Würzburg. 8. März, p. 26. In: Gesammelte und hinterlassene Schriften zur Anatomie und Physiologie des Auges, ed. O. Becker, vol. 1, p. 340 (published 1872), Leipzig: Engelmann

403. MÜLLER, H.: Anatomische Beiträge zur Ophthalmologie. Albrecht v. Graefes Arch. Ophthal. **4**(2), 1–40 (1858)

404. MÜLLER, J.: Amaurose nach Tubenruptur. Zbl. Gynäk. **75**, 1601–1609, 1953

405. NAFFZIGER, H.C.: Progressive exophthalmos. Bull. Amer. Coll. Surg. **40**, 33–39 (1955)

406. NELSON, M.G., WEAVER, J.A.: A case of Addisonian Pernicious Anaemia presenting with optic atrophy, iron-deficiency anaemia and pigmentation of the skin. Irish J. med. Sci. **6**(365), 229–233 (1956)

407. NETTLESHIP, E.: Embolism of central artery of retina—microscopical examination. Roy. Lond. ophthal. Hosp. Rep. **8**, 9–20 (1874)

408. NEUMANN, E., HYAMS, S.W.: Intermittent glaucomatous excavation. Arch. Ophthal. (Chic.) **90**, 64–66 (1973)

409. NIEDERMEIER, S.: Betrachtungen zur Frage der vasogenen Glaukomkomponente. Albrecht v. Graefes Arch. Ophthal. **158**, 303–309 (1957)

410. NORDMANN, J.: In discussion of paper on "Probleme bei der Diagnose und Therapie des Glaukoms" by W. Leydhecker. Docum. Ophthal. **10**, 230–232 (1956)

411. NORDMANN, J.: Au sujet de quelques questions fondamentales concernant le glaucome. Ann. Oculist. (Paris) **193**, 17–27 (1960)

412. O'DAY, D., CROCK, G., GALBRAITH, J.E.K., PAREL, J.M., WIGLEY, A.: Fluorescein angiography of normal and atrophic discs. Lancet **1967|II**, 224–226

413. OGAWA, K.: Über die kavernöse Degeneration des Sehnerven. Arch. Augenheilk. **72**, 10–20 (1912)

414. PAGANI, L.: Sull'arterite temporale. Rass. Ital. Ottal. **27**, 444–462 (1958)

415. PAILLAS, J., CHRISTOPHE, L.: Les thromboses de la carotide interne et de ses branches. Rev. méd. Liège **10**, 302–308 (1955)

416. PAILLAS, J.E., GUILLOT, P., Duplay, J.: Six observations de neuropapillites aigües etc. Bull. Soc. Ophtal Fr. 202–210 (1949)

417. PALM, E.: The ocular crisis of the temporal arteritis syndrome (Horton). Acta ophthal. (Kbh.) **36**, 208–243 (1958)

418. PALM, E.: Optico-retinal ischemia in cases of occult temporal arteritis (Abstract). Acta ophthal. (Kbh.) **42**, 501–502 (1964)

419. PARRY, T.G.W., LASZLO, G.C.: Herpes zoster ophthalmicus—two rare manifestations. Brit. J. Ophthal. **27**, 465–467 (1943)

420. PARSONS-SMITH, G.: Ophthalmic manifestations of temporal arteritis. Brit. J. Ophthal. **36**, 615–625 (1952)

421. PARSONS-SMITH, G.: Sudden blindness in cranial arteritis. Brit. J. Ophthal. **43**, 204–216 (1959)

422. PASTEUR, V.R., BLAMOUTIER, P., MAWAS, L., HAMBURGER, J.: Accès de migraine ophtalmique suivis d'une hémorragie rétinienne. Ann. Méd. **42**, 132–137 (1937)

423. PATON, L.: The trigeminal and its ocular lesions. Brit. J. Ophthal. **10**, 305–342 (1926)

424. PAUFIQUE, L., ETIENNE, R.: Le diagnostic des névrites retrobulbaires. Gaz. méd. Fr. **58**, 1007–1011 (1951)

425. PAUFIQUE, L., ETIENNE, R.: Les symptomes neuro-végétatifs oculaires dans les discopathies cervicales. Sém. Hôp. (Paris) **55**, 2294 (1954)

426. PAUFIQUE, L., GIRARD, P.F., ETIENNE, R.: Discopathies cervicales et névrites optiques. Bull. Soc. franç. Ophtal. **63**, 90–97 (1950)

427. PAYNE, R.W.: Causes of the grossly elevated erythrocyte sedimentation rate. Practitioner **200**, 415–417 (1968)

428. PEARS, M.A., PICKERING, G.W.: Changes in the fundus occuli after haemorrhage. Quart. J. Med. **29**, 153–178 (1960)

429. PENZOLDT, F.: Über Thrombose (autochthone oder embolische) der Carotis. Dtsch. Arch. klin. Med. **28**, 80–93 (1881)

430. PERGENS, E.: L'amourose et l'amblyopie après hématémèse. Ann. Oculist. (Paris) **115**, 5–32 (1896)

431. PESTALOZZI, D., MARTENET, A.C.: Zur Kasuistik der Arteritis temporalis mit Augenbeteiligung (Bericht über II Fälle). Ophthalmologica (Basel) **141**, 155–180 (1961)

432. PELTOLA, P.: Temporal arteritis. Ann. med. intern. Fenn. **36**, 112–123 (1947)

433. PETERS, W.: Über die Neuritis optici arteriosklerotischer Genese. Klin. Mbl. Augenheilk. **132**, 363–377 (1958)

434. PICKARD, R.: Cavernous optic atrophy and its relation to glaucoma. Brit. J. Ophthal. **9**, 385–398 (1925)

435. PICKARD, R.: The perioptic atrophic ring and its relationships. Brit. J. Ophthal. **30**, 437–445 (1946)

436. PIETROWA, N.: Lesions of the fundus in peripheral vessel diseases. Pol. Arch. Med. Wewnet. **28**, 716–718 (1958) Cit. Ophthal. Lit. (Lond.) **12**, 741 (1958)

437. PINCUS, F.: Über Sehstörungen nach Blutverlust. Albrecht v. Graefe's Arch. Ophthal. **98**, 152–170, 1919

438. PINCUS, J.H., GROVE, I., MARINO, B.B., GLASER, G.E.: Studies on the mechanism of action of diphenylhydantoin. Arch. Neurol. **22**, 566–571 (1970)

439. PINES, N.: Retinitis nephritica or albuminurica. Brit. J. Ophthal. **15**, 75–101 (1931)

440. PINKHAM, R.A.: The ocular manifestations of the pulseless syndrome. XVII Conc. Ophthal., 1954. Canada, United States of America. Acta vol. **I**, 348–366 (1954)

441. PIPER, H.F. VON, UNGER, L.: Hemianopsia horizontalis inferior bei akuten Durchblutungsstörungen des Sehnerven. Ophthalmologica (Basel) **134**, 169–180 (1957)

442. PONTE, F.: La pseudo-papillite vasculaire artério-scléreuse. G. ital. Oftal. **17**, 170–191 (1964)

443. POPPEN, J.L.: Intractable exophthalmos in thyroid disease. Postgrad. Med. **14**, 130–133 (1953)

444. PRIESTLY-SMITH: Reflex amblyopia and thrombosis of the retinal artery. Ophthal. Rev. **3**, 1–17 (1884)

445. PRÖLL: Über Sehstörungen nach Blutverlust. Inaugural-Dissertation, Freiburg, 1907

446. PUPPEL, E.: Sehstörungen nach Genitalblutungen. Mschr. Geburtsh. Gynäk. **65**, 351–358 (1924)

447. RADOVICI, A., LASCO, F.: L'hémiplégie alterne optico-pyramidale par thrombose carotidienne. Presse méd. **56**, 573–574 (1948)

448. RAEHLMANN, E.: Über Sklerose der Netzhautarterien als Ursache plötzlicher beiderseitiger Erblindungen. Fortschr. Med. (Berl.) **7**, 928–938 (1889)

449. RAUBITSCHEK, E.: Über alternierende Papillitis bei Albuminurie. Klin. Mbl. Augenheilk. **52**, 457–464 (1914)

450. RAYNAUD, M.: Nouvelles recherches sur la nature et le traitement de l'asphyxie locale des extrémités. Arch. gén. Méd. **23**, 189–206 (1874)

451. REDSLOB, E.: Glaucome sans hypertension et excavation glaucomateuse. Ann. Oculist. (Paris) **177**, 323–340 (1941)

452. REDSLOB, E.: Le glaucome primaire vu à travers son anatomie pathologique. Ann. Oculist. (Paris) **188**, 781–826 (1955)

453. REDSLOB, E.: Le problème de l'atrophie du nerf optique dans le glaucome chronique. Ann. Oculist. (Paris) **190**, 261–267 (1957)

454. REESE, A.B., CARROLL, F.D.: Optic neuritis following cataract extraction. Amer. J. Ophthal. **45**, 659–662 (1958)

455. REESE, A.B., McGAVIC, J.S.: Relation of field contraction to blood pressure in chronic primary glaucoma. Arch. Ophthal. (Chic.) **27**, 845–850 (1942)

456. REESE, T.S., KARNOVSKY, M.J.: Fine structural localization of a bloodbrain barrier to exogenous peroxidase. J. Cell Biol. **34**, 207–217 (1967)

457. RINTELEN, F.: Über arteriosklerotische Opticusatrophie. Ophthalmologica (Basel) **111**, 285–290 (1946)

458. RINTELEN, F.: Zur Kenntnis der Leitungsstörungen des Fasciculus opticus, insbesondere der "Apoplexia papillae." Ophthalmologica (Basel) **141**, 283–289 (1961)

459. RISER, FELGINES, GAYRAL, GÉRAUD, RIBAUT: L'amaurose posthémorragique. Rev. Oto-neurooftal. **23**, 175–181 (1951)

460. RIZZINI, V., FRASSINETI, A.: Un cas d'artérite temporale à issuefatale. Ophthalmologica (Basel) **130**, 178–186 (1955)

461. ROBERTSON, K.: Temporal or giant cell arteritis. Brit. med. J. **1947 II**, 168–170

462. RODENHÄUSER, J.H.: Über pathologisch-anatomische Augenveränderungen bei generalisierter Riesenzellarteriitis. Klin. Mbl. Augenheilk. **145**, 414–429 (1964)

463. RØNNE, H.: Sehnenervenleiden nach Blutverlust. In: Kurzes Handbuch der Ophthalmologie, ed. F. Schieck and A. Bruckner, vol. 5, p. 702–704. Berlin: Springer 1932

464. RÖTTH, A. VON: Ein Fall von Schüller-Christianscher Krankheit. Klin. Mbl. Augenheilk. **92**, 675 (1934)

465. ROTH, A.M., FOOS, R.Y.: Surface structure of the optic nerve head. Amer. J. Ophthal. **74**, 977–985 (1972)

466. RUCKER, C.W.: circulatory disorders. Trans. Amer. Acad. Ophthal. Otolaryng. **60**, 60–62 (1956)

467. RUSSELL, R.W.R.: Giant-cell arteritis. Quart. J. Med. **28**, 471–489 (1959)

468. RUSSELL, R.W.R., EARL, C.J.: Loss of vision from cranial arteritis without other symptoms. Brit. J. Ophthal. **48**, 619–621 (1964)

469. RYAN, H.: Total blindness from temporal arteritis. Med. J. Aust. **47**, 978–979 (1960)

470. SALZMANN, M.: The anatomy and histology of the human eyeball in the normal state, its development and senescence, p. 94. Translator: E.V.L. Brown, Chicago: Chicago University Press 1912

471. SANDERS, M.D.: Ischaemic papillopathy. Trans. ophthal. Soc. U.K. **91**, 360–386 (1971)

472. SANNA, M.: Angio- e neuroscotometria nel glaucoma cronico semplice. Boll. Oculist. **29**, 111–122 (1950)

473. SANNA, M.: Le Pseudopapilliti vascolari. Riv. otoneuro-oftal. (B. Aires) **33**, 449–470 (1958)

474. SAURAUX, H., MURAT, J.P.: Les pseudo-papillites d'origine vasculaire. Ann. Oculist. (Paris) **200**, 1–19 (1967)

475. SARIN, L.K.: Carotid artery disease and papilledema. J. Maine med. Ass. **51**, 48–49 (1960)

476. SAVORY, M.: In Sorsby, A., Systemic ophthalmology, 2 nd ed., p. 500. St. Louis: Mosby 1958

477. SCHIMEK, R.A., NEWSOM, S.R.: Restoration of vision in temporal arteritis by retrobulbar injections of steroids. Amer. J. Ophthal. **62**, 693–696 (1966)

478. SCHMELZER: Zur Thromboangiitis obliterans am Auge. Klin. Mbl. Augenheilk. **98**, 389 (1937)

479. SCHMIDT, M.: Intracranial aneurysms. Brain **53**, 489–540 (1930)

480. SCHNABEL, J.: Das glaukomatöse Sehnervenleiden. Arch. Augenheilk. **24**, 273–292 (1892)

481. SCHNABEL, J.: Die Entwicklungsgeschichte der glaukomatösen Exkavation. Z. Augenheilk. **14**, 1–22 (1905)

482. SCHNABEL, W.J.: Klinische Daten zur Entwicklungsgeschichte der glaukomatösen Exkavation. Z. Augenheilk. **19**, 335–346 (1908)

483. SCHNAUDIGEL, O.: Die kavernöse Sehnervenentartung. Albrecht v. Graefes Arch. Ophthal. **59**(2), 344–359 (1904)

483a. SCHNEIDER, H.A., WEBER, A.A., BALLEN, P.H.: The visual prognosis in temporal arteritis. Ann. Ophthal. **3**, 1215–1230 (1971)

484. SCHNEIDER, R.W., GARDNER, W.J.: Correction of malignant exophthalmos by transection of the pituitary stalk after unsuccessful orbital decompression. (Abstract), J. clin. Endocr. **14**, 830 (1954)

485. SCOTT, G.I.: Traquair's clinical perimetry, 7th ed., p. 187–188. London: Kimpton 1957

486. SCOTT, G.I.: Optic disc oedema. Trans. ophthal. Soc. U.K. **87**, 733–753 (1967)

487. SCOTT, T., MAXWELL, E.S: Temporal arteritis. Internat. Clin. **2**, 220–223 (1941)

488. SEESE: Dissertation Jena, 1914. Cit. by Wolff, 1935

489. SEGAL, P., ADAMCZEWSKA, Z., KRAWCZYK, Z.: Some eye symptoms in thrombosis of the internal carotid artery. (Polish). Klin. Oczna **31**, 1–9 (1961)

490. SEITZ, R.: Über die Pathogenese des Verschlusses der Netzhautarterien. Ber. dtsch. ophthal. Ges. **64**, 321–328 (1961)

491. SHAFFER, R.N.: The role of astroglial cells in glaucomatous disc cupping. Docum. ophthal. **26**, 516–525 (1969)

492. SHAFFER, R.N., HETHERINGTON, J.: The glaucomatous disc in infants. A suggested hypothesis for disc cupping. Trans. Amer. Acad. Ophthal. Otolaryng. **73**, 929–935 (1969)

493. SHAKIB, M., CUNHA-VAZ, J.G.: Studies on the permeability of the bloodretinal barrier: IV. Exp. Eye Res. **5**, 229–234 (1966)

494. SHANNON, E.W., SALOMON, J.: Bilateral temporal arteritis with complete loss of vision. J. Amer. med. Ass. **127**, 647–649 (1945)

495. SHEEHAN, B., HARRIMAN, D.G.F., BRADSHAW, J.P.P.: Polyarteritis nodosa with ophthalmic and neurological complications. Arch. Ophthal. (Chic.) **60**, 537–547 (1958)

495a. SHIMIZU, K.: Arterial and venous occlusions of the retina. Abstracts, IX Intern. Cong. Angiology, Florence, Italy. Minn. Cardioang. **22**, 137–138 (1974)

496. SHIMIZU, K., SANO, K.: Pulseless disease. J. Neuropath. clin. Neurol. **1**, 37–47 (1951)

497. SHINKLE, C.E.: Raynaud's disease involving retina. J. Amer. med. Ass. **83**, 355–356 (1924)

498. SIEGERT, P.: Akute Ischämie der Papille bei Arteriitis cranialis (temporalis). Klin. Mbl. Augenheilk. **120**, 254–273 (1952)

499. SIEGRIST, A.: Die Gefahren der Ligatur der großen Halsschlagadern für das Auge und das Leben des Menschen. Albrecht v. Graefes Arch. Ophthal. **50**, 511–646 (1900)

500. SIMMONS, R.J., COGAN, D.G.: Occult temporal arteritis. Arch. Ophthal. (Chic.) **68**, 8–18 (1962)

501. SINGER, K.: Über Sehstörung nach Blutverlust. Beitr. Augenheilk. **6**, 1–30 (1904)

502. SINGH, S., DASS, R.: The central artery of the retina. I. Origin and course. Brit. J. Ophthal. **44**, 193–212 (1960)

503. SINGH, S., DASS, R.: The central artery of the retina. II. A study of its distribution and anastomoses. Brit. J. Ophthal. **44**, 280–299 (1960)

504. SJÖGREN, H.: A study in pseudoglaucoma (glaucoma without hypertension). Acta ophthal. (Kbh.) **24**, 239–294 (1946)

505. SKILLERN, P.G., LOCKHART, G. III: Optic neuritis and uncontrolled diabetes mellitus in 14 Patients. Ann. intern. Med. **51**, 468–475 (1959)

506. SMITH, C., GREENE, P.B.: Ocular complications of temporal arteritis. Amer. J. Ophthal. **32**, 685–690 (1949)

507. SMITH, J.L., ISRAEL, C.W., HARNER, R.E.: Syphilitic temporal arteritis. Arch. Ophthal. (Chic.) **78**, 284–288 (1967)

508. SMITH, J.L.: Editor's note. Miami Neuro-ophthal. Symp. Proc. IV, ed. J.L. Smith, p. 156. St. Louis: Mosby 1968

508a. SMITH, J.L.: In: Neuro-ophthalmology symposium of the University of Miami and the Bascom Palmer Eye Institute. **VII**, ed. J.L. Smith and J.S. Glaser, p. XI. St. Louis: Mosby 1973

509. SMITH, R.J.H.: Clinical glaucoma, p. 154–155. London: Cassell 1965

510. SMITH, V.H.: Pressure changes in the ophthalmic artery after carotid occlusion—an experimental study in rabbit. Brit. J. Ophthal. **45**, 1–26 (1961)

511. SPENCER, W.H., HOYT, W.F.: A fatal case of giant-cell arteritis (temporal or cranial arteritis) with ocular involvement. Arch. Ophthal. (Chic.) **64**, 862–867 (1960)

512. SPROUL, E.E.: A case of temporal arteritis. N.Y. J. Med. **42**, 345–346 (1942)

513. STEELE, E.J., BLUNT, M.J.: The blood supply of the optic nerve and chiasma in man. J. Anat. (Lond.) **90**, 486–493 (1956)

514. STENSAAS, L.J., Stensaas, S.S.: Astrocytic neuroglial cells, oligodendrocytes, and microgliacytes in the spinal cord of the toad. Z. Zellforsch. Mikrosk. Anat. **86**, 184–213 (1968)

515. STIEF, A. VON: Zur Histopathologie des Sehnerven bei der Arteriosklerose und bei der senilen Demenz. Z. Augenheilk. **70**, 41–52 (1930)

516. STOCK, W.: Über kavernöse Sehnervenatrophie bei Myopie. Klin. Mbl. Augenheilk. **46**(1), 342–358 (1908)

517. STOCK, W.: Entstehung der lakunären Atrophie beim Glaukom. Klin. Mbl. Augenheilk. **78**, 61–63 (1927)

518. SUGAR, H.S., WEBSTER, J.E., GURDJIAN, E.S.: Ophthalmologic findings in spontaneous thrombosis of the carotid arteries. Arch. Ophthal. (Chic.) **44**, 823–832 (1950)

519. SVANE-KNUDSEN, P.: Bilateral ophthalmic arteritis as part of the temporal arteritis syndrome. Acta ophthal. (Kbh.) **38**, 708–712 (1960)

520. SVANE-KNUDSEN, P.: Ocular changes in periarteritis nodosa. Ungeskr. Laeg. **123**, 229–232 (1961) Cit. from Ophthal. Lit. (Lond.) **15**, 123 (1961)

521. SWIETLICZKO, J., DAVID, N.J.: Fluorescein angiography in experimental ocular hypertension. Amer. J. Ophthal. **70**, 351–363 (1970)

522. SZYMANSKI, J., WLADYCZKO, S.: Jaskra prosta doswiadczalna. Klin. oczna **3** 145–150, (1925)

523. TAKAYASU, M.: Strange Central retinal vascular changes (Japanese) Acta Soc. Ophthal. Jap. **12**, 554–555 (1908)

524. TAPTAS, J.N.: Rachis cervico-dorsal et pathologie carotidienne. Sém. Hôp. Paris 149–152, 1950

525. TENG, C.C.: Glaucomatous cupping. Amer. J. Ophthal. **58**, 379–407 (1964)

526. TERRIEN, F.: Amaurose post-hémorragique. Arch. Ophtal. (Paris) **39**, 263–269 (1921)

527. TERRIEN, F., RENARD, G.: Atrophie optique et hématémèse. Rev. Oto-neuro-ophtal. **8**, 41–45 (1930)

528. TERSON, A.: Les troubles visuels graves après les hématémèses et les metrorragies. Sém. méd. 245 (1894)

529. TERSON, A.: Atrophies partielle des nerfs optiques à la suite d'une hématémèse. Rev. gén. clin. thérap. (Paris) **11**, 819–821 (1897)

530. TERSON, A.: Sur la pathogénie et le traitement des doubles visuels après les pertes de sang. Ann. Oculist. (Paris) **159**, 23–65 (1922)

531. THEOBALD, S.: A case of atrophy of the optic nerves following haemorrhage from the stomach, with a consideration of the causes of post-haemorrhagic blindness. Amer. J. Ophthal. **16**, 145–152 (1899)

532. THEODOSSIADIS, G.P.: Über die Vaskularisation in der Regio praelaminaris der Papilla Optica. Klin. Mbl. Augenheilk. **158**, 646–652 (1971)

533. THOMAS, H.M., WOODS, A.C.: Progressive exophthalmos following thyroidectomy. Bull. Johns. Hopk. Hosp. **59**, 99–113 (1936)

534. TIDY, H.L.: Loss of vision following haemorrhage. Brit. med. J. **1941 I**, 774–776

535. TOPILOW, A., BISLAND, T.: Diabetes mellitus as a cause of papillitis. Amer. J. Ophthal. **35**, 855–858 (1952)

536. TOWNES, D.E., BLODI, F.C.: The diagnostic value of temporal arteritis biopsy. Trans. Amer. ophthal. Soc. **66**, 33–44 (1968)

537. TRAQUAIR, H.M.: The nerve-fibre bundle defect. Trans. ophthal. Soc. U.K. **64**, 3–23 (1944)

538. TRONCOSO, M.U.: An. Oftal. **4**, 97, 135, 167 (1902) Cit. by Evans, 1939

539. TOUSSAINT, D., KUWABARA, T., COGAN, D.G.: Retinal vascular patterns—II. Human retinal vessels studies in three dimensions. Arch. Ophthal. (Chic.) **65**, 575–581 (1961)

540. TÜRK, W.: Arterieller Collateralkreislauf bei Verschluss der großen Gefässe am Aortenbogen durch deformierende Aortitis. Wien. klin. Wschr. **14**, 757–763 (1901)

541. UHTHOFF, W.: Beiträge zu den Sehstörungen und Augenhintergrundsveränderungen bei Anaemie. Ber. dtsch. ophthal. Ges. Heidelberg **43**, 204–212 (1922)

542. UHTHOFF, W.: Über Sehnervenveränderungen bei Arteriosklerose. Klin. Mbl. Augenheilk. **70**, 399 (1923)

543. UHTHOFF, W.: Zu den entzündlichen Sehnerven-Affektionen bei Arteriosklerose (Atherosklerose). Ber. dtsch. ophthal. Ges. Heidelberg **44**, 196–208 (1924)

544. UYAMA, Y.: Über das Vorkommen der sogenannten Thromboangiitis obliterans am Auge unter Berücksichtigung anatomischer Untersuchungen. Albrecht v. Graefes Arch. Ophthal. **137**, 438–446 (1937)

545. VAIL, D.: Pseudo-glaucoma: a nutritional disease of the optic nerve. Quart. Bull. Northw. Univ. med. Sch. **27**, 74–77 (1953)

546. VEASEY, C.A.: Report of two unusual complications of Herpes zoster ophthalmicus; (a) acute retrobulbar neuritis (neuritis axialis); (b) acute glaucoma. Arch. Ophthal. (N.Y.) **48**, 364–367 (1919)

547. VEASEY, C.A., VEIRS, E.R.: Acute ischemic papilledema and optic atrophy. Tex. St. J. Med. **62**, 40–41 (1966)

548. WAGENER, H.P.: Temporal arteritis and loss of vision. Amer. J. med. Sci. **212**, 225–228 (1946)

549. WAGENER, H.: Retinal lesion in lupus erythematosus. Amer. J. med. Sci. **211**, 240–244 (1946)

550. WAGENER, H.P.: Amaurosis fugax. Amer. J. med. Sci. **224**, 229–236 (1952)

551. WAGENER, H.P., GIPNER, J.F.: Arterial spasm in production of occlusion of branches of central artery of the retina. Amer. J. Ophthal. **10**, 650–657 (1927)

552. WAGENER, H., HOLLENHORST, R.W.: The ocular lesion of temporal arteritis. Amer. J. Ophthal. **45**, 617–630 (1958)

553. WALDECK, H.J.S.: Post-haemorrhagic optic atrophy as complication of severe epistaxis. J. Laryng. **74**, 491–492 (1960)

554. WALKER, C.B., CUSHING, H.: Studies of the optic nerve in association with chiasmal lesions. Arch. Ophthal. (N.Y.) **45**, 407–437 (1916)

555. WALSH, F.B., HOYT, W.F.: Clinical neuro-ophthalmology, 3rd ed., p. 1178–1182, 1358, 1607, 1802–1835, 1862, 1918–1921. Baltimore: Williams and Wilkins 1969

556. WALSH, F.B., SMITH, G.W.: The ocular complications of carotid angiography: the ocular signs of thrombosis of the internal carotid artery. J. Neurosurg. **9**, 517–537 (1952)

557. WEBER, A.: Ein Fall von partieller Hyperämie der Chorioidea bei einem Kaninchen. Albrecht v. Graefes Arch. Opththal. **2**, abt 1, 133–157 (1855)

558. WECKER, L. DE: Le faux glaucome. Ann. Oculist (Paris) **116**, 249–262 (1896)

559. WEEKERS, R.: Le glaucome incomplet. Contribution à l'étude du glaucome sans hypertension. Ophthalmologica (Basel) **104**, 316–331 (1942)

560. WEISS, K.E.: Amaurosis fugax durch Krampf der Retinalgefässe. Ber. dtsch. ophthal. Ges. Heidelberg **38**, 205–209 (1912)

561. WERNER, L.: On vascular and other retinal changes associated with general disease. Trans. ophthal. Soc. U.K. **33**, 9–30 (1913)

562. WERNER, S.C.: Prednisone in emergency treatment of malignant exophthalmos. Lancet **1966 II**, 1004–1007

563. WESTHOFF, ZIEGLER: Cit. by Theobald, 1899

564. WHITEFIELD. A.G.W., BATEMAN, M., COOKE, W.T.: Temporal arteritis. Brit. J. Ophthal. **47**, 555–566 (1963)

565. WHITEFIELD, A.G.W., COOK, W.T., JAMESON-EVANS, P., RUDD, C.: Temporal arteritis and its treatment with cortisone and ACTH. Lancet **1953 I**, 408–412

566. WHITING, M.: Optic atrophy following haemorrhage from the alimentary tract. Trans. ophthal. Soc. U.K. **49**, 144–154 (1929)

567. WILBRAND, H., SAENGER, A.: Die Neurologie des Auges. In: Handbuch für Nerven- und Augenärzte, vol. 3, part 2. Wiesbaden: Bergmann 1906

568. WILLIAMSON, D., RACHMAN, I.: Mpilo Hospital Staff Clinical Meeting, Case No. 29. Cent. Afr. J. Med. **10**, 114–116 (1964)

569. WINIWARTER, F. VON: Über eine eigenthümliche Form von Endarteriitis und Endophlebitis mit

Gangrän des Fusses. Langenbecks Arch. klin. Chir. **23**, 202–226 (1879)

570. WOLFF, E.: The causation of amblyopia following gastric and other haemorrhages. Trans ophthal. Soc. U.K. **55**, 342–349 (1935)

571. WOLFF, E.: Some aspects of the blood supply of the optic nerve. Trans. ophthal. Soc. U.K. **59**, 157–162 (1939)

572. WOLFF, E.: Schabel's cavernous atrophy. Trans. ophthal. Soc. U.K. **67**, 133–140 (1947)

573. WOLFF, E.: The anatomy of the eye and orbit, 3rd ed., p. 265–272. London: Lewis 1948

574. WOLFF, J.: Beiträge zur Ultrastruktur der Kapillaren in der normalen Großhirnrinde. Z. Zellforsch. Mikrosk. Anat. **60**, 409–431 (1963)

575. WOLTER, J.R.: The human optic papilla. Amer. J. Ophthal. **44**, 48–65 (Oct. pt. 2) (1957)

576. WOLTER, J.R., PHILLIPS, R.L.: Secondary glaucoma in cranial arteritis. Amer. J. Ophthal. **59**, 625–634 (1965)

577. WYLLIE, A.M., McLEOD, D., CULLEN, J.F.: Traumatic ischaemic optic neuropathy. Brit. J. Ophthal. **56**, 851–853 (1972)

578. YATES, P.O.: Cerebral pathology following carotid spasm. Proc. roy. Soc. Med. **47**, 606–608 (1954)

579. YOUNESSIAN, S.: L'ERG dans l'artérite temporale. Ophthalmologica (Basel) **143**, 288–290 (1962)

580. ZIEGLER, E.: Zur Kenntnis der Entstehung der Amaurose nach Blutverlust. Beitr. path. Anat. **2**, 57–72 (1887)

581. ZIMMERMAN, L.E.: Histology and pathology of the outflow channels. In: Symposium on Glaucoma. Trans. N. Orleans Acad. Ophthal., 1967, p. 1–30. St. Louis: Mosby

582. ZIMMERMAN, L.E., DE VENECIA, G., HAMASAKI, D.I.: Pathology of the optic nerve in experimental acute glaucoma. Invest. Ophthal. **6**, 109–125 (1967)

Subject Index

Handbook of Sensory Physiology

Editorial Board:
H. Autrum, R. Jung,
W.R. Loewenstein,
D.M. MacKay, H.L. Teuber

Distribution rights for
India: UBS, Delhi

Prices are subject to change
without notice

**Springer-Verlag
Berlin
Heidelberg
New York**

**Vol. 1: Principles of
Receptor Physiology**
Editor: W.R. Loewenstein
262 figures. XII, 600 pages
1971
ISBN 3-540-05144-9
Cloth DM 168,–
ISBN 0-387-05144-9
(North America)
Cloth US $53.30

This is an authoritative
book dealing with basic
chemical and physical
mechanisms of receptor
action and with the
question of how nerve
connections are made in
sensory systems.

**Vol. 7: Part 1:
Photochemistry of Vision**
Editor: H.J.A. Dartnall
296 figures. XII, 810 pages
1972
ISBN 3-540-05145-7
Cloth DM 238,–
ISBN 0-387-05145-7
(North America)
Cloth US $75.50

An integrated, complete
and authoritative account
of the pigments used in
vision, treated from the
various standpoints of
photochemistry, photo-
biology, zoology, ecology,
and anatomy.

Part 2:
**Physiology of
Photoreceptor Organs**
Editor: M.G.F. Fuortes
342 figures. X, 765 pages
1972
ISBN 3-540-05743-9
Cloth DM 244,–
ISBN 0-387-05743-9
(North America)
Cloth US $77.40

A reference handbook
including basic information
and advanced articles
dealing with the properties
of photoreceptor cells
and the organization of
photoreceptor organs.

Part 3:
**Central Processing of
Visual Information**
Editor: R. Jung

A: Integrative Functions
and Comparative Data
208 figures. XI, 775 pages
1973
ISBN 3-540-05769-2
Cloth DM 248,–
ISBN 0-387-05769-2
(North America)
Cloth US $101.70

B: Visual Centers in the
Brain
216 figures. 1973
ISBN 3-540-06056-1
Cloth DM 248,–
ISBN 0-387-06056-1
(North America)
Cloth US $91.80

The two parts of volume
7/3 give a complete
presentation of the brain
physiology of vision.

Part 4:
Visual Psychophysics
Editors: D. Jameson,
L.M. Hurvich
297 figures. X, 812 pages
1972
ISBN 3-540-05146-5
Cloth DM 248,–
ISBN 0-387-05146-5
(North America)
Cloth US $101.70

The volume consists of a
series of chapters by
specialists on the psychophysics of vision and
treats the fundamental
characteristics of the
visual system as revealed
by psychophysical studies.

G. Eisner
**Biomicroscopy of the
Peripheral Fundus**
An Atlas and Textbook
Foreword by H. Goldmann
Drawings by W. Hess
121 partly colored figures
IX, 191 pages. 1973
ISBN 3-540-06374-9
Cloth DM 128,–
ISBN 0-387-06374-9
(North America) Cloth $54.30
Distribution rights for Japan:
Maruzen Co. Ltd., Tokyo

**Information Processing
in the Visual Systems
of Arthropods**
Symposium held at the Dapart-
ment of Zoology, University
of Zurich, March 6-9, 1972
Editor: R. Wehner
263 figures. XI, 334 pages. 1972
ISBN 3-540-06020-0 DM 46,–
ISBN 0-387-06020-0
(North America) $14.80

K. Motokawa
**Physiology of Color and
Pattern Vision**
137 figures, 26 tables. 283 pages
1970
ISBN 3-540-04977-0
Cloth DM 88,–
ISBN 0-387-04977-0
(North America) Cloth $22.90
Published by Igaku Shoin Ltd.,
Tokyo. Distribution rights for
all countries excluding East Asia:
Springer-Verlag

**Biochemistry
and Physiology of Visual
Pigments**
Symposium held at Institut
für Tierphysiologie, Ruhr-
Universität Bochum/W. Germany
August 27-30, 1972
For the Organizing Committee,
Editor: H. Langer
202 figures. XIII, 366 pages
1973
ISBN 3-540-06204-1
Cloth DM 50,–
ISBN 0-387-06204-1
(North America) Cloth $11.80

**Springer-Verlag
Berlin
Heidelberg
New York**

Journals

**Albrecht
von Graefes Archiv
für klinische
und experimentelle
Ophthalmologie**
Albrecht von Graefe's Archive
for Clinical and Experimental
Ophthalmology
Editorial Board: F.C. Blodi
(Managing Editor), J. Böck,
D.G. Cogan, R.A. Crone,
E. Engelking,
G. Meyer-Schwickerath
(Managing Editor), H.K. Müller,
F. Rintelen, E. Schreck
(Managing Editor), W. Straub
(Managing Editor), C. Thomas

Ophthalmology
**Zentralblatt für die gesamte
Ophthalmologie
und ihre Grenzgebiete**
Zugleich Referatenteil zu
Albrecht von Graefes Archiv
Editors: J. Babel, G. Bietti,
E. Engelking, W. Jaeger, O. Käfer,
W. Kreibig (Managing Editors),
G. Meyer-Schwickerath,
J.K. Müller, J. Nordmann,
A. Pillat, H. Sautter, E. Schreck
Sample copies as well as
subscription and
back-volume information
available upon request.
Please address:
Springer-Verlag
Werbeabteilung 4021
D 1000 Berlin 33
Heidelberger Platz 3
or
Springer-Verlag
New York Inc.
Promotion Department
175 Fifth Avenue
New York, N.Y. 10010

Prices are subject to change
without notice